Every part of this soil is sacred.
Every hillside, every valley, every plain and grove
Has been hallowed by some sad or happy event
In days long vanished.
—Chief Seattle

I think I know now the secret of making the best person.
It is to live in the open air and sleep with the earth.
—Walt Whitman

OTHER BOOKS BY LEONARD M. ADKINS

Hike Virginia South of US 60: 51 Hikes from the Cumberland Gap to the Atlantic Coast

50 Hikes in Maryland: Walks, Hikes, and Backpacks from the Allegheny Plateau to the Atlantic Ocean

50 Hikes in West Virginia: From the Allegheny Mountains to the Ohio River

Hiking and Traveling the Blue Ridge Parkway: The Only Guide You Will Ever Need, Including GPS, Detailed Maps, and More

Wildflowers of the Appalachian Trail
(Joe Cook and Monica Sheppard, Photographers)

Wildflowers of the Blue Ridge and Great Smoky Mountains
(Joe Cook, Photographer)

The Best of the Appalachian Trail: Day Hikes
(with Victoria and Frank Logue)

The Best of the Appalachian Trail: Overnight Hikes
(with Victoria and Frank Logue)

All About the Appalachian Trail (for ages 9–13)

Nature of the Appalachian Trail: Your Guide to Wildlife, Plants, and Geology

Images of America: Along the Appalachian Trail: Georgia, North Carolina, and Tennessee

Images of America: Along the Appalachian Trail: Massachusetts, Vermont, and New Hampshire

Images of America: Along the Appalachian Trail: New Jersey, New York, and Connecticut

Images of America: Along the Appalachian Trail: West Virginia, Maryland, and Pennsylvania

Images of America: Along Virginia's Appalachian Trail

Postcards of America: Along Virginia's Appalachian Trail

Maryland: An Explorer's Guide

West Virginia: An Explorer's Guide

Adventure Guide to Virginia

The Caribbean: A Walking and Hiking Guide

HIKE VIRGINIA

· NORTH OF US 60 ·

51 HIKES FROM THE ALLEGHENY MOUNTAINS TO THE CHESAPEAKE BAY

LEONARD M. ADKINS

MENASHA RIDGE PRESS
Your Guide to the Outdoors Since 1982
an imprint of AdventureKEEN

HIKE VIRGINIA NORTH OF US 60

51 Hikes from the Allegheny Mountains to the Chesapeake Bay

Published by Menasha Ridge Press
Distributed by Publishers Group West
Printed in China
First edition, first printing

Substantial portions of material in this guide were in a prior work published by the author.

Library of Congress Cataloging-in-Publication Data
Names: Adkins, Leonard M., author.
Title: Hike Virginia north of US 60 : 51 hikes from the Allegheny Mountains to the Chesapeake Bay / Leonard M. Adkins.
Description: First edition. | Birmingham : Menasha Ridge Press, An imprint of AdventureKEEN, [2023] Includes index.
Identifiers: LCCN 2022036955 (print) | LCCN 2022036956 (ebook) | ISBN 9781634043489 (pbk.) ISBN 9781634043496 (ebook)
Subjects: LCSH: Hiking—Virginia—Guidebooks. | Walking—Virginia—Guidebooks. Backpacking—Virginia—Guidebooks. | Trails—Virginia—Guidebooks. | Virginia—Guidebooks.
Classification: LCC GV199.42.V8 A353 2023 (print) | LCC GV199.42.V8 (ebook) DDC 796.5109755—dc23/eng/20220805
LC record available at https://lccn.loc.gov/2022036955
LC ebook record available at https://lccn.loc.gov/2022036956

Cover design: Scott McGrew
Text design: Annie Long
Cover photo: © Jon Bilous/Shutterstock
Interior photos: Leonard M. Adkins, except where noted
Cartography: Scott McGrew
Project editor: Holly Cross
Proofreader: Emily Beaumont
Index: Potomac Indexing, LLC

MENASHA RIDGE PRESS
An imprint of AdventureKEEN
2204 First Ave. S., Ste. 102
Birmingham, Alabama 35233
800-678-7006, fax 877-374-9016

Visit menasharidge.com for a complete listing of our books and for ordering information. Contact us at our website, at facebook.com/menasharidge, or at twitter.com/menasharidge with questions or comments. To find out more about who we are and what we're doing, visit blog.menasharidge.com.

SAFETY NOTICE Though the author and publisher have made every effort to ensure that the information in this book is accurate at press time, they are not responsible for any loss, damage, injury, or inconvenience that may occur while using this book—you are responsible for your own safety and health on the trail. The fact that a hike is described in this book does not mean that it will be safe for you. Always check local conditions (which can change from day to day), know your own limitations, and consult a map. Also note that many water sources are identified for hikers' convenience, but this is not an endorsement of their purity. All water should be treated before consuming.

For information about trail and other closures, check the "Contact" listings in the hike profiles.

AN INVITATION TO THE READER Over time trails can be rerouted and signs and landmarks altered. If you find that changes have occurred on the routes described in this book, please let us know so that corrections may be made in future editions. The author and publisher also welcome other comments and suggestions. Email: habitualhiker@verizon.net.

Dedication

In memory of Leonard Wilson Adkins, who understandingly said to me,
"I know you need to go hiking, son, so go."

Hike Virginia North of US 60 Overview

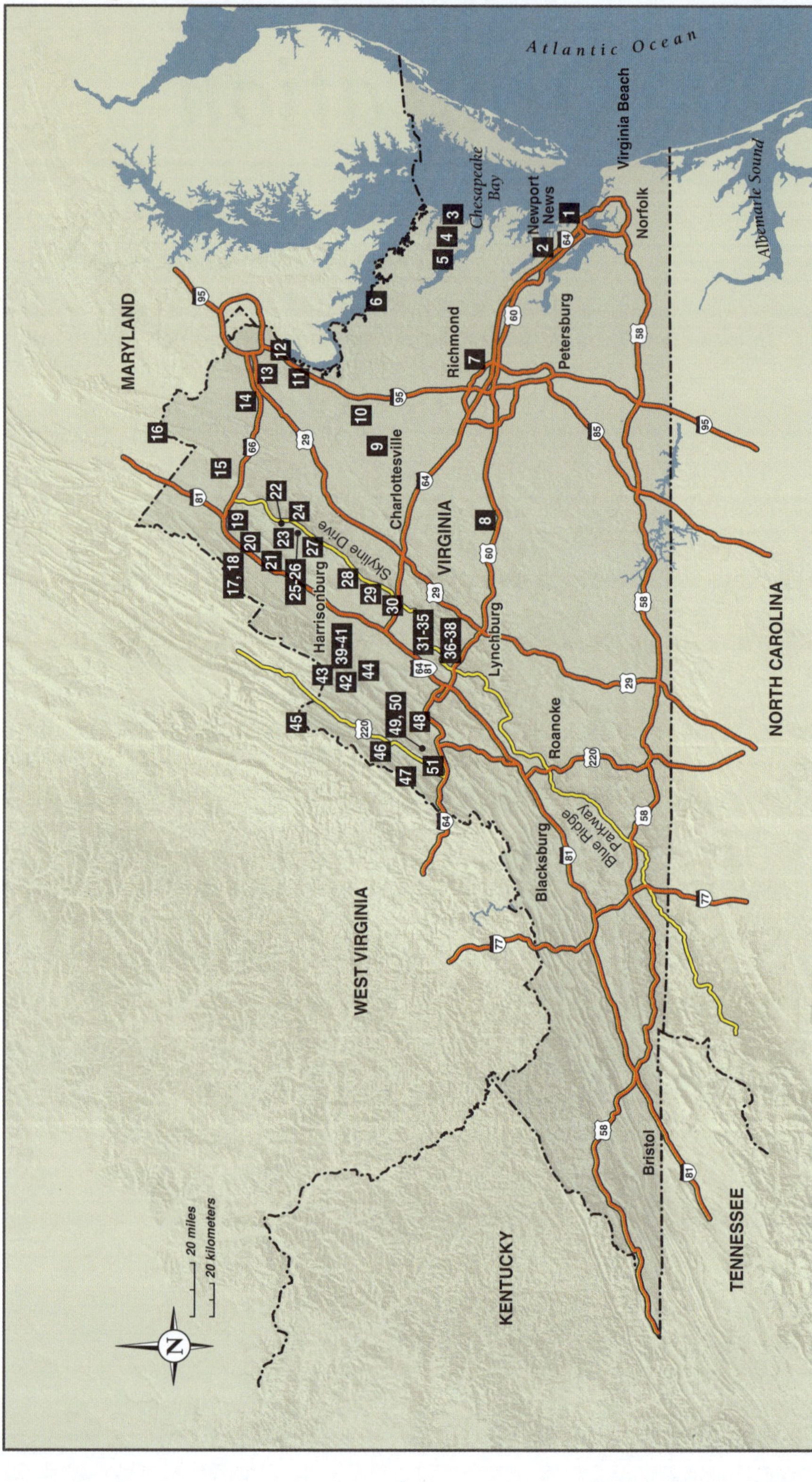

Contents

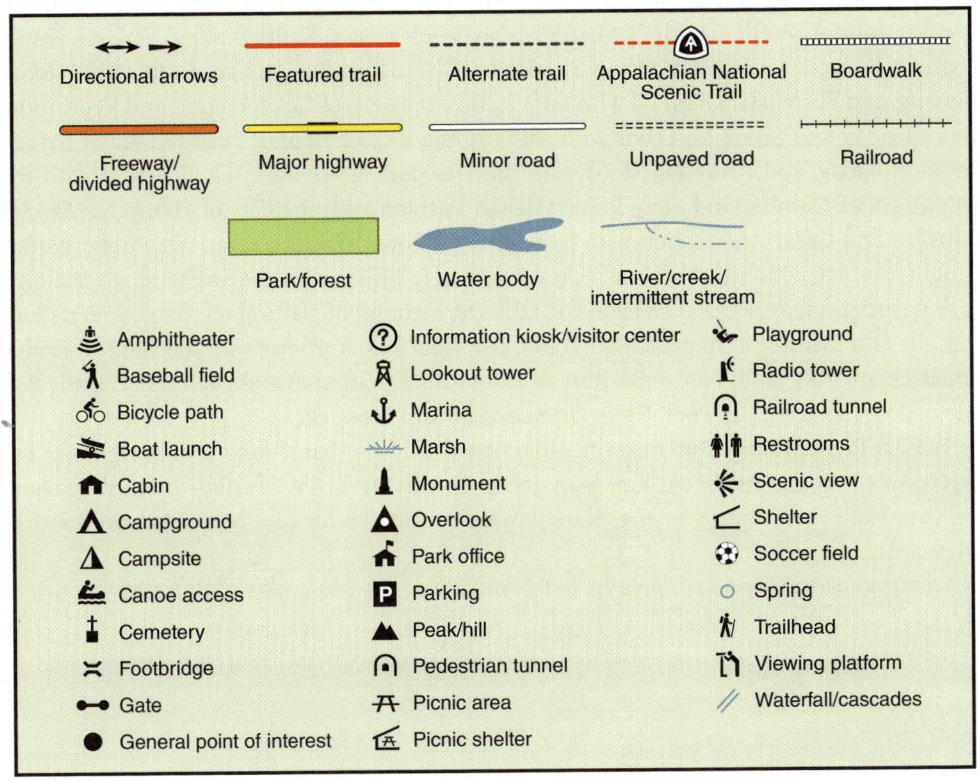
Directional arrows
Featured trail
Alternate trail
Appalachian National Scenic Trail
Boardwalk
Freeway/ divided highway
Major highway
Minor road
Unpaved road
Railroad
Park/forest
Water body
River/creek/ intermittent stream
Amphitheater
Baseball field
Bicycle path
Boat launch
Cabin
Campground
Campsite
Canoe access
Cemetery
Footbridge
Gate
General point of interest
Information kiosk/visitor center
Lookout tower
Marina
Marsh
Monument
Overlook
Park office
P
Parking
Peak/hill
Pedestrian tunnel
Picnic area
Picnic shelter
Playground
Radio tower
Railroad tunnel
Restrooms
Scenic view
Shelter
Soccer field
Spring
Trailhead
Viewing platform
Waterfall/cascades

Acknowledgments

My name may be on the front cover of this book, but I owe a debt of gratitude to all of the people who willingly devoted time, energy, and expertise in seeing that the information presented is as complete and accurate as possible:

Bob Tennyson, Bud Risner, Douglas H. Graham, James Hunt, Dave Benavitch, Dawn Coulson, Sharon Mohney, Ronald Swann, David Rhodes, Wade L. Bushong, Cynthia Snow, Stephanie Chapman, Krissy Sherman, Eric Freels, Lilith Milam, and John Coleman with the U.S. Forest Service; Emond Raus, Michael Andrus, Steve Bair, Donald Pfanz, Deanne Adams, Bob Hickman, Janet Stombock, James Burgess, Stephanie Pooler, Matt Graves, Arthur C. Webster III, Bert Dunkerly, Henry P. Elliott, and Donald W. Campbell with the National Park Service; Melissa Rudacille, Howard Morrison, Stephen Paull, Karen Michaud, and the staff of Shenandoah National Park; Tim Vest, Scott Shanklin, Paul Billings, Shawn Spencer, John A. Reffit, Charli Conn, Steve Davis, Jeff Foster, Kathy Budnie, Vanessa Lewis, Kenneth Benson, Jess Lowry, David Stapleton, Alison Weddle, Zachary R. Bradford, Mark Herring, and Forrest Gladden III with the Virginia Division of Conservation and Recreation; Vance Coffey and Shannon Lewis with the Virginia Department of Forestry; Kristi Barber, Becky Holliday, and Andy Lunsford with the Newport News Park; H. B. Radar with the Volunteers of Cumberland State Forest; Calvin Pearson with the City of Hampton; Darrell Winslow and Carol Ann Cohen with NOVA; Glen Rowe with the Lancaster Public Works; Vaughn Stanley with Stratford Hall Plantation; Greta Miller with the Shenandoah National Park Association; Rebecca O. Wilson with the Department of Natural Heritage; J. E. Raynor with the Old Dominion Appalachian Trail Club; Nancy D. Anthony with the Natural Bridge Appalachian Trail Club; Henry Bashore of Kilmarnock, Virginia; and good trail friends Bob Ellenwood, Pat Love, Bill Foot, Steve Gomez, and Ann Messick.

Carl Taylor, Robin Dutcher, and Gretchen Gordon—thank you for helping make my foot travels become this book. Kathleen, John, Timmy, and JAY Yelenic—thanks for opening your home and family to me. Nancy Adkins—thanks for life, Mom. Laurie—thanks for sharing life with me.

A thunderous round of applause to the builders and maintainers of all trails!

Introduction

Only a person traveling by foot can truly appreciate the natural beauty to be found in Virginia. The two flower scars evident on a tiny red partridgeberry or the rich aroma and cool temperatures of an evergreen forest will be overlooked by those passing through in an automobile. Virginia's most impressive waterfalls are accessible only to someone who is willing to put forth a bit of effort to reach them, and the majestic serenity of a golden sunset shining on distant mountains is made all the more inspiring when you know you have reached the viewpoint under your own power. Only by walking on a quiet beach will you be permitted to study etchings in the sand that mark the movements of a ghost crab or have the time to watch the swooping silhouette of an osprey outlined by a silvery glow reflecting off salt water.

The topography of the northern portion of Virginia, stretching from the craggy summits of the Allegheny Mountains to the soft shores of the Chesapeake Bay, provides some of the widest variety of hiking terrain and sights to be found in any of the Middle Atlantic states. In the eastern part of the commonwealth—the coastal plain where land meets salt water—you will often find yourself hiking up and down minor changes in elevation and walking past herons and egrets as they fish in small swamps, brackish ponds, and slow-moving streams. The Piedmont in central Virginia is characterized by gently rolling land that will lead you into grassy meadows for open views almost as often as you will be treading in mixed hardwood forests. Influenced by narrow mountains and their spreading spur ridges, trails in the Blue Ridge and Massanutten Mountains either follow the rises and falls of fluctuating mountain crests or descend past quickly flowing streams and waterfalls into small valleys and coves. The mountains of western Virginia are the least populated, and it is here that you will find the most rugged yet isolated and quiet hiking and have the best chance of viewing the state's abundant wildlife.

This book was originally envisioned as a guide to 51 hikes throughout the entire state. It soon became apparent, however, that by trying to incorporate so much area, I would actually be limiting myself, and you, by having to reject and ignore far too many places deserving of your hiking time and attention. By concentrating on only about half the state, it is possible to include many of the most enjoyable and rewarding hikes in the northern part of Virginia. With descriptions of more than 360 miles of pathways, this book offers hikes for every degree of physical stamina and time constraint. Best of all, no matter where you happen to be at any given moment (north of US 60), you are never going to be more than a 30- to 45-minute drive away from one of the hikes.

Like most guidebooks, this one will tell you where the hikes are and how to follow the pathways, and it will point out the plants, animals, and birds you may see along the way. It differs from many guides, however, in that it also contains interpretive information; by using it you will not be hiking "blind." Not only will you be informed where to turn left, right, and so forth, but you will also receive background information on the

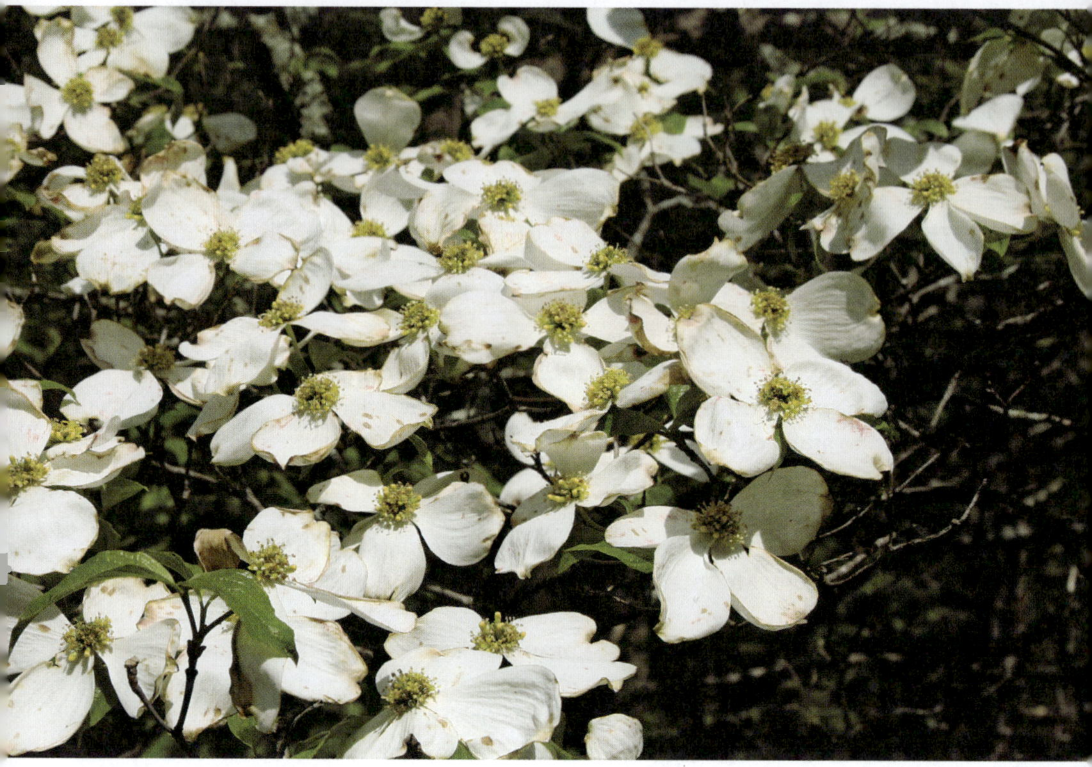

Dogwood in full bloom

plants, animals, and natural and human history or issues facing a certain area. You will come to understand why the pink lady's slipper grows in such an exotic shape, what animal likes what types of foods, and how to tell what an animal has recently eaten. You'll learn to look for signs that show whether a bear or a turkey inhabits an area. You will also be able to determine why human history has left its mark on the land and what caused certain events to occur. There is, of course, much more to be learned than can be presented in this book. To help you gain an even greater awareness, enjoyment, and understanding of your surroundings, I urge you to read (and possibly carry) some additional books and field guides. (See "Suggested Readings and Field Guides" on page 228.)

Birds singing early in the morning, flowers opening wide to soak in the noontime sun, and owls hooting in the evening make it worthwhile to walk the same trail at different times of the day. Also, a trail walked in late spring is certainly going to be a different experience when you return to hike it in the fall. Therefore, be willing to visit an area more than once, and don't limit your outdoor activities to just one or two seasons; hiking in Virginia can be a year-round activity. Of course, you must be prepared for sudden changes in the weather, but even on the highest mountains in Virginia there are numerous days when winter temperatures reach into the 50s and 60s.

To paraphrase Will Rogers, I've never met a trail I didn't like. My wish is that this guidebook conveys to you the sense of excitement, joy, wonder, peace, and contentment that can only be found in the freedom of traveling the natural world by foot. Virginia awaits—go do some exploring!

How to Use This Book

This book includes a wide variety of hikes—ranging from pleasant strolls on nearly level ground to challenging, several-day backpacking trips over rugged terrain—so that everyone, regardless of their hiking experience or level of physical stamina, can choose an excursion that best fits their schedule, lifestyle, or expectations. The headings at the beginning of each hike were designed to give you—at a quick glance—an overview of what to expect.

GPS lists the coordinates for each hike's trailhead in decimal degrees.

I arrived at the **total distance** for each hike by walking with a surveyor's measuring wheel. If you compare some of my distances to those of other guidebooks or information from the forest service, state parks, or other sources, you may notice some discrepancies. Most often these sources give distances from a beginning trailhead, not taking into account how far you must walk to reach that trailhead. In order to give you as true a picture as possible of how far you are actually going to walk, I measured the hike from the point you leave your automobile to where you are able to return to it.

A *one-way* hike is just that—you walk in one direction, ending the hike at a different point from where you started. A one-way hike necessitates a car shuttle. On a *round-trip,* you go to your destination and then return by way of the same route. On a *circuit* hike, which represents the vast majority of the hikes presented in this book, you will take a circular route to return to your starting point, rewalking little, if any, of the same trail or trails.

Hiking time is the minimum amount of time that it would take a person of average ability to do a trip at a leisurely pace. Some of you may go faster, a few of you slower. Begin with some of the shorter hikes and compare your time with those stated. This way you can approximate how long it should take you to do the more extended excursions. Do keep in mind that the stated time does not account for any rest breaks, meals, resupplying for water, or sightseeing and nature study, and that in hiking, it is not how fast you go, but how much you enjoy the trip. Robert Louis Stevenson may have said it best: "To travel hopefully is a better thing than to arrive."

Vertical rise is probably the best way to determine how strenuous a hike will be. It represents the sum total of all the uphill hiking you will do and is not, as most other guides provide, just the difference in elevation between the lowest and highest point of a hike. This rise was determined using information from United States Geological Survey (USGS) maps.

This book includes a detailed map for each outing and will be sufficient to use to complete each hike. However, in the **maps** category, additional maps are identified that are available for each hike if you wish to obtain more detailed information. These include the appropriate USGS 7.5-minute series topographic maps (of which several may be needed for just one outing), the National Geographic Trails Illustrated map (if available for the particular hike), and the hand-out maps (most often free of charge) that are available at the appropriate contact stations, visitor centers, or agency offices.

Some maps mark the trails in the national forest with the official forest service inventory numbers, so to help you orient yourself, I have included these numbers in brackets (e.g., {FS 621}) in the hike descriptions. I have also used the initials FSR to refer to forest service roads (which are usually unpaved). Be aware that trails in the national forest may not be as well maintained or marked as those in the national, state, or regional parks.

"The Hike at a Glance" section describes the milestones in each route.

Please do not dismiss a hike or an area as being beyond your capabilities because you are intimidated by its length, time, or vertical rise. Because I enjoy walking so much, I have often described one of the longest and most meandering hikes to be taken in a particular area. Yet many places have numerous side trails or alternate routes you could take in order to shorten a hike. A good example is the Tuscarora Overlook hike in Douthat State Park. I describe a trip of more than 9 miles with a vertical rise of more than 2,000 feet, but there are so many interconnecting trails in the park that you could take a very rewarding circuit hike of about 3 miles, with only a minimal change in elevation. Study maps and my descriptions and you will find that this is the case in many places.

Advice and Precautions

WATER

It is always wise to carry water no matter the length of your outing. A good rule is to hydrate before your hike, carry (and drink) 16 ounces of water for every mile you plan to hike, and hydrate again after your hike. On overnight trips you may have to depend on a stream or spring, but the rise in the number of people visiting the natural areas of Virginia has brought about an increase of giardia, a water-borne parasite. Water can also become tainted by viruses, bacteria, and man-made pollutants.

Boiling could make stream or spring water potable, but a portable purifier is more convenient and, possibly, more effective. Be aware that a filter only removes bacteria, while a purifier is also capable of eliminating viruses. Since they cost about the same, the wiser move would be to purchase a purifier (even though it will probably weigh a little more).

Please note: For your convenience, water sources are identified in a number of the hike descriptions, but this is not an endorsement of their purity. Water from all sources should be treated before drinking!

SNAKES

Only four snakes in Virginia are venomous. The **copperhead** and **timber rattlesnake** are found throughout most of the region, while the **cottonmouth** (sometimes called water moccasin) inhabits eastern Virginia and a small part of central Virginia. The very eastern part of the state is within the range of the **canebrake rattlesnake** (considered by many to be the same species as the timber rattler), but sightings have been almost nonexistent within the last few decades. It would be wise to learn how to identify all four of these pit vipers.

Do remember that the outdoors is a snake's natural habitat and that it has as much right, if not more, to be there as you do. Please refrain from killing any snake; just walk around it, giving it a wide berth, and continue on your way.

Important: All snake bites may contain bacteria, so seek medical attention as soon as possible for any bite.

BLACK BEARS

Virginia is home to thousands of black bears. Although it is exceedingly rare for a black bear to attack a human, you must remember that they are wild animals and do not like to be approached at close range. Do not try to feed a bear. Not only does this endanger you, it also endangers the bear. Once a bear becomes used to close human contact, it may begin wandering into campsites or housing developments looking for handouts. This often results in the bear having to be destroyed by the authorities.

INSECTS

Warm weather brings **no-see-ums, gnats, fleas, sand fleas, deerflies, mosquitoes, ticks,** and more. Although the mountains have their fair share, the lowlands, marshes, and beaches of central and eastern Virginia can be nearly swarming with them at times. Bring lots of repellent on any hike from late spring to mid-autumn. (And remember that one of the pleasures of hiking during the colder months is the absence of insects.)

Recent years have seen a rise in the reported cases of Lyme disease, a bacterial infection transmitted by the bite of the deer tick. Check yourself for ticks after each outing, remembering that the thing you are looking for could be as small as the period at the end of this sentence.

PLANTS

Poison ivy is found just about everywhere in Virginia. Learn how to identify it, as it can grow in a number of forms. The most common is a woody shrub of up to 2 feet high that grows in large patches, often lining or overtaking pathways. Just as likely, it will grow as a hairy, root-covered vine that clings to the trunk of a tree, climbing far up into the branches. All parts of the plant contain the poison urushiol and can give you an itchy rash; this is true even in winter, when it appears to be dead.

Not as prevalent, but certainly present, **poison oak** is most often found in sandy soil habitats. As its name suggests, its leaflets resemble the leaves of an oak tree, but they are fuzzy. **Poison sumac** occurs most notably in the eastern part of Virginia. Unlike the low-standing poison ivy, poison sumac can grow to be 25 feet tall and has compound leaves with an odd number of leaflets. The upper side of the leaflets is shiny green, while the underside is lighter and has small hairs.

Poison ivy photo: Tom Watson

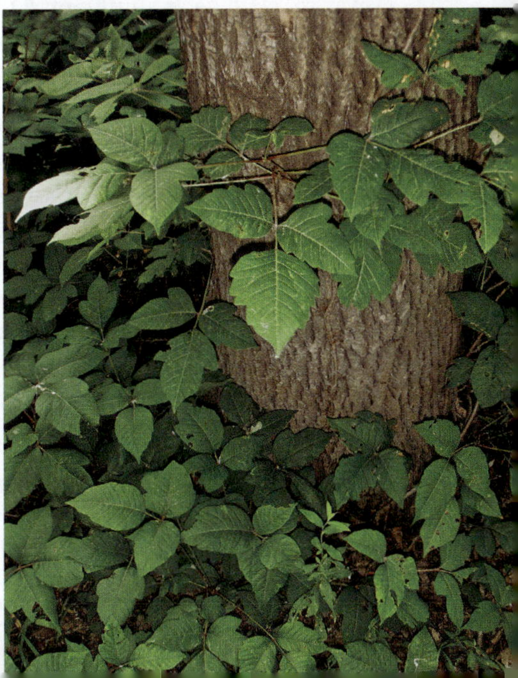

Trumpet creeper or vine is most often found in the lowlands. Also known as cow itch, it can cause contact dermatitis.

Stinging nettle will grow in large carpets and encroach upon pathways that are not well maintained. Brushing up against the plant may cause your skin to itch for the rest of the day.

Hogweed is an invasive plant that was first found in the United States in the early 1900s. It is a member of the carrot family, looks somewhat like Queen Anne's lace, and can grow to more than 14 feet tall. Touching it can cause skin blisters so severe as to create permanent scars and blindness if it gets in the eye. Definitely learn how to identify this one.

SUN

The consensus in the medical community is that you should apply a high-strength sunblock whenever you will be outdoors for extended periods of time—any time of year.

HUNTING

Due to the abundance of wildlife, hunting is extremely popular in Virginia, even in the more populated counties. Hunting seasons usually run from early fall into January, and again for part of the spring. Dates vary from year to year and place to place, so check with local authorities. During hunting season, it may be best to hike in a group; do not venture forth without wearing some kind of blaze-orange clothing. If you are hunting (or fishing), be sure to obtain the proper licenses and check into local regulations.

UNATTENDED VEHICLES

There is always the possibility of theft and vandalism to cars left unattended at trailheads, so it is wise to leave your valuables at home. If you must bring valuables with you, take them with you when you go hiking, or stash them out of sight and lock the car.

A way to avoid a car shuttle on a one-way hike, as well as the problems associated with leaving an automobile overnight, is to have someone drop you off at the trailhead and pick you up when you have finished.

PROPER CLOTHING AND EQUIPMENT

As with any outdoor pursuit, you need to be ready for abrupt fluctuations in the weather. Warm and sunny summer days may become cold and rainy within minutes. Also, do not be surprised if a pleasant spring or fall day changes to one with sleet or snow.

Because people are caught off guard on days such as this, when the temperature dips into the low 60s and 50s, **hypothermia**—one of the leading causes of hiker and camper deaths—may strike. Be prepared by carrying raingear and an insulating layer of clothing, such as a wool sweater or synthetic jacket, in your day pack. Layering is a more effective means of keeping warm than wearing one thick garment, so carry several items of clothing.

In addition to the above, your pack should include a first aid kit, flashlight, knife, compass, toilet paper, and waterproof matches. Be prepared for possible cool nights even in the summer.

It is not necessary to subject your feet to the tortures of heavy-duty boots to enjoy hiking in Virginia. Unless you have ankle or foot problems, comfortable tennis, walking, or running shoes will probably suffice for most of the hikes—especially the shorter ones in the eastern half of the state. Lightweight hiking boots or shoes should be sufficient for journeys into the mountains and on overnight trips.

Applying moleskin or a similar product (available at most pharmacies and outdoors outfitters) immediately at the first sign of a "hot spot" will help prevent blisters from developing.

These are just the basics you should know about foot travel in areas removed from the mainstream. Obviously it is not the intent of this guidebook to be a hiking or backpacking primer, so I suggest you solicit advice from backpacking acquaintances, trail club members, and outdoors outfitters. I am a firm believer in supporting your neighborhood outdoors outfitter instead of mail-order companies. Not only will the local folks help fit and adjust your equipment and be there if you have any questions, but some shops rent hiking and camping equipment, enabling you to try something before you decide to buy it.

HIKING AND CAMPING ETIQUETTE

Endorsed by almost every organization connected with the outdoors, the **Leave No Trace Seven Principles** have been developed to protect a fragile natural world from increased usage. (Leave No Trace Seven Principles © by the Leave No Trace Center for Outdoor Ethics: lnt.org.)

Plan Ahead and Prepare

- Know the regulations and special concerns for the area you'll visit.
- Prepare for extreme weather, hazards, and emergencies.
- Schedule your trip to avoid times of high use.
- Visit in small groups. Split larger parties into groups of 4–6.
- Repackage food to minimize waste.
- Use a map and compass to eliminate the use of marking paint, rock cairns, or flagging.

Travel and Camp on Durable Surfaces

- Durable surfaces include established trails and campsites, rock, gravel, dry grasses, and snow.
- Protect riparian areas by camping at least 200 feet from lakes and streams.
- Good campsites are found, not made. Altering a site is not necessary.

In popular areas:

- Concentrate use on existing trails and campsites.
- Walk single file in the middle of the trail, even when wet or muddy.
- Keep campsites small. Focus activities in areas where vegetation is absent.

In pristine areas:

- Disperse use to prevent the creation of campsites and trails.
- Avoid places where impacts are just beginning.

Dispose of Waste Properly

- Pack it in, pack it out. Inspect your campsite and rest areas for trash or spilled foods. Pack out all trash, leftover food, and litter.
- Deposit solid human waste in catholes dug 6–8 inches deep at least 200 feet from water, camp, and trails. Cover and disguise the cathole when finished.
- Pack out toilet paper and other hygiene products.
- To wash yourself or your dishes, carry water 200 feet away from streams or lakes and use small amounts of biodegradable soap. Scatter strained dishwater.

Leave What You Find

- Preserve the past: examine, but do not touch, cultural or historic structures and artifacts.
- Leave rocks, plants, and other natural objects as you find them.
- Avoid introducing or transporting nonnative species.
- Do not build structures or furniture or dig trenches.

Minimize Campfire Impacts

- Campfires can cause lasting impacts to the backcountry. Use a lightweight stove for cooking and enjoy a candle lantern for light.
- Where fires are permitted, use established fire rings, fire pans, or mound fires.
- Keep fires small. Only use sticks from the ground that can be broken by hand.
- Burn all wood and coals to ash, put out campfires completely, then scatter cool ashes.

Respect Wildlife

- Observe wildlife from a distance. Do not follow or approach wildlife.
- Never feed animals. Feeding wildlife damages their health, alters natural behaviors, and exposes them to predators and other dangers.
- Protect wildlife and your food by storing rations and trash securely.
- Control pets at all times, or leave them at home.
- Avoid wildlife during sensitive times: mating, nesting, raising young, or winter.

Be Considerate of Other Visitors

- Respect other visitors and protect the quality of their experience.
- Be courteous. Yield to other users on the trail.
- Step to the downhill side of the trail when encountering pack stock.
- Take breaks and camp away from trails and other visitors.
- Let nature's sounds prevail. Avoid loud voices and noises.

For further information, *The Green Guide to Low-Impact Hiking and Camping* by Laura and Guy Waterman is an excellent resource, providing details on not only the "how" of making little or no impact on the environment but also the "why."

HIKES AT A GLANCE

	REGION/HIKE	DISTANCE (in Miles)	VERTICAL RISE	VIEWS	GOOD FOR KIDS	WATERFALLS	CAMPING	HISTORY
	CHESAPEAKE BAY AND EASTERN VIRGINIA							
1	Grandview Nature Preserve *Chesapeake Bay shoreline*	5.0	0	W	✔	–	–	–
2	Newport News Park *Easy terrain; Civil War site*	5.6	130	W	–	–	D	✔
3	Hughlett Point Natural Area Preserve *Optional mile-long beach walk*	2.1	10	W	✔	–	–	–
4	Hickory Hollow Natural Area Preserve *Swamp exploration; wildflowers*	3.0	130	–	✔	–	–	–
5	Belle Isle State Park *Hike beside Rappahanock River*	5.0	30	W	✔*	–	D	–
6	The Northern Neck *Horsehead Cliffs fossil; Washington's birthplace*	4.0	370	W	✔*	–	D	✔
	CENTRAL VIRGINIA							
7	Cold Harbor *Civil War trenches*	1.0	100	–	✔	–	–	✔
8	Willis River Trail *Most rugged hike in the Piedmont; for the experienced hiker*	15.3	700	–	–	–	–	–
9	Lake Anna State Park *In the rolling woodlands of the Piedmont*	12.9	660	W	–	–	D	–
10	Spotsylvania *Site of major Civil War battle*	5.3	240	–	–	–	–	✔
11	Prince William Forest Park *Streams and isolation close to D.C.*	13.5	400	–	–	–	D, B	✔
12	Mason Neck State Park *Turtles, eagles, muskrats, and ducks*	2.7	50	W	✔	–	–	–
13	Bull Run–Occoquan River *Hike along streams most of the way*	11.0	3,180	W	–	–	–	–
14	Manassas National Battlefield Park *Site of two major Civil War battles*	5.5	390	–	–	–	–	✔
15	Sky Meadows State Park *Best view of the Piedmont*	5.4	1,460	M	✔*	–	B	–
16	Split Rock *Views of Shenandoah and Potomac Rivers*	5.2	950	W, M	–	–	–	✔
	BLUE RIDGE AND MASSANUTTEN MOUNTAINS							
17	Little Sluice Mountain and Cedar Creek *Mountains along Virginia–West Virginia border*	12.7	2,080	M	–	–	B	–
18	Big Schloss *Excellent views and interesting rock outcrops*	4.4	710	M	–	–	B	–
19	Signal Knob *Has become popular with mountain bikers*	10.4	2,220	M	–	–	B	–
20	Woodstock Observation Tower *Very easy walk with great views*	0.3	50	M	✔	–	–	–
21	Duncan Knob *Off-trail scramble to view*	8.5	2,240	M		–	B	–
22	Marys Rock *Views extend almost 360 degrees*	3.6	1,240	M	✔	–	–	–
23	Stony Man *Shenandoah Valley view*	3.5	760	M	✔*	–	–	–

KEY TO TABLE ABBREVIATIONS		
W = water views	D = developed camping available	* = for kids with stamina
M = mountain views	B = backcountry camping available	

HIKES AT A GLANCE *(continued)*

	REGION/HIKE	DISTANCE (in Miles)	VERTICAL RISE	VIEWS	GOOD FOR KIDS	WATERFALLS	CAMPING	HISTORY
	BLUE RIDGE AND MASSANUTTEN MOUNTAINS *(continued)*							
24	**Old Rag** *Arduous with rock scrambles, but extremely popular*	9.2	2,380	M	–	–	–	–
25	**Cedar Run and Whiteoak Canyon** *Almost continuous waterfalls*	8.0 or 9.3	2,560	–	–	✔	B	–
26	**Hawksbill** *High point of Shenandoah National Park*	2.8	740	M	✔	–	B	–
27	**Rapidan Camp** *President Hoover's mountain retreat; small streams*	7.4	1,480	–	–	–	B	✔
28	**Rocky Mountain, Brown Mountain, and Rockytop** *Two-day hike into isolated valley*	20.0	4,000	W, M	–	–	B	–
29	**Riprap Hollow** *Waterfall and swimming hole*	9.6	2,260	M	–	✔	B	–
30	**Blue Ridge Tunnel** *Dark, dripping tunnel almost a mile long*	2.3 or 4.6	300 or 480	–	✔	–	–	✔
31	**Whetstone Ridge** *Less used than many other trails; rugged ridgeline walk*	11.8	4,500	M	–	–	B	–
32	**White Rock Falls and Slacks Overlook Trail** *Along the Blue Ridge Parkway*	5.0	1,050	W	–	✔	B	–
33	**Sherando Lake** *Nice break from noisy campground*	1.6	280	M	✔		D	–
34	**Saint Mary's Wilderness** *Two-day hike with remote campsites*	17.5	2,400	–	–	✔	B	–
35	**Crabtree Falls** *Strenuous, but 1.5 miles of waterfalls*	5.8	1,520	W, M	✔ *	✔	B	–
36	**Appalachian and Mau-Har Trails** *Has everything that makes hiking worthwhile*	26.1	7,000	M	–	✔	B	–
37	**Mount Pleasant** *A protected National Scenic Area*	5.5	1,400	M	–	–	B	–
38	**Cole Mountain** *High mountain meadow*	5.8	1,320	M	–	–	B	–
	WESTERN VIRGINIA							
39	**North River Gorge** *Nine river fords*	4.5	40	–	–	–	B	–
40	**Todd Lake Recreation Area and Trimble Mountain** *Circuit hike of Trimble Mountain*	3.8	1,120	M	–	–	D, B	–
41	**Wild Oak National Recration Trail** *Three days with ups and downs, but also long ridges*	27.2	7,550	M	–	–	B	–
42	**Ramseys Draft** *Popular wilderness; fords and possible overgrown trails*	8.5	1,080	M	–	–	B	–
43	**Shenandoah Mountain** *Easiest long hike in Virginia mountains; snowshoeing*	10.6	1,400	M	–	–	B	–
44	**Elliott Knob and Falls Hollow** *Great sunrise and sunset spot*	9.0	2,060	M	–	✔	B	–
45	**Laurel Fork** *Most isolated hike; fords and possible overgrown trail*	14.0	2,300	–	–	✔	B	–
46	**Hidden Valley** *Trout fishing on side streams*	4.3	100	W	–	–	D, B	–
47	**Lake Moomaw** *Lakeshore camping*	6.6	1,700	W	–	–	B	–
48	**Rich Hole Wilderness** *Accessible; lightly traveled; signs of black bears*	5.8	980	M	–	–	B	–
49	**Douthat State Park: Beards Mountain** *Explore a mountaintop environment*	7.1	1,360	M	–	–	D	–
50	**Douthat State Park: Tuscarora Overlook** *Two waterfalls and a grand overlook*	9.6	2,180	M	–	✔	D	–
51	**Dry Run** *Secluded stream with campsites*	9.7	1,640	–	–	–	B	–

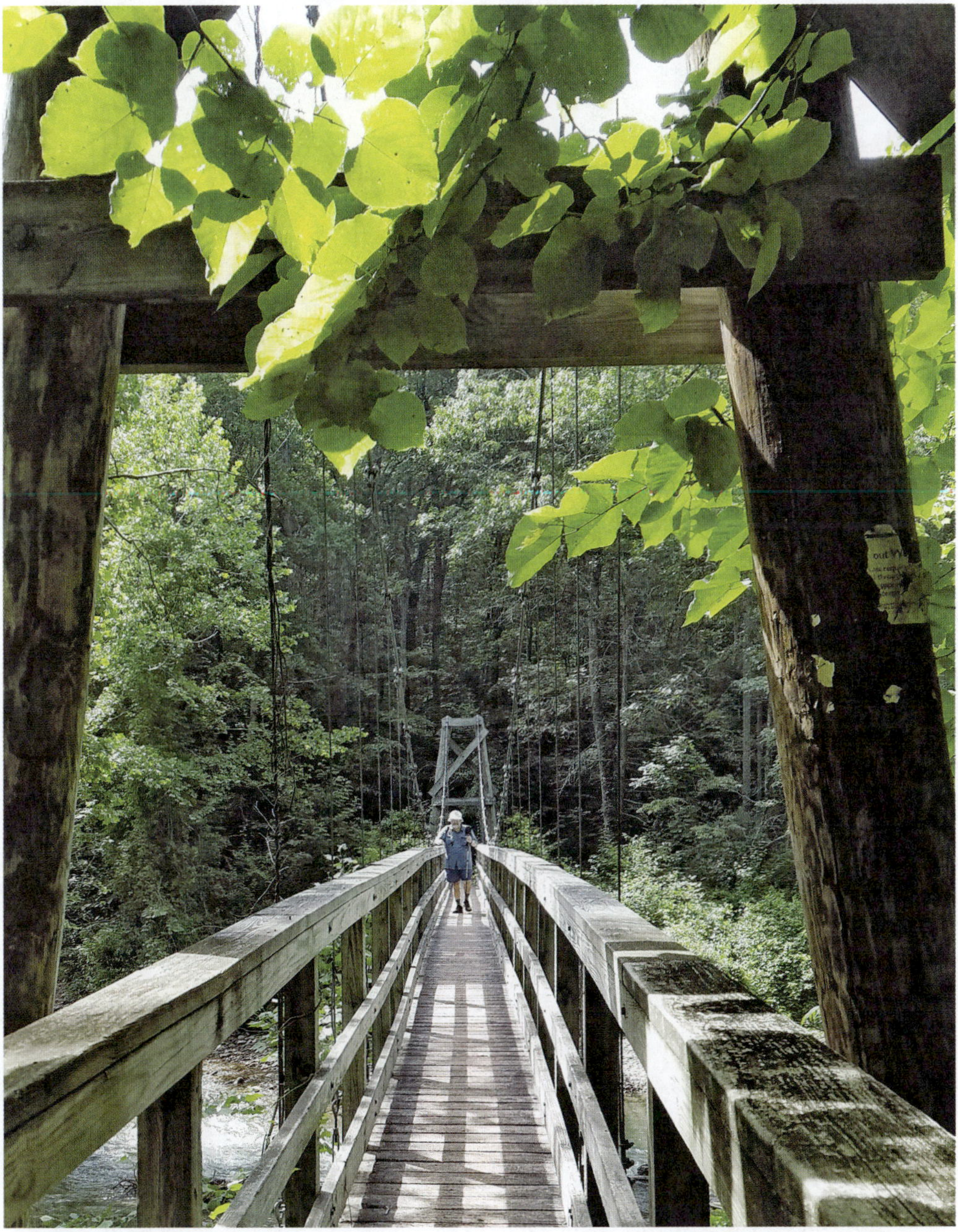

The Jackson River swinging bridge

KEY TO TABLE ABBREVIATIONS		
W = water views	D = developed camping available	* = for kids with stamina
M = mountain views	B = backcountry camping available	

Chesapeake Bay and Eastern Virginia

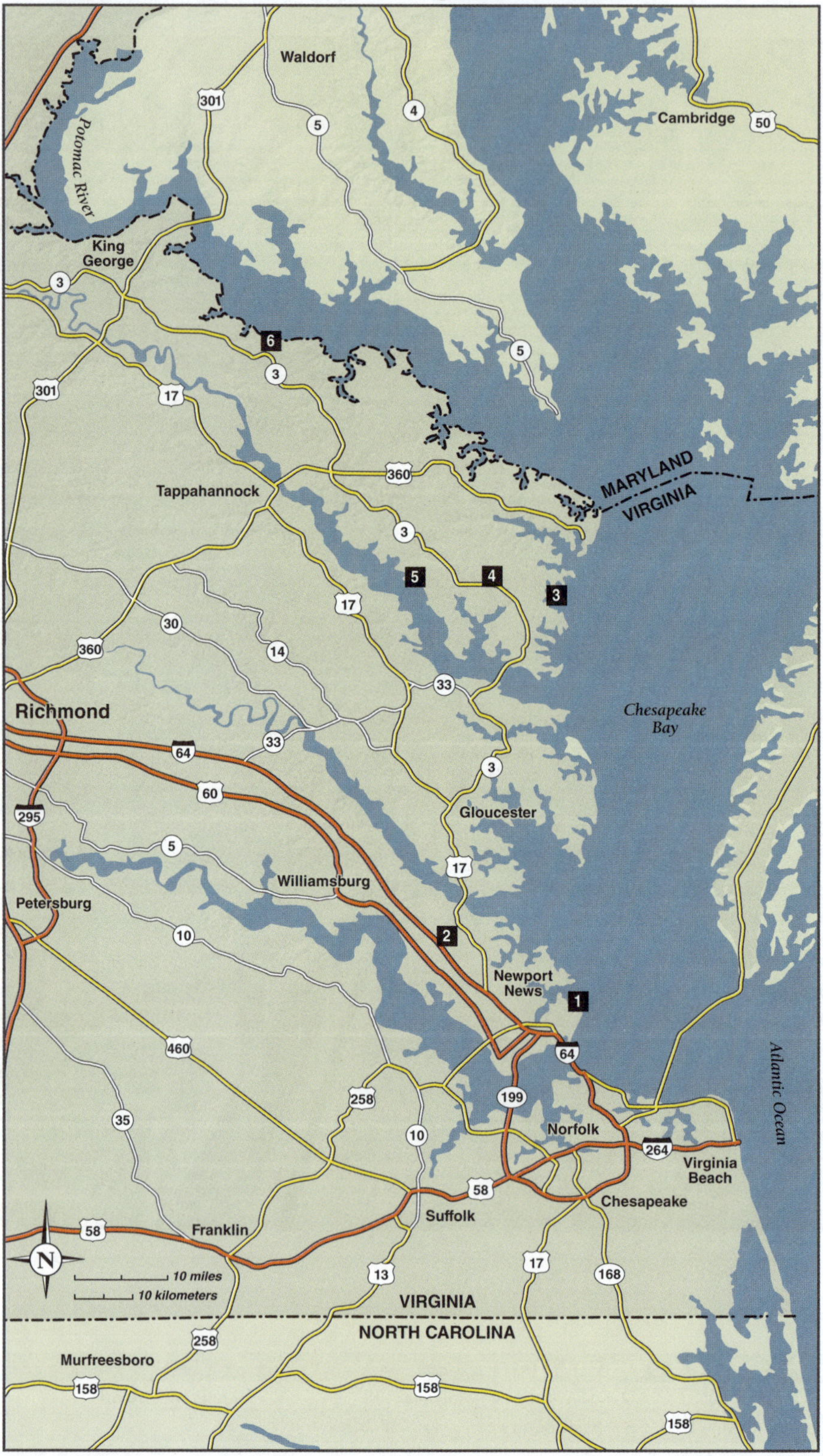

Chesapeake Bay and Eastern Virginia

Grandview Nature Preserve

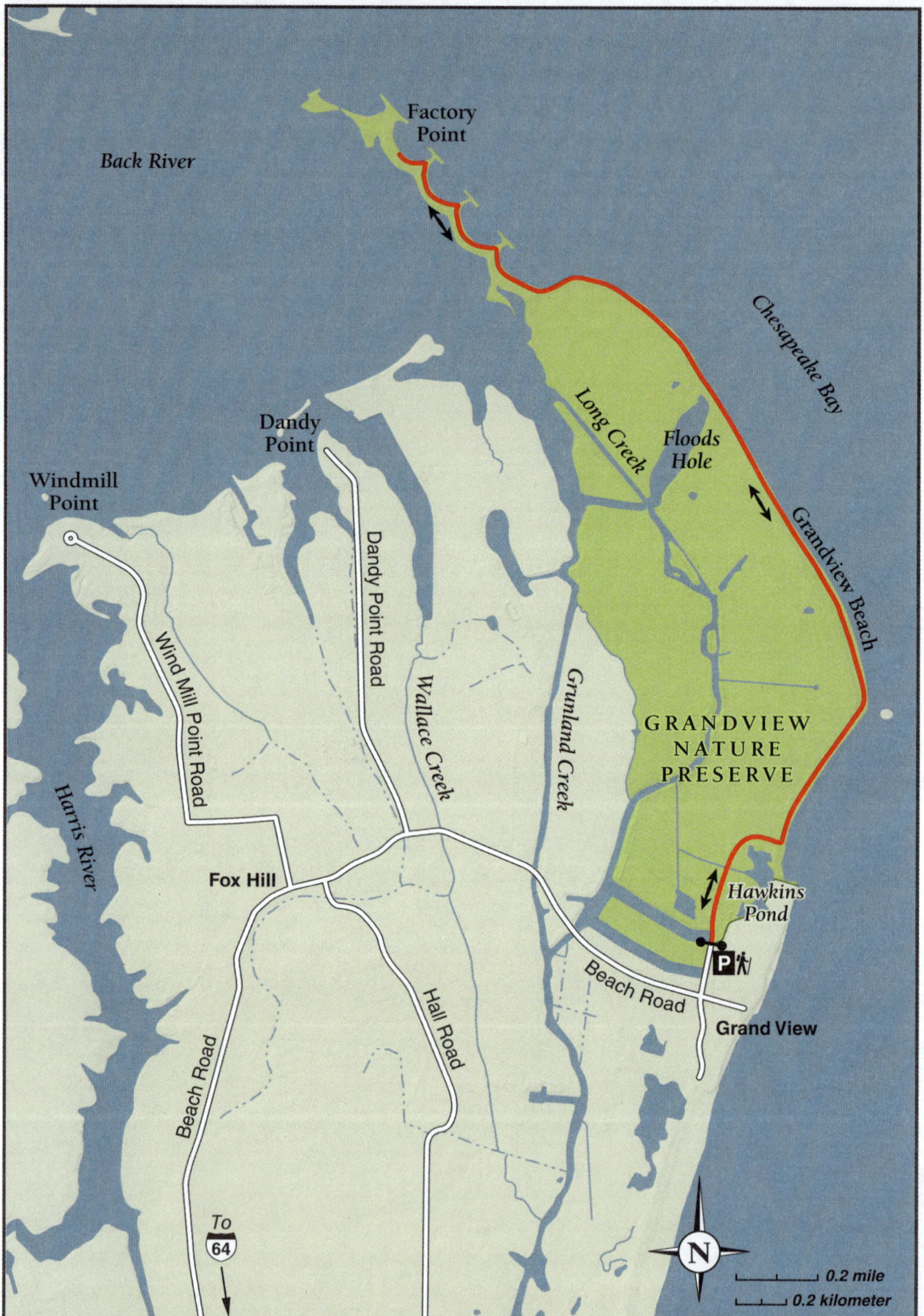

1 Grandview Nature Preserve

- **GPS:** N37.0791832 W76.2775342
- **TOTAL DISTANCE (round-trip):** 5.0 miles
- **HIKING TIME:** 2.5 hours
- **VERTICAL RISE:** None
- **MAP:** USGS *Hampton*
- **CONTACT:** Hampton Parks, Recreation, and Leisure Services
  22 Lincoln St.
  Hampton, VA 23669; 757-727-8311
  hampton.gov/1187/Parks-Recreation

The Hike at a Glance

0.4 Turn left onto the beach

0.7 Round a corner of the beach

1.7 Large dunes; shortly thereafter walk onto a narrow spit of land

2.5 Sign denoting area behind it closed in the warmer months; retrace steps

5.0 Return to automobile

The Chesapeake Bay, America's largest bay, is the catch basin for a far-reaching drainage system that covers 64,000 square miles. Snowmelt that begins its downstream journey near Cooperstown, New York, meets and mingles in the bay with rainwater that fell on the higher elevations of the Allegheny Mountains on the central West Virginia–Virginia border. The bay is considered an estuary, a body of water where tidal movements bring salt water upstream, where it comes into contact with the fresh water being carried toward the ocean by river currents.

There are many other estuaries throughout the world, such as Puget Sound in Washington, Cook Inlet in Alaska, and the fjords of Norway, but none of them are nearly as productive as the Chesapeake Bay. Millions of pounds of seafood are harvested from the bay each year, including large percentages of America's supply of blue crabs and oysters. A number of conditions combine to make the bay this productive. Probably the two most important factors are the large amounts of fresh water coming into the bay and the vast acreage of marshlands surrounding the bay, which provides an abundance of detritus and other nutrients. These wetlands are home to numerous shorebirds and are also major stopping-over and resting areas on the Great Atlantic Flyway for migratory waterfowl, including a wide array of ducks, swans, and Canada geese.

Although the Chesapeake Bay has about 4,000 miles of shoreline—more than the entire US Pacific coast (excluding Alaska)—a large percentage of it is privately owned, heavily developed, or both. It is our good fortune that the city of Hampton has set aside a few miles of that shoreline as the Grandview Nature Preserve, where you and I can walk on a secluded beach, far removed from hordes of sunbathing vacationers, carnival-atmosphere boardwalks, high-rise condominiums, or busy shipping yards. Here, in a place of relative quiet, we can study the bay's waters, shoreline, and marshes at our leisure, or just sit peacefully on the sand.

Be aware that the preserve has no restroom facilities or potable water. Note, too, especially if you're hiking in the cooler months, that the winds around the bay can teach your body the meaning of a windchill factor. There is no shade in the preserve, so be ready for the glare of the sun hitting from above and reflecting off the water beside you and the sand underneath your feet. Regulations prohibit visitors from being in the preserve after sunset.

DIRECTIONS To reach the preserve, take I-64 Exit 263 in Hampton onto US 250N/VA 134S/Mercury Boulevard and drive 3.2 miles to make a left onto Fox Hill Road. Continue straight onto Silver Isle Boulevard in an additional 2.9 miles, but just 0.1 mile later turn left onto Beach Road and follow it for 2.7 miles to make a left onto State Park Road. Park your automobile at the end of the street, being sure to obey the posted regulations.

Route Description

Walk through the gate, and immediately to the right you may see several turtles basking in the sun on and around Hawkins Pond. At dawn or dusk, you might see a raccoon searching for a meal at the pond, and despite all the houses and other developments in the area, deer have been spotted roaming about on the preserve. Arrive at the beach in 0.4 mile and turn to your left (to the right is private property in a few yards), enjoying, as the name of this place suggests, a grand view of the Chesapeake Bay. Huge cargo ships often go slowly by, for the Norfolk–Hampton area is one of the busiest ports in the world. Off in the distance you may be able to make out the Chesapeake Bay Bridge-Tunnel, built in 1965 at a cost of $200 million. The bridge-tunnel spans the mouth of the bay—a distance of 18 miles—joining southeast Virginia with the Delmarva Peninsula. A trip across the bridge-tunnel to the peninsula is worthwhile; Jay Abercrombie thoroughly covers some good hikes in this area, which most people tend to overlook, in his book *Weekend Walks on the Delmarva Peninsula*.

Continue walking and doing a bit of beachcombing. You will find the shells of the jackknife clam, known locally as a razor clam because of its resemblance to the old-fashioned shaving razor. You might happen to see a few live ones wash up on the beach, but they are such fast burrowers that they will quickly disappear, making them next to impossible to dig up. The clams use a strong foot to anchor themselves in the sand as they send up siphons to feed on plankton and detritus floating about in the water.

Various body parts of the blue crab may be spread over the sand. In addition to being a favorite food of the shorebirds, blue crabs are one of the most important seafood species of the bay. Commercial watermen catch millions of pounds annually, with the same amount also estimated to be caught by weekend crabbers. The crabs bury themselves in the mud and become dormant in the winter, emerging as soon as the water temperature rises a few degrees. You will find large numbers of female crabs here in late summer, as they move into this area from the north so that their young will be released into the more saline water found near the mouth of the bay. The interesting lives of blue crabs are described in superbly entertaining and nontechnical detail in William Warner's *Beautiful Swimmers: Watermen, Crabs, and the Chesapeake Bay* ("beautiful swimmers" is the English translation of the blue crab's Latin name, *Callinectes sapidus*).

The dune on your left was formed when sand, blown about by winds off the bay, became trapped in bits of beach debris. As the winds continued to blow more sand onto and over the dune, wind- and salt-resistant vegetation established itself and helped stabilize the dune.

Rounding a corner of the beach at 0.7 mile, look for brown pelicans resting on rocks in the water. Pelicans were once on the decline around the bay, but they have made a remarkable comeback since the banning of the pesticide DDT. It is now common to be able to watch one use its 90-inch wingspan to build up speed for a spectacular dive into the water. The cartoons you watched in your childhood may have convinced you that a pelican uses its pouch to carry fish, but in reality the pouch is primarily employed as a device to scoop the fish out of the water.

Looking back onto the beach, you'll see that the sand is dotted by small holes with scratch marks in front of them. These are the homes of small ghost crabs. If you wait and watch long enough, one of them will make a mad dash for the water because they have to wet their gills on a periodic basis. Sadly for them, this is when they often become a meal for a circling gull or tern. In addition to the crab holes, that string of tan capsules you find on the beach is a collection of whelk eggs. Many times the capsules do not hatch and, if you break them open, you'll find tiny whelk shells inside, identical to those of adults.

Rounding another curve in the beach, you will notice the dune has become large enough to develop sand "cliffs," but by the time you have walked 1.7 miles, the dune will have disappeared and you can look out across the inland marsh where herons and egrets wade in search of food. At about this spot, the waves become larger and louder because the land no longer slopes gently into the water but rather drops steeply into the bay. Shortly thereafter, you will arrive on a narrow spit of land, which has some interesting history.

This spit existed until the late 1990s when a violent storm that blew in from the northeast breached the land, creating a small channel and separating the tip of the spit from the mainland. It remained this way until bulkheads were constructed around 2010, which allowed sand to build up and rejoin everything together again. The spit has now become a popular place for boaters to have picnics. At 2.5 miles, you should come to a sign that will inform you that the land behind it is closed to visitors during the warmer months of the year. This is to protect migratory birds—primarily oystercatchers, black skimmers, and least terns—during their nesting season.

Turn around and stroll back to your car, delighting in the sunshine, the salty breeze, the antics of passing seagulls, and the discovery of other sights, sounds, and small treasures you may have missed on the way out.

While in this area you should consider driving over to the City of Hampton's Sandy Bottom Nature Park (accessible from I-61 Exit 261A). A stroll along the several miles of pathways there will take you through lake edge, marsh, streamside, and forest habitats.

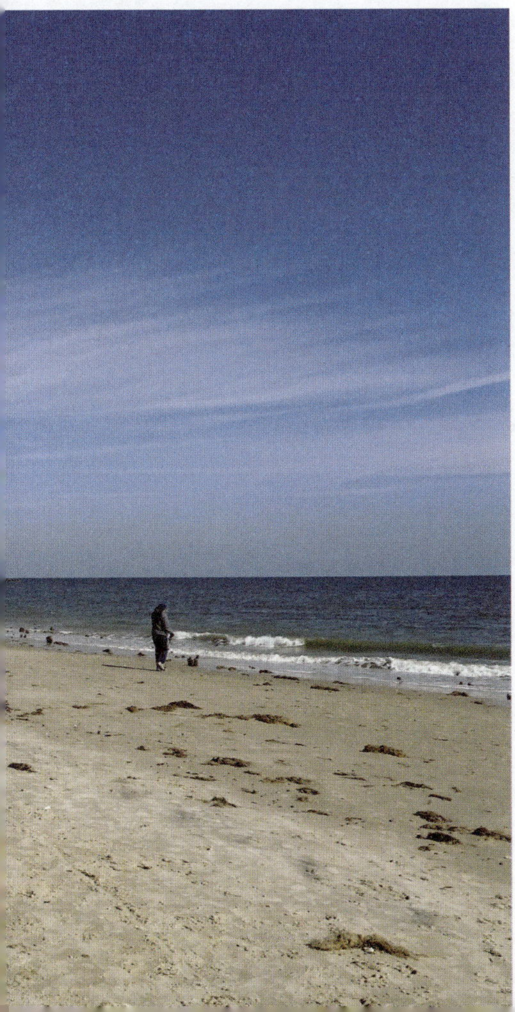

The preserve may be lightly visited on a late fall day.

Newport News Park

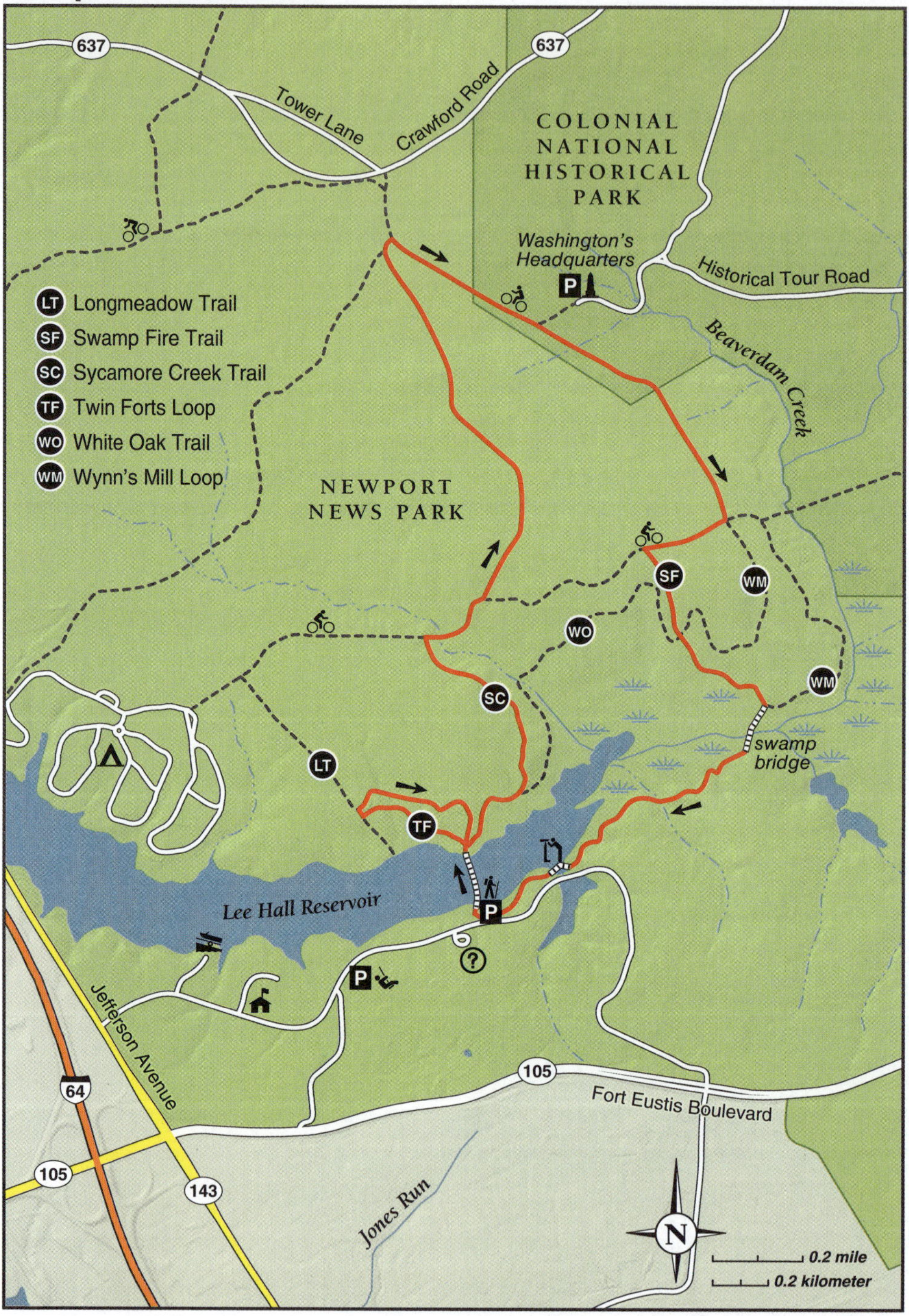

2 Newport News Park

- **GPS:** N37.1826327 W76.5365394
- **TOTAL DISTANCE (circuit):** 5.6 miles
- **HIKING TIME:** 3.0 hours
- **VERTICAL RISE:** 130 feet
- **MAPS:** USGS *Yorktown; Newport News Park* map
- **CONTACT:** Newport News Park
  13560 Jefferson Ave.
  Newport News, VA 23603-1104
  757-888-3333
  nnva.gov/894/Parks-Squares-Plazas

The Hike at a Glance

0.0 Cross bridge over Lee Hall Reservoir; at far end turn left onto Twin Forts Loop

0.4 Go right at four-way intersection; 100 feet later stay right to continue on Twin Forts Loop

0.8 Left onto White Oak Nature Trail

1.1 Left onto Sycamore Creek Trail

1.5 Right onto Bikeway

1.7 Left onto unmarked wide roadway

2.6 Road comes in from left, but continue a few feet to make a right onto Bikeway

3.6 Bear left onto ungraveled roadbed

3.7 Turn right onto Wynn's Mill Loop; soon come to Swamp Fire Trail and turn left to cross footbridge

4.5 Another section of Wynn's Mill Loop comes in from left; keep right, cross Swamp Bridge and keep right at its far end

5.1 Observation deck

5.6 End of hike

Golden Gate Park in San Francisco and Central Park in New York may be more famous than the Newport News Park, but these and other municipal parks often contain amusement rides, zoos, bandstands, and other highly developed areas spread out and connected by networks of paved roadways. With approximately 8,000 mostly wooded acres, Newport News Park is one of the country's largest city-owned parks to provide hikers with multiple miles of walking routes through dense forests, well removed from automobiles and the resulting din of traffic noise—all the more amazing when you realize the park sits within the confines of one of Virginia's most heavily populated areas.

In order to meet the diverse recreational needs of so many people, the park provides bicycle and boat rentals, an archery range, a 36-hole golf course and driving range, picnic shelters, an arboretum, an interpretive center, an excellent seasonal schedule of naturalist-conducted programs, playgrounds, concessions, and a campground with close to 200 sites. Yet, all of these facilities are concentrated on just a few hundred acres, and approximately 40 miles of pathways and fire roads can lead visitors away from intensely used areas around Lee Hall Reservoir and through dark stands of loblolly pine, by overgrown reminders of wars past, and into lushly green and quiet swamplands. The official state transportation map of Virginia may show this as metropolitan property, but you are in for a most decidedly un-urban walk. Park personnel and volunteers have inventoried in excess of 70 spring flowers; more than 100 summer and fall blossoms; at least 60 tree types; various shrubs, vines, and other plants; and so much wildlife that it takes an eight-page pamphlet just to list all of the native species. Take a look at the total vertical rise you're going to experience while on this hike of more than 5 miles and you will know you're in for an easy stroll over gentle terrain.

DIRECTIONS Take I-64 Exit 250B in Newport News onto VA 105 East, drive for less than 0.2 mile, and make a left onto VA 143. In 0.5 mile, turn right into the park and continue about 1 mile to the Discovery Center, where you can obtain maps and other information about the park, which is open year-round.

Route Description

You can leave your car either at the center or in the parking area across the road from it. Begin by crossing the bridge over Lee Hall Reservoir, which is open for the fishing of catfish, largemouth bass, northern pike, crappie, chain pickerel, bluegill, and white and yellow perch. At the far end of the bridge, bear left to follow the left branch of the Twin Forts Loop, where you'll see the first of many mounds and trenches that made up the Confederate lines of defense during the Civil War's Battle of Dam Number One. The dam, now covered by the waters of the reservoir, is still visible from the footbridge you just crossed.

At the beginning of 1862, the Union strategy of the peninsula campaign was for Major General George B. McClellan's Army of the Potomac to swiftly defeat the Confederate forces on the peninsula and move on to capture Richmond before it could be fortified. At this time the war was still in its early stages and the Union felt the fall of Richmond would depress Southern resolve and bring about a speedy conclusion to the rebellion. Preparing for the impending attack, the Confederates constructed, with the supplementary labor of slaves from nearby plantations, a series of fortifications (known as breastworks because soldiers could fire from the trenches but still be protected to the breast by the high mounds) stretching across the peninsula. Following a failed attempt to make it past the Warwick River on April 5, the Army of the Potomac was again repulsed on April 16 by soldiers entrenched behind the breastworks close to Dam Number One.

Some of the old breastworks found at other sites in Virginia have deteriorated to the point of being barely distinguishable, but the ones you'll see throughout your hike in the park are remarkably well preserved, many coming close to retaining their original shape and size. Please refrain from walking on any of them.

After the two skirmishes, McClellan halted frontal assaults in favor of large artillery bombardments. After suffering several weeks under the Union barrage, the Confederates retreated—not quite in defeat, as they had gained a month's worth of valuable time for Richmond to fortify and reinforce.

At 0.3 mile, the trail swings away from the reservoir to cross a creek beside the high mounds of the breastworks. When you come to the four-way intersection at 0.4 mile, the pathway straight ahead goes to the campground while the Longmeadow Trail to the left heads back to the reservoir. You need to continue right for 100 feet before making another right and continuing on the Twin Forts Loop, walking on the other side of the breastworks you've been observing.

At 0.8 mile, the route will have returned you to the bridge, where you'll make a left onto the White Oak Nature Trail. People who have been to Florida or the Caribbean may be reminded of mangroves when looking at the vegetation in the shallow waters of the reservoir. On the dry land, the mixed forest of oak, hickory, and loblolly pine has an intermediate story of holly, pawpaw, and dogwood, with very little undergrowth. Make a left onto the Sycamore Creek Trail at 1.1 miles, reaching the well-maintained Bikeway at 1.5 miles. To the left, it is about 0.7 mile to the campground; turn right into a younger forest of smaller trees. Be alert at 1.7 miles, where the Bikeway curves to the right; you want to take the unmarked but wide roadway to the left, where the undergrowth suddenly expands into hundreds of blueberry bushes, which are abundant throughout the park. A road comes in from the left at 2.6 miles, but you want to keep to the right for a few more feet to make a right onto the Bikeway and enter a small portion of the Colonial National Historical Park.

The historical park commemorates the battle of Yorktown and the surrender of Lord Cornwallis to General George Washington. (The park is connected by way of the 20-plus-mile Colonial Parkway—passing through Colonial Williamsburg—to the site of Jamestown, the first permanent English settlement in the New World.) Honeysuckle and poison ivy vines

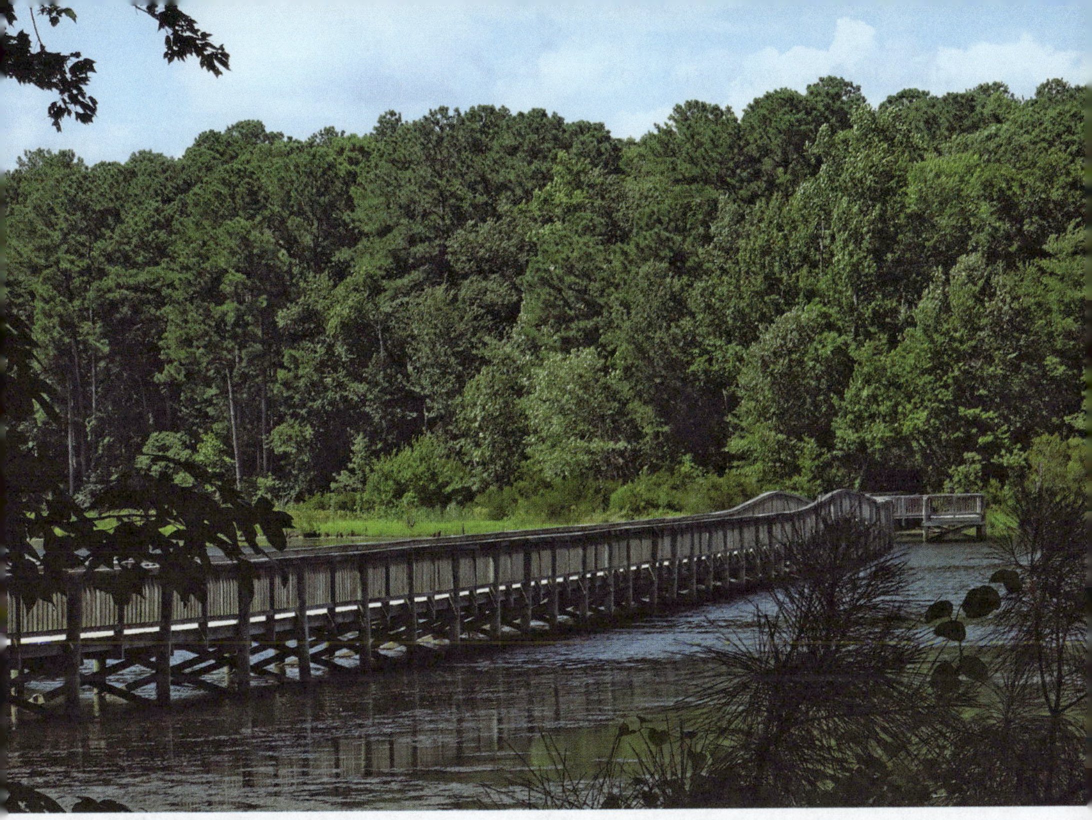

Lee Hall Reservoir is open for fishing.

are draped over the trees where a road to the left leads approximately 500 feet to Washington's Yorktown headquarters. Continuing right on the Bikeway, you'll return to the confines of Newport News Park; bear left onto an ungraveled roadbed when the Bikeway makes a 90-degree turn at 3.6 miles.

Turn right onto Wynn's Mill Loop (which has habitat for the cottonmouth snake, so be alert) at 3.7 miles, making sure, 100 feet beyond that, to turn right again. The maze of a multitude of breastworks going off in different directions must have required hundreds of hours of backbreaking labor to construct. Coming to the Swamp Fire Trail, turn left, soon crossing a small footbridge. Five-lined skinks are often seen skittering across the bridge in search of insects. The young skinks have five well-defined lines along their backs and bright-blue tails, but the characteristics fade and become less obvious with age. As defense mechanisms, the skink has a detachable tail as well as a bite powerful enough to draw blood.

Another section of the Wynn's Mill Loop comes in from the left at 4.5 miles; you want to keep right, heading onto the Swamp Bridge and into a radically different environment of lush summer greenery. Mixed in with the swamp's dense tangle of vegetation is arrow arum, differentiated from other arrowhead-shaped plants by its distinctive long green sheath, or spathe, surrounding tiny flowers that grow on a fleshy spike known as a spadix by botanists. Spotted turtles, aptly named for the yellow dots on their head, neck, and shell, are sometimes seen basking in warm sunshine on logs floating in the swamp. Although they may not appear so as they leisurely slide into the water when disturbed, spotted turtles are amazingly intelligent creatures and have shown an ability to correctly negotiate elaborate mazes.

At the far end of the bridge, make a right, coming to an observation platform at 5.1 miles.

Looking to your right, you'll see where the lake meets the swamp, and it is in this zone of transition that Canada geese, tundra swans, and a variety of ducks make their winter homes. Continue along the trail, cross a footbridge that parallels the paved road, and stay along the reservoir shoreline to the end of the hike at 5.6 miles.

If you haven't had your fill of easy hiking on nearly flat tidewater terrain, there are still miles of pathways and fire roads you can use to explore the thousands of acres in a less frequently visited part of the park across VA 105. Personnel at the Discovery Center can supply you with the information you'll need.

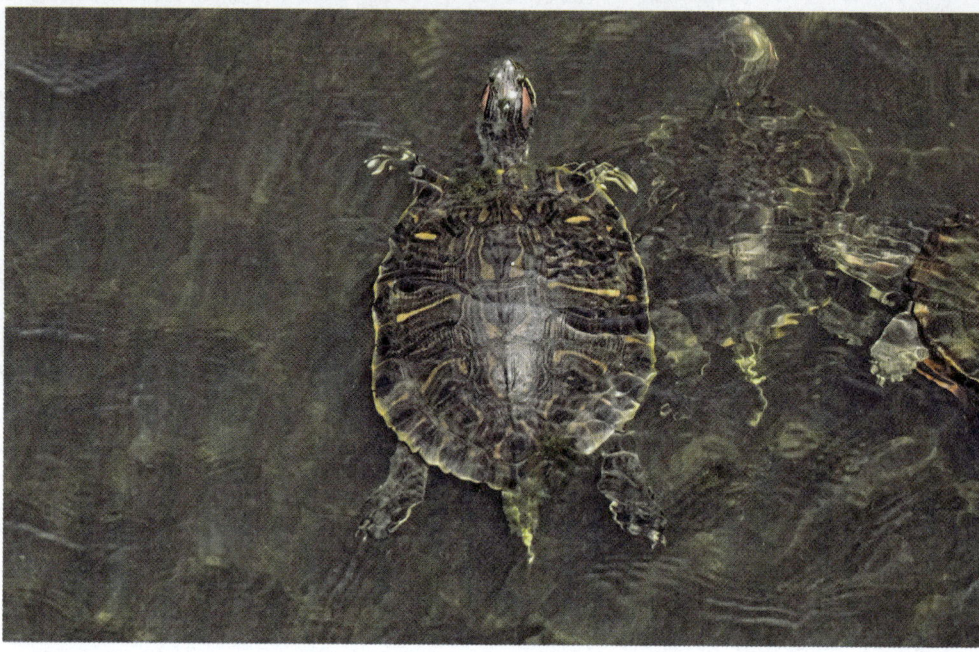

Dozens of turtles live in the reservoir.

3 Hughlett Point Natural Area Preserve

- **GPS:** N37.7418722 W76.3174065
- **TOTAL DISTANCE (circuit):** 2.1 miles
- **HIKING TIME:** 45 minutes
- **VERTICAL RISE:** 10 feet
- **MAP:** USGS *Fleets Bay*
- **CONTACT:** Division of Natural Heritage
  600 E. Main St., 24th Floor
  Richmond, VA 23219
  804-786-7951
  dcr.virginia.gov/natural-heritage/natural-area-preserves/hughlett

The Hike at a Glance

0.15 Right onto woods road

0.4 Left onto side trail to observation deck; retrace steps to woods road and turn left

0.9 Observation deck; left turn onto beach a few feet later

1.8 Make left onto trail into woods; turn left onto woods road and a few feet later make right onto trail back to parking area

2.1 Return to your automobile

Like Belle Isle State Park (see Hike 5), the Hughlett Point Natural Area Preserve is a gift Virginians gave themselves by voting for the 1992 Parks and Recreational Facilities Bond. The U.S. Fish and Wildlife Service also provided funds to help purchase the 204-acre tract in order to protect the rare northeastern beach tiger beetle and the occurrences of Chesapeake Bay salt marshes, beaches, and dunes.

Enclosed on three sides by the waters of Ingram Cove, Dividing Creek, and the Chesapeake Bay, and rising no more than 10 feet above sea level, the preserve in many places is more marsh than it is dry land. Plants that find a favorable home here include needle rush, salt meadow hay, switchgrass, common reed, cordgrass, and marsh elder. The inland marshes are bordered by wax myrtle, whose berries begin forming in August and develop a white, waxy dust that was used in former times to make bayberry candles. But it is not just the berries that have a pleasant scent; rubbing just about any part of the plant will produce the familiar fragrance. Areas just slightly lower in elevation produce the right conditions for cattails to survive.

DIRECTIONS From VA 3 in Kilmarnock, in the main part of town, turn northeast onto VA 200 and follow it 4.3 miles to a right turn onto VA 606. In another 2.1 miles, make a right onto VA 605. The parking area for the preserve is on the left in an additional 2.0 miles. No visitor's or parking fee is charged, but be aware that it is a day-use area only. Pets must be on a leash at all times.

Route Description

Enter the preserve by taking the boardwalk into a forest dominated by loblolly pine trees, where you might see a gray fox splashing through shallow, tannin-stained water in pursuit of an early morning meal. The mounds of what appear to be dirt covered by rich vegetation are actually the decaying piles of wood debris left over from the last time this area was logged, several decades ago. Look closely and you may find that tracks made by heavy logging equipment are slowly disappearing into the soft soil.

Intersect a woods road at 0.15 mile and turn right; the Chesapeake Bay is visible through the vegetation to the left. To appreciate as much of what the preserve has to offer as possible, turn left onto a side trail at 0.4 mile to follow it out to an observation deck overlooking a large marsh and the bay. Note that the deck you are standing upon is built with recycled plastic; maybe one of your old soda bottles contributed

Hughlett Point Natural Area Preserve

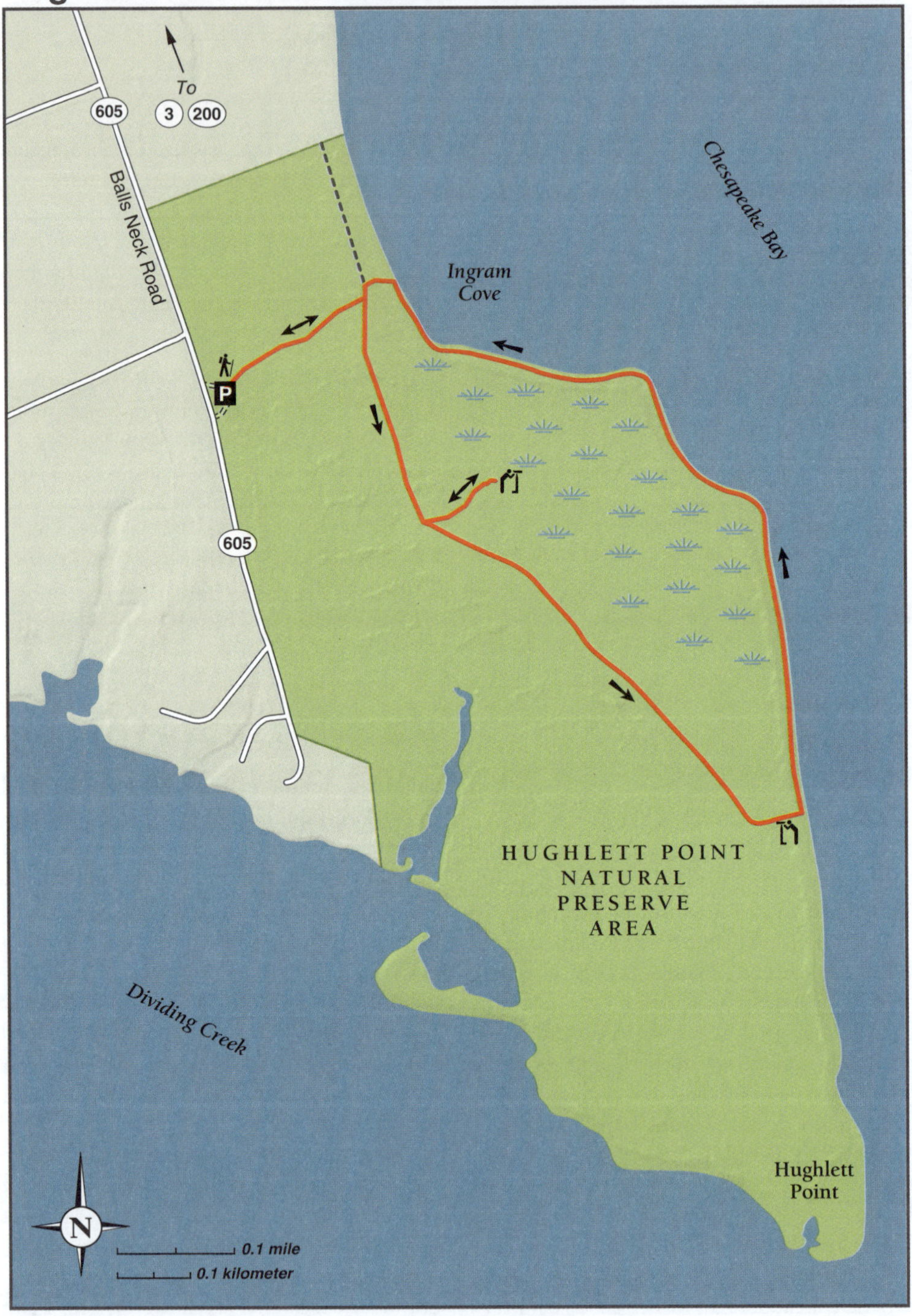

to this "lumber" and helped save a tree from being destroyed.

From the vantage point of the deck, the Chesapeake Bay and its accompanying shoreline look much as they did at the time of Captain John Smith's explorations in the early 1600s. Reminders of the modern world may be a large ship passing by on the horizon, or the smoke from the menhaden processing plant in Reedville to the north. Menhaden, herring that can grow up to 14 inches in length and distinguished by silver sides marked with large dark spots below a bluish upper portion, are caught in large quantities in the bay. Most often turned into fertilizer, the fish may also be included in pet foods or nutritional supplements.

Return to the main trail and turn left, soon passing a possible wet-weather small pond on the right at 0.7 mile. The route swings to the left at 0.9 mile, coming to another observation deck. The cattail-lined marsh here has been known to be a good place to watch ospreys and bald eagles on the wing. In addition to providing nourishment and home-building material for muskrats, cattails help stabilize soil along the edge of the marsh.

You will arrive at the beach, the home of the northeastern beach tiger beetle, less than 300 feet later. The beetle begins its life by crawling out of the egg its parent laid in the sand. Spending the first two years of its life in the larval stage, it grows to 5/8 inch in length and has noticeable humps on its back, as well as large jaws like the adult. It survives by waiting at the mouth of a 4- to 10-inch burrow for prey to come along and be snatched by the powerful jaws. With russet-green heads and black markings on white backs, the adults are only two-thirds of an inch long. They can often be seen during the warmer months, hopping across the sand

In a natural process, Chesapeake Bay is gradually eroding the shoreline.

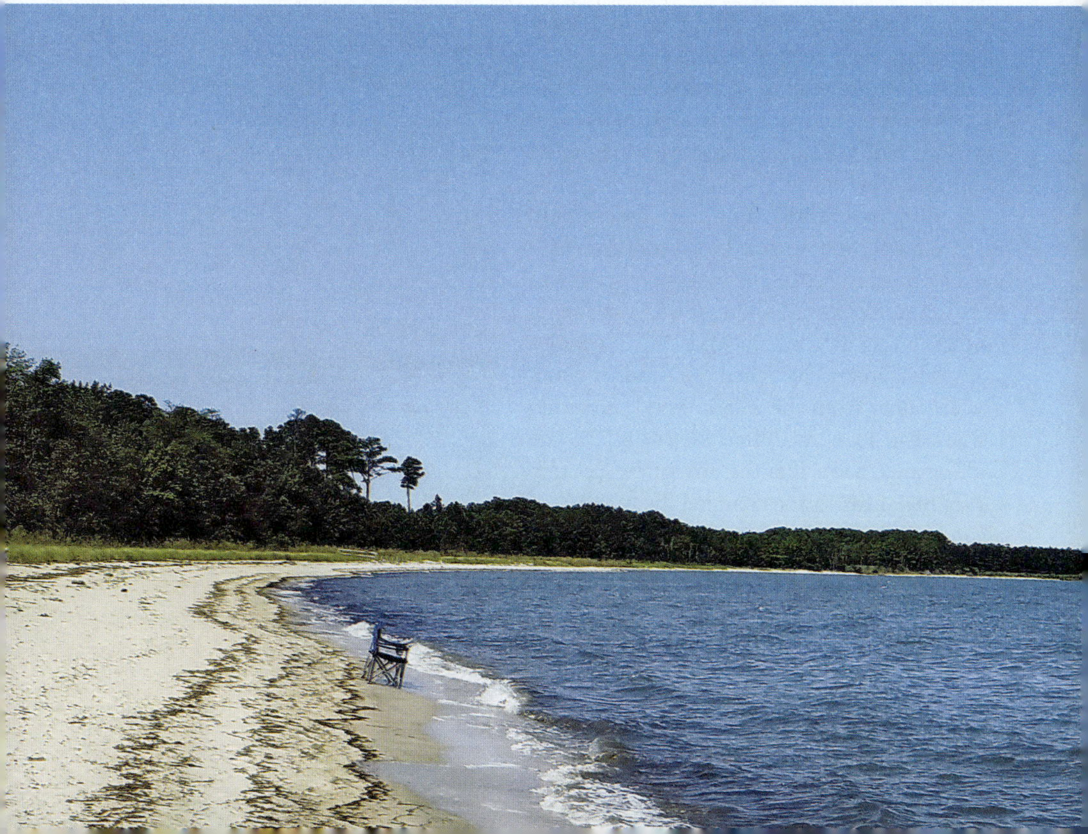

in search of food. At one time these beetles inhabited much of the shoreline around the Chesapeake Bay, but waterfront development, increased human foot traffic on their sandy home, and the effects of pollutants have caused their numbers to decrease dramatically. There are only a few places left in Virginia and Maryland where they are known to exist.

It's time to take a break, so dip your feet into the water (although swimming is prohibited), and sit back to enjoy the sun and the sand. One of the most enjoyable activities in the Chesapeake Bay is to go crabbing by becoming what the locals call a "chicken necker." This is done by attaching a chicken neck (or any other bony piece of meat) to a string and casting it a few feet out into the water. Gradually pull the string in when you feel a tug on it. With luck, a crab will be hanging tenaciously onto the bait, and you can slip a net under it before you lift it out of the water. Be careful of the claws when you turn the net over to gently shake the crab out! No license is required for recreational crabbing in Virginia, but I suggest you follow the example of a Maryland law and throw back all crabs less than 5 inches from shell point to shell point.

You have the option of extending the hike by a little more than 1 mile (round-trip) by turning right and walking southward to Hughlett Point and a bit beyond—all of which is public land. To continue with this hike description, turn left and follow the beach northward—maybe. This is a landscape that is constantly in flux. When I first came here, it was possible to do this outing as a circuit hike. Then a major storm blew in and breached the sand, creating a wide outlet from the inland pond, meaning visitors had to retrace their steps back to the parking area. Soon after the turn of the 21st century, a major hurricane changed the beachfront again and reclosed the outlet. However, the last time I was here that situation had changed once more. There was a new outlet, but it was not so wide that it could not be waded across. (You may, however, not want to do this if the tide is going out, as the current is quite swift. In addition, signs periodically posted discourage crossing due to deep mud or other hazards.)

If you are able to continue with the circuit hike, enjoy the quiet of your surroundings, comb the beach for hidden treasures, or keep a lookout for some of the area's wildlife. At one time of year or another, deer, river otter, herons, scoters, egrets, rails, loons, American black ducks, and tundra swans have all been seen along this shoreline.

Be watching for the unmarked trail to the left at 1.8 miles that will bring you back to the woods road, where you will turn left, walk a few yards, and then turn right to rewalk the original portion of the trail on which you started the journey, returning to your car at 2.1 miles.

Take in the beauty at Hughlett Point.

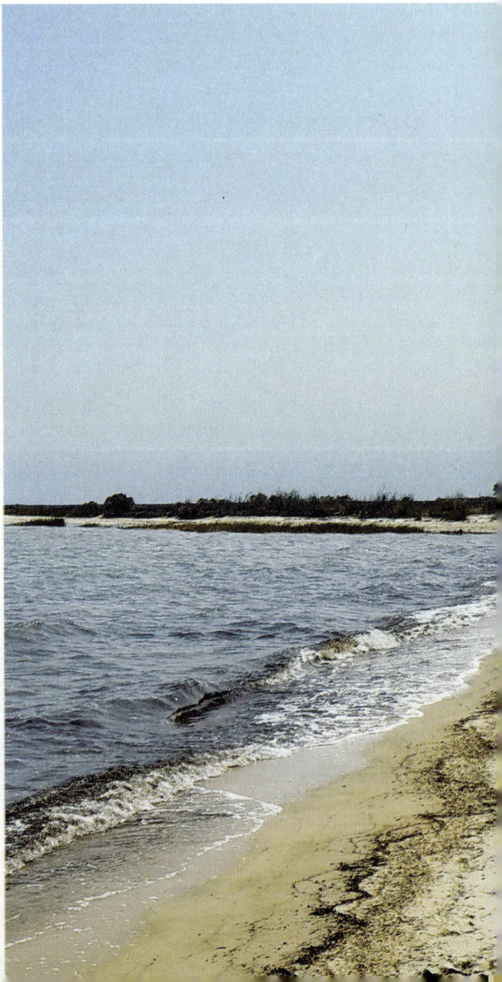

4 Hickory Hollow Natural Area Preserve

- **GPS:** N37.7721713 W76.4440805
- **TOTAL DISTANCE (circuit):** 3.0 miles
- **HIKING TIME:** 1.5 hours
- **VERTICAL RISE:** 130 feet
- **MAP:** USGS *Lancaster*
- **CONTACT:** Division of Natural Heritage
  600 E. Main St., 24th Floor
  Richmond, VA 23219
  804-786-7951
  dwr.virginia.gov/vbwt/sites/hickory-hollow-nature-trail

The Hike at a Glance

0.2 Right onto green-blazed Tom Teeples Trail

0.7 Right onto white-blazed trail; 300 feet later make a right onto Ann Messick Trail

1.0 Cabin Swamp; retrace steps to main trail

1.2 Right onto main trail; 200 feet later onto red-blazed Overlook Trail

2.0 Right onto main trail

2.2 Keep left to stay on main trail; bypass side trails

2.9 Make right onto road trail

3.0 Return to parking area

The existence of a marked trail system in the Hickory Hollow area of Lancaster County is proof that the efforts of one person can enhance the lives of many people. Although a number of state, civic, and environmental organizations contributed donations and volunteer efforts, county forester Henry Bashore is generally acknowledged as the person who made an idea into a reality. Not only did he help coordinate the groups' efforts and persuade the county bureaucracy to open Hickory Hollow to the public, he also spent his own time and funds developing, building, and maintaining the trail system. This is surely a lesson to those of us who feel one person alone cannot make a difference.

From 1780, the first year of recorded ownership, to 1877, the approximately 200 acres of Hickory Hollow changed hands several times and were used for a variety of purposes, notably for timber or farming. In 1877, Lancaster County purchased the property and maintained a poor farm on it until 1905. The process of reforestation has allowed the timber to be harvested numerous times, the last in 1962.

Much of this hike is on old logging roads, making the walk moderately easy. Wildflowers are plentiful. Among them are trout lily, cranefly orchids, violets, pygmy pipe, and horsetail. Flying squirrels begin their acrobatics in the early evening, and ovenbirds, with their familiar *teacher, teacher, teacher* call, are more often heard than seen.

DIRECTIONS To reach the trailhead, follow VA 3 for 0.9 mile eastward from the Lancaster County Courthouse. Make a left onto VA 604, turning into the parking area on the left in 0.3 mile.

Route Description

Begin by taking the trail beside the bulletin board to an old road into the woods. The large holes in the ground next to the road are known as borrow pits. Soil, rock, and clay were "borrowed" from these spots to aid in building a level roadbed. Walk past the aqua-and-white-blazed trail to the left in less than 0.1 mile; you will return this way. Pink lady's slippers usually begin lining the roadside sometime in April. Although their numbers may appear to be more than adequate here in Hickory Hollow, this plant is becoming rarer every year in Virginia. Watch your step and please don't dig one up to replant at home. Besides, like other orchids, the lady's slipper will grow only when certain fungi are present in soil around its roots. If soil and weather conditions aren't conducive to the fungus, the lady's slipper will not survive. Remember the axiom to follow

Hickory Hollow Natural Area Preserve

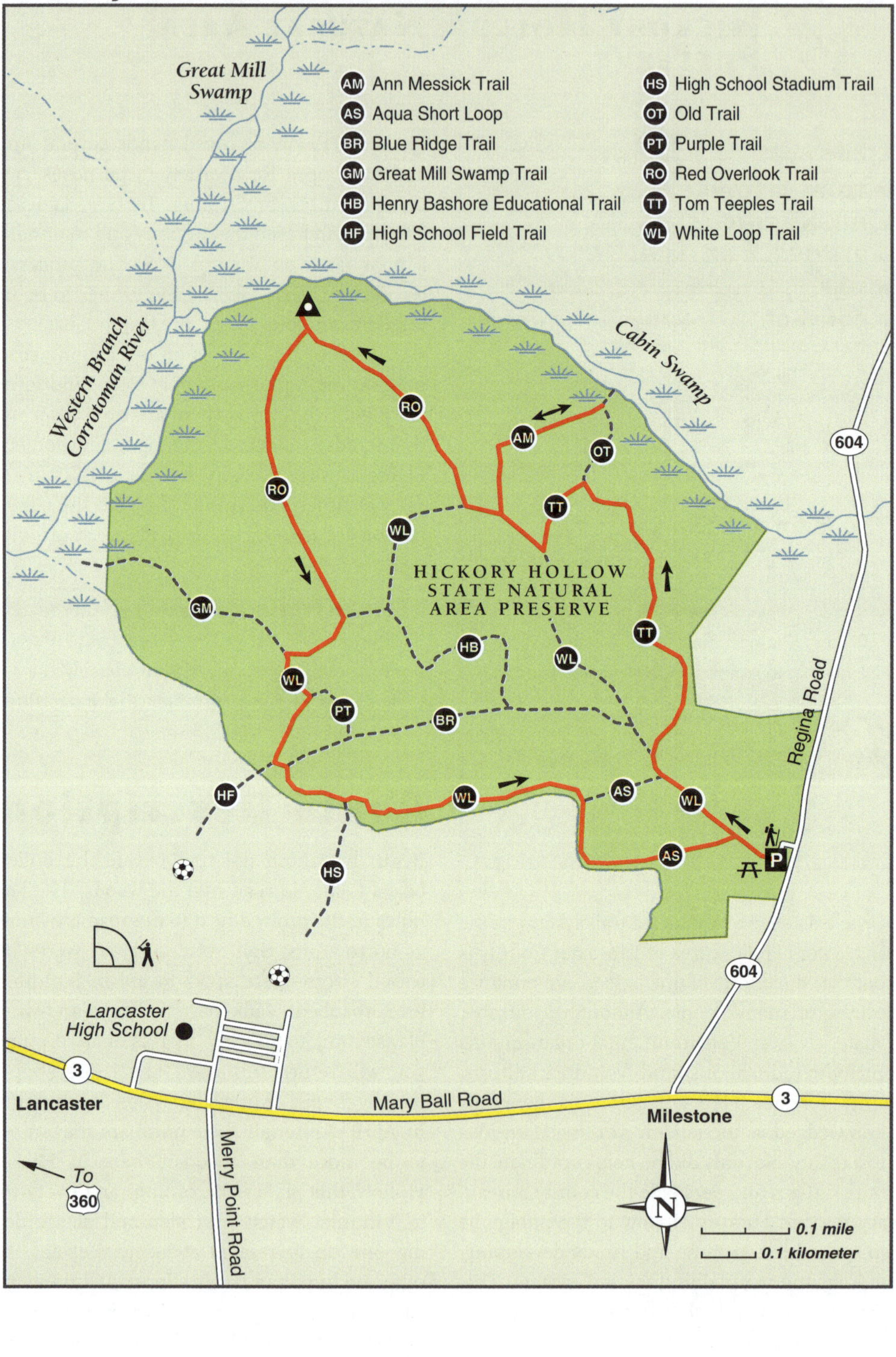

while on any hike: "Take only pictures; leave only footprints."

Pass another aqua-blazed trail to the left at 0.2 mile, and turn right onto the green-blazed Tom Teeples Trail, an old woods road that quickly fades to a trail, just 15 feet later. Swing to the right onto another woods road at 0.4 mile, but be alert just 600 feet later, as the road ends and your route swings to the left. Pass a picnic table and bench at 0.6 mile, and be sure to turn left onto a woods road less than 300 feet later. Arrive at the main, white-blazed trail at 0.7 mile, turn right, and, in less than 300 feet, turn right onto the yellow-blazed Ann Messick Trail, which makes a sharp right turn at 0.8 mile and descends.

The beginning of a 200-foot-long boardwalk marks your arrival in Cabin Swamp at 1.0 mile. Enjoy this quiet place, which is so intensely green and lush during the warm months that it may make other parts of the forest seem sparse and dull in comparison. Skunk cabbage, jack-in-the-pulpit, spring beauty, wild ginger, marsh marigold, and false hellebore grow among dozens of other wildflowers. Freshwater clams have been seen next to the pennywort in the small streams, and the call of great horned owls often echoes through the woods.

Retrace your steps back to the main white-blazed trail at 1.2 miles, turn right, and, in less than 200 feet, bear right onto the red-blazed Overlook Trail that gradually descends through a forest with many loblolly pine and beech trees. The trail makes a sharp left at 1.5 miles, but, for the moment, keep right for 250 feet to arrive at an overlook of another portion of Cabin Swamp. Return to the intersection, turn right, and, making use of an old fire break, follow the trail as it descends into, and ascends out of, a narrow stream valley that has a wonderful sense of isolation.

Turn right onto the main white-blazed trail at 2.0 miles, coming to an intersection with the brown-blazed Great Mill Swamp Trail at 2.1 miles. The latter route descends for 0.3 mile to the edge of the swamp and is a nice side trip if you wish to take it, but this hike description continues by keeping left on the main,

Observing Cabin Swamp

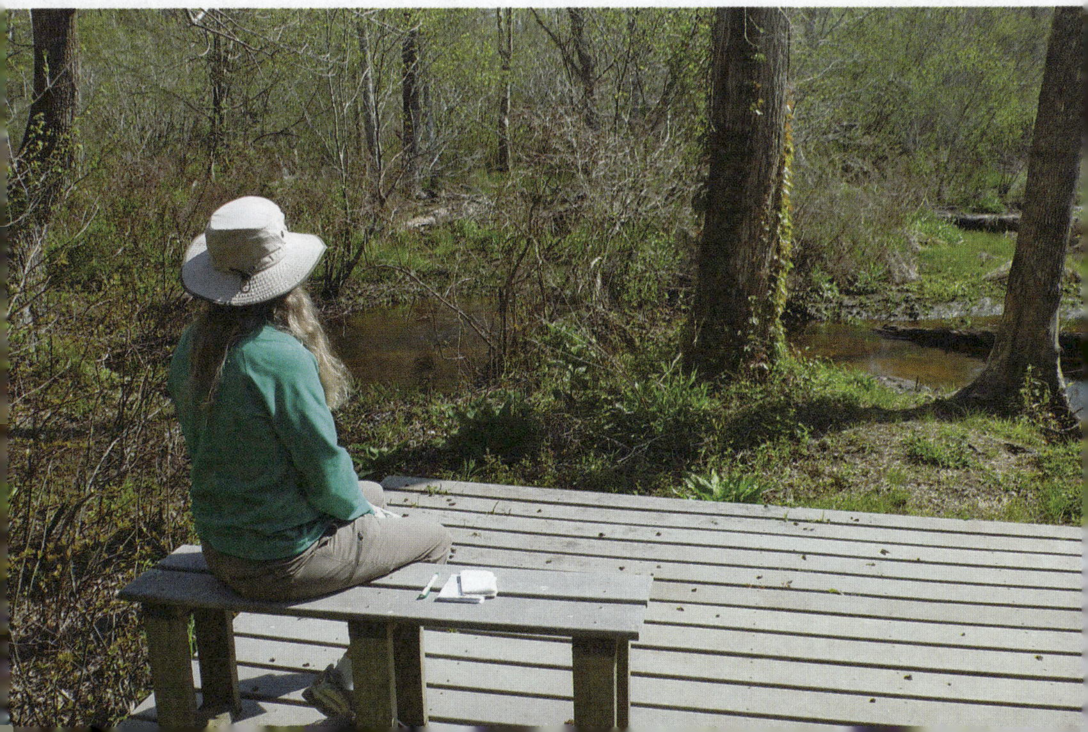

white-blazed trail. A purple-blazed trail comes in from the left 300 feet later; keep right and make an abrupt descent, coming to another intersection at 2.2 miles. The unmarked trail to the right ascends to Lancaster High School. You want to turn left and ascend, but in less than 100 feet, pay attention—your journey does not follow the blue-blazed Ridge Trail to the left, but rather bears right to continue on the white-blazed route.

Because you are now on a trail instead of an old road, the hike takes on a more rustic feeling, as you walk through an open beech forest next to a creek (bypassing another trail to the right that also leads to the school). Passing in and out of laurel tunnels, the trail goes by heartleaf, running cedar, and partridgeberry that make up the ground cover. Come to an intersection at 2.6 miles. The main road/trail on which you started this hike is a couple hundred feet to the left via the aqua-blazed trail; however, in order to enjoy the walk for a few minutes longer, keep right. The loblolly pines have dropped so many needles onto the understory that it looks to be festooned by thousands of thin brown icicles. Come to the road/trail at 2.9 miles, and make a right to return to the parking area in less than 500 feet.

You should be aware that in the late 1990s, many residents of Lancaster County (rallied by local citizens Henry Bashore and Ann B. Messick) fought short-sighted government officials who were trying to develop an industrial park on Hickory Hollow lands. The residents' nearly tireless efforts were fruitful. Grants and donations, including $150,000 from the Virginia Land Conservation Foundation, were raised to purchase and protect the land. Hickory Hollow is now administered by the Northern Neck Audubon Society with assistance from the Virginia Department of Conservation and Recreation's Natural Heritage Program. If you have enjoyed your hike here, be sure to let the county officials know.

This boardwalk leads into lush, tranquil Cabin Swamp.

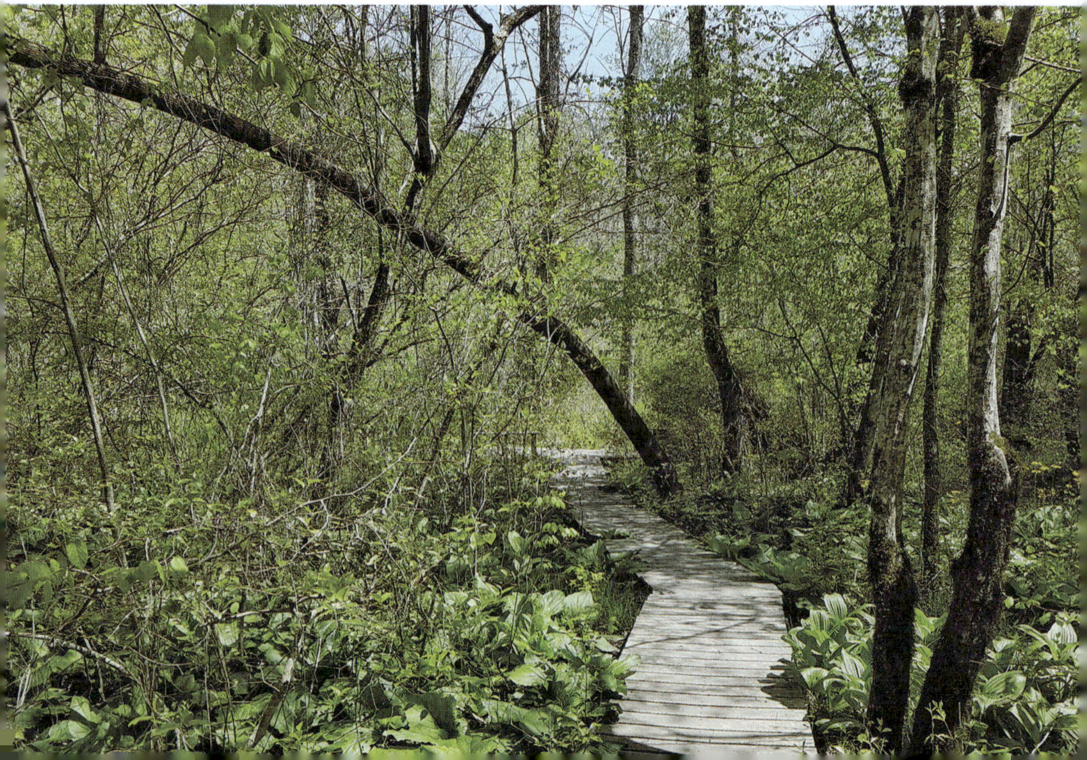

5 Belle Isle State Park

- **GPS:** N37.7734926 W76.5924604
- **TOTAL DISTANCE (round-trip):** 5.0 miles
- **HIKING TIME:** 2.75 hours
- **VERTICAL RISE:** Less than 30 feet
- **MAPS:** USGS *Lively; Belle Isle State Park* map
- **CONTACT:** Belle Isle State Park
1632 Belle Isle Road
Lancaster, VA 22503
804-462-5030
dcr.virginia.gov/state-parks/belle-isle

The Hike at a Glance

0.2 Left to observation blind; then return to main route and turn left

0.5 Turn left onto Watch House Trail

0.8 Bypass Neck Fields Trail coming in from the right; few feet later make left onto mowed pathway

1.1 Turn left onto Watch House Trail

1.4 left onto Neck Fields Trail

1.7 Left off of Neck Fields Trail

2.5 Left onto Neck Fields Trail

3.2 Brewer's Point; turn around and head back on Neck Fields Trail

4.4 Left onto Watch House Trail

4.6 Bypass Mud Creek Trail; turn right onto Porpoise Creek Trail

5.0 End of hike

The Tidewater area of Virginia has always had fewer places in which the public could walk or hike when compared to other parts of the commonwealth. So, it was a sad day in 1999 when two of its best trails located on private forest lands were closed—one was located beside the Corrotoman River in Lancaster County and the other one was near West Point in New Kent County. Thanks to hard work by local volunteers, those pathways have now been reopened, though they are now shorter in length and travel through areas diminished in acreage.

Earlier in the same decade, Virginians were foresighted enough to see that occurrences similar to this—coupled with the rapid spread of the modern world—threatened their ability to recreate in the natural world. Approving the Parks and Recreational Facilities Bond in 1992, the citizens authorized the commonwealth to expend state funds for the purpose of bringing more acreage into the public domain (and upgrading facilities at existing sites).

Bounded by water on three sides, 890-acre Belle Isle State Park was the first parcel of land to be purchased with the bond money. Archaeological evidence has shown that this small tract along the northern side of the Rappahannock River has been inhabited for approximately 1,000 years. The temporary camps of Native Americans who seasonally visited the area became the settlements of Algonquin-speaking peoples who moved inland from the coast. In turn, they were replaced by the Moraughtacunds, part of the Powhatan tribe, who were living in the region when colonists arrived.

The newcomers from the Old World soon turned the riverside acreage into a large and thriving plantation. Soon after the Civil War, the land was sold off into several parcels, and by the late 1900s was threatened with the possibility of becoming a waterfront community until the state purchased it in 1993.

The state park offers picnic areas; a campground and a backcountry canoe-in campsite; overnight accommodations in a Georgian-style mansion and guest house; an accessible boardwalk and fishing pier; bicycle, kayak, and canoe rentals; a motorboat launch; and a cartop launch. Rockfish, croaker, spot, and flounder are found in the waters around the park. The interpretive programs include canoe trips onto the river and into the creeks and marshes. Led by park personnel and volunteer naturalists, the guided paddle journeys focus on the ecology and fragility of the area. Making use

Belle Isle State Park

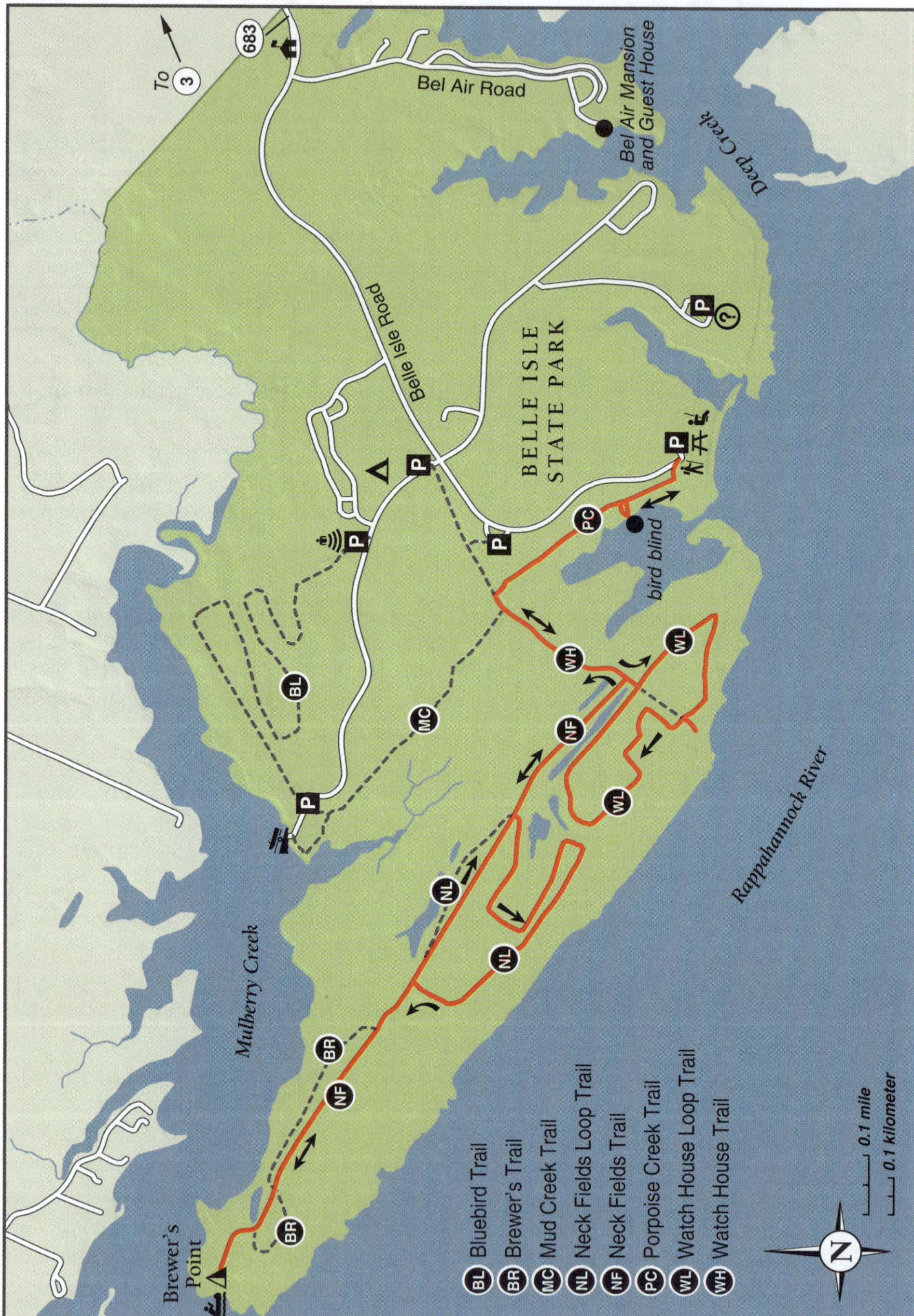

of innovative conservation practices to reduce pollution runoff into the Chesapeake Bay, some of the land is still open fields.

Following old farm roads, a network of trails provides the opportunity to walk by these fields and out to vistas overlooking the Rappahannock River and Mulberry Creek. Most of the pathways are also open to bicyclists and equestrians. Pets must be on a leash at all times.

DIRECTIONS Drive northward from Kilmarnock on VA 3 for 10.0 miles to Lively. Turn westward and follow VA 201 for 3.3 miles, then turn right onto VA 354. An additional 3.2 miles brings you to a left turn onto VA 683. The contact station is 0.7 mile down this road, the camp store is 0.8 mile farther, and the playground area where you leave your car is an additional 0.5 mile.

Route Description

Walk from the parking lot to the fence overlooking the broad Rappahannock River, more than 3 miles wide at this point. This is a great place to be in early morning as the sun spreads its glow across the water. After enjoying the view, walk next to the woods to begin following the Porpoise Creek Trail, an old road.

Turn left onto a small pathway into the woods at 0.2 mile and come to an enclosed blind overlooking a small backwater area of the river. Staying inside this small hut built by volunteers of a local conservation organization, and being quiet as long as possible, increases your chances of observing great blue herons, ducks, geese, and other waterfowl. Small ripples moving across the water in a zigzag fashion could indicate a snake gliding to the opposite shore. You may also see the head of a muskrat bobbing up and down as it swims to its tunnel home in the bank. Boosted by partially webbed hind feet, these amphibious members of the rodent family are able to swim forward or backward and have been known to stay submerged for more than 10 minutes at a time.

Return to the main trail and turn left, walking between woods and field. Pass through a windrow at 0.5 mile and come to a T-intersection beside another field. Turn left onto the Watch House Trail. The Mud Creek Trail comes in from the right a few feet later; keep left on the Watch House Trail—the only bit of dryness separating two wetlands—with a view of the Rappahannock River to the left.

The Neck Fields Trail comes in from the right at 0.8 mile; keep left. Just 100 feet later, turn left onto a mowed pathway, the Watch House Loop. Your perspective onto the Rappahannock River changes as you continue along.

Intersect and turn left onto the Watch House Trail at 1.1 miles, passing through a stand of towering loblolly pine trees and coming to the edge of the river. More than 100 years ago, an oyster watch house stood close to 100 feet offshore to ensure that thieves did not sneak in to harvest the fruits of the oyster beds. A later watch house was built on the point of land you are now standing upon. As did those throughout the Chesapeake Bay, the oysters here began to dwindle in numbers in the 1970s due to nonpoint pollution and disease.

Return inland along Watch House Trail to bear left onto the Neck Fields Trail, a wide country lane bordered by loblolly trees, at 1.4 miles. For a bit of a change from walking the old farm roads, turn left onto a mowed pathway, the Neck Fields Loop, at 1.7 miles. Tracks in the soft soil attest to an abundance of deer in the park, while the pond visible through the trees may harbor ducks, geese, egrets, and herons. While you may see some great blue herons in Virginia all year long, others fly as far north as Ontario for the summer and migrate to Virginia's Northern Neck—or points farther south—for the winter. At 2.3 miles, come to an intersection of woods roads and bear to the right. Songbirds may serenade you in the early morning, while vultures, crows, and hawks wing their way across the open sky.

Intersect the Neck Fields Trail at 2.5 miles and turn left. As you pass by the Brewer's Trail (whose mowed pathway is an additional walking option), private homes along Mulberry Creek are barely visible through the vegetation to the right at 2.8 miles. Be sure to stay on the main route to come to its end at the canoe-in campsite on Brewer's Point at 3.2 miles. You certainly deserve a break, so bring the snacks out of the day pack and enjoy the sights and sounds. A small fishing boat may pass by, causing small waves to lightly splash upon the shore, while an osprey may drop to the water, rising a few moments later with a fish grasped in its talons. Bald eagles have been seen winging past this point.

When you are ready to return, follow Neck Fields Trail back to Watch House Trail at 4.4 miles. Turn left and bypass Mud Creek Trail on the left at 4.6 miles. (If you wish to extend the hike, you could follow Mud Creek Trail to another point overlooking the Mulberry River, a round-trip of a little more than 0.5 mile.)

Making a right turn onto the Porpoise Creek Trail less than 200 feet later will return you to the playground area at 5.0 miles.

For a whimsical diversion before heading home after the hike, drive back to Lively and turn right onto VA 3. In Lancaster Court House make a right onto VA 604 and drive for several miles. The Merry Point Ferry, one of the few remaining river ferries in Virginia, will shuttle you across the West Branch of the Corrotoman River. Although this is a utilitarian boat, the ride across the river can be a scenic and enjoyable one as you watch waterfowl and other birds fly above the river. To return to VA 3 after the ferry ride, take VA 604 to Ottoman, where you will make a right onto VA 354. Watch for a right turn onto VA 201 to bring you to back to Lively.

View from Brewer's Point

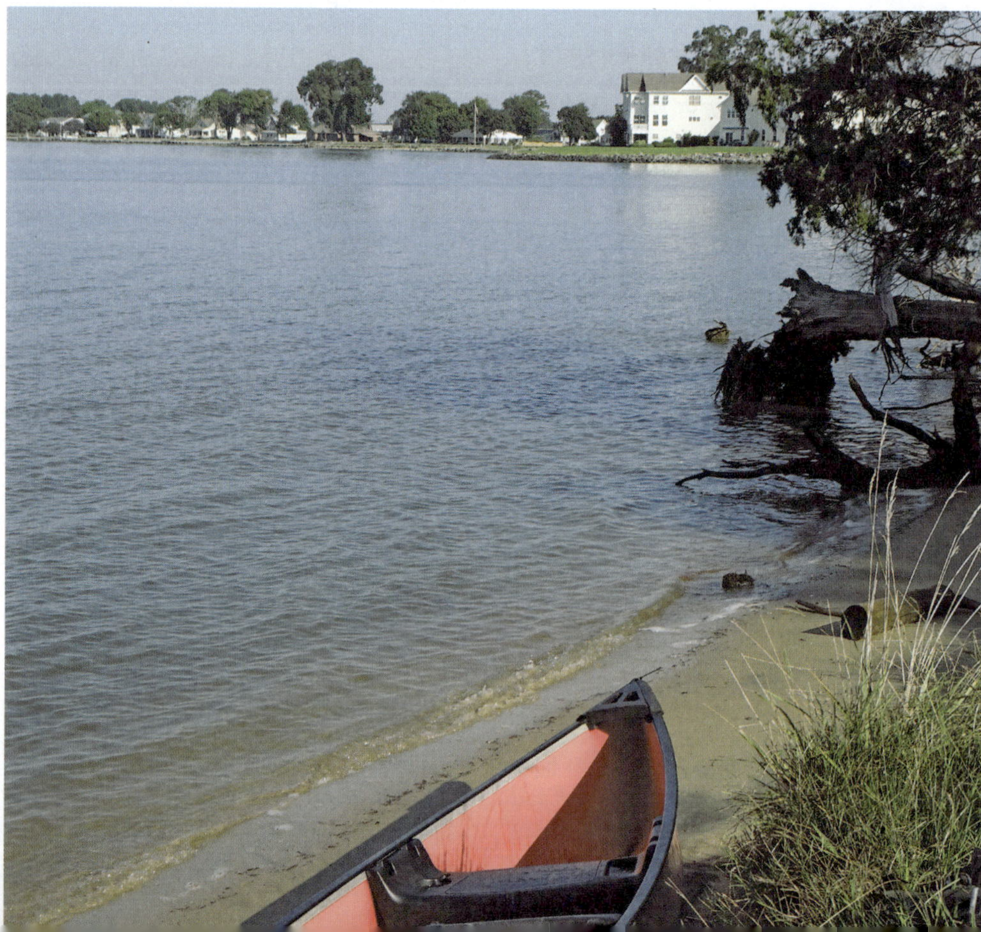

6 The Northern Neck

- **GPS:** N38.1696993 W76.8634969
- **TOTAL DISTANCE (circuit):** 4.0 miles
- **HIKING TIME:** 2.0 hours
- **VERTICAL RISE:** 370 feet
- **MAPS:** USGS *Stratford Hall* and *Colonial Beach South; Westmoreland State Park* map
- **CONTACT:** Westmoreland State Park
  145 Cliff Road
  Montross, VA 22520
  804-493-8821
  dcr.virginia.gov/state-parks/westmoreland

The Hike at a Glance

0.7 Take trail left to beach; then retrace steps to Big Meadow Trail and turn left

1.0 Turkey Neck Trail comes in from right, stay left

1.2 Beaver Dam Trail comes in from right, stay left

2.1 Other end of Beaver Dam Trail comes in from right, stay left. Soon another branch of Turkey Neck Trail comes in from right, stay left

2.4 Another branch of Turkey Neck Trail comes in from right; stay left, go through campground, cross park road, turn right, and, in a few feet, turn left onto Laurel Point Trail

3.2 Right onto Rock Spring Pond Trail

3.8 Left onto park road, follow it to right turn onto road leading to visitor center

4.1 Return to your automobile

Driving east on VA 3 from I-95 Exit 130 at Fredericksburg will bring you onto the Northern Neck, a wide peninsula between the Potomac and Rappahannock Rivers. The land took on its present form some 5,000–6,000 years ago after glaciers from the last Ice Age melted, raising sea levels enough to form the Chesapeake Bay and cover the Susquehanna River floodplain. The area can be a lesson in the history of America's earlier days, and three sites—one federal, one state, and one private—have trails coursing through them that let you study that time period from a pedestrian's point of view. Fees of some kind are collected at each location.

DIRECTIONS About 36 miles east of I-95 at Fredericksburg is the George Washington's Birthplace National Monument located off of VA 3. After passing through Oak Grove on VA 3, look for a sign directing you to make a left turn onto VA 204 to reach the grounds of the monument in approximately 2 miles. Washington was born here on February 22, 1732. The property, once known as Pope's Creek Plantation and now called Wakefield, was Washington's home for the first three years of his life. Walking the small network of trails past numerous sites will help you gain insight into the life of America's first president and the era in which he lived. The Memorial House, built in the 1930s, is typical of 18th-century plantation homes of the area. Also built in the 1930s, the Kitchen House stands on the site of the original kitchen. Nearby, the park service manages some of the more than 500 acres of the monument as a demonstration and working farm, using the agricultural technology of the 1700s. Other portions of the trail network have interpretive signs that discuss the natural, as well as human, history of the land. Pets are required to be on a leash.

From Washington's birthplace continue driving east on VA 3 for 5.0 miles to bypass the entrance to Westmoreland State Park for the moment. Just 0.6 mile beyond it is a left turn onto VA 214, which leads to Stratford Hall. Like Wakefield, Stratford Hall was once part of an enormous tract patented by Nathaniel Pope in the 1650s. In 1716, Colonel Thomas Lee purchased about 4,000 acres and built what became home to several generations of one of Virginia's premier families. Among the most famous of the famous to live here were Richard

The Northern Neck

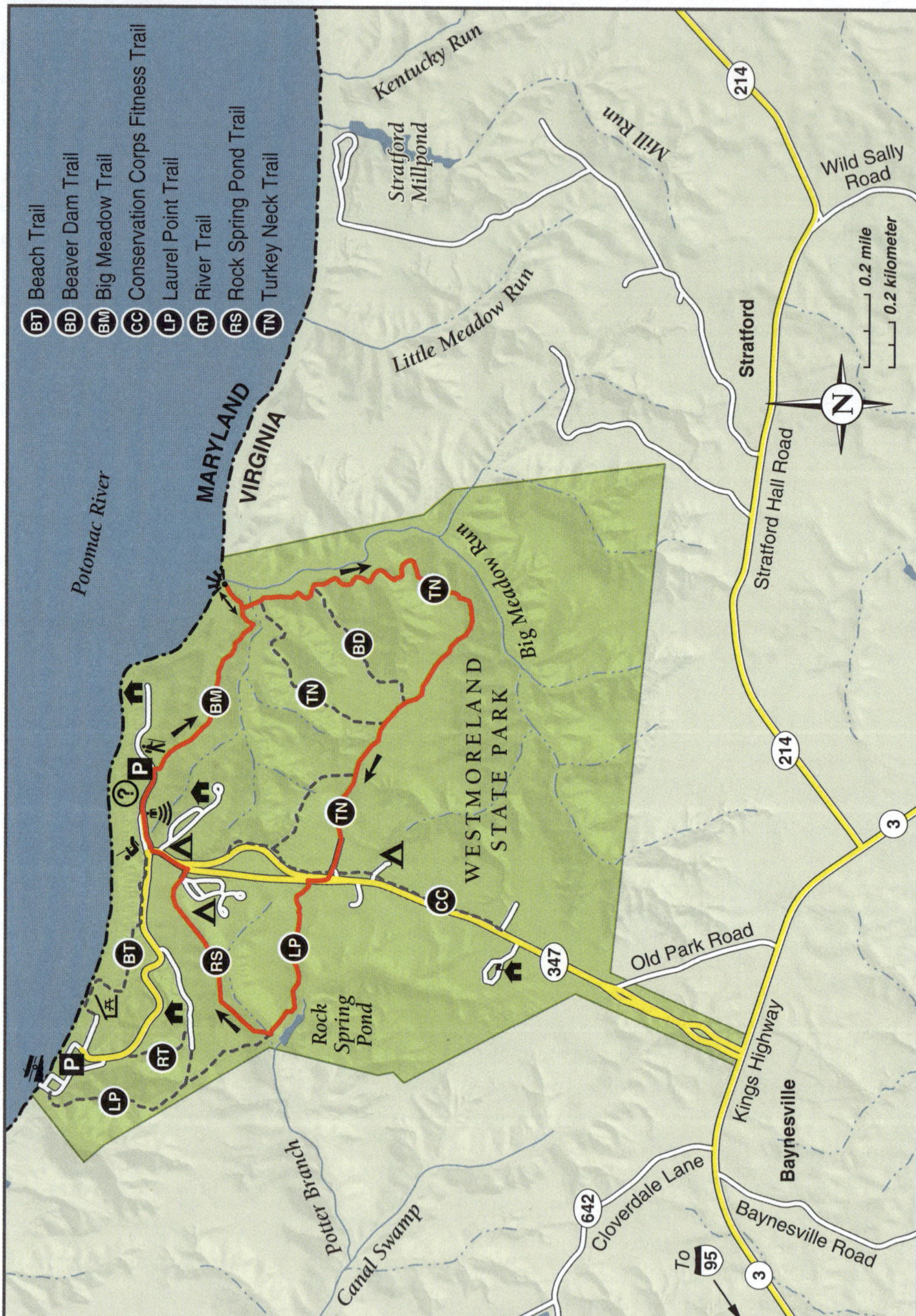

Henry Lee and Francis Lightfoot Lee, both signers of the Declaration of Independence, and the Confederate States' military leader during the Civil War, Robert E. Lee. Privately owned, the 1,500-plus acres are operated as a plantation much as it would have been during Robert E. Lee's lifetime. Livestock graze in open meadows, and fields are cultivated by traditional methods. By taking a 2- to 3-mile circuit hike on a system of interconnecting pathways, you can tour the H-shaped Great House, pass through reforested acres of hardwoods, watch the reconstructed mill grind grains, overlook the broad Potomac River, and visit the spring that supplied water (and a means of refrigeration) for the plantation.

After the visit to Stratford Hall, return to VA 3, turn right, and go 0.7 mile to make a right turn into Westmoreland State Park. Follow the main park road for 1.7 miles to turn right onto the road leading a few hundred feet to the visitor center and the parking area.

Route Description

The Commonwealth of Virginia purchased approximately 1,300 acres (at $11.50 an acre) in 1933 to develop Westmoreland State Park, which was once a part of Stratford Hall. The Civilian Conservation Corps (CCC) built most of the still-existing structures and roadways. Westmoreland, one of Virginia's original six state parks, now has rental cabins, several campgrounds, a camp store and conference center overlooking the river, a picnic area and shelters, an Olympic-size swimming pool, and boat rentals available at a dock on the river. Like all of Virginia's state parks, Westmoreland offers interpretive programs throughout the heavy tourist season.

Ever since the park opened in 1936, one of its great attractions has been the fossils found on the river beaches. Visitors have discovered the skeletal remains of crocodiles, stingrays, porpoises, turtles, whales, sharks, and other marine life that lived in the Miocene Sea some 15 million years ago. Be sure to ask about the tides at the visitor center; the river overtakes the beach below Horsehead Cliffs at high tide.

The trails of Westmoreland will bring you into a woods that has not been timbered since the beginning of the 20th century, making the forest a wonderland of exceptionally large-trunked trees towering over sparse undergrowth. Opossums, raccoons, weasels, mink, river otters, beavers, foxes, squirrels and various other rodents, wild turkeys, deer, turtles, snakes, and frogs have all been seen by hikers at one time or another. Yellow Swamp and Big Meadow are good introductions to coastal-plain marshes.

Enjoy the view along the Potomac River from the visitor center. Across the 6-mile-wide river is southern Maryland. There is also the possibility of sighting an osprey or bald eagle on the wing.

After looking at the visitor center's displays, start the hike on the Big Meadow Trail. Enter the woods on an 1890s logging road, where dogwoods and pawpaws are part of the understory. In late fall the pawpaw trees, among the last to lose their leaves, add various tones of yellow to an otherwise brown and gray forest.

At 0.7 mile, make a left onto the short trail leading you onto the beach, a great place to learn more about the makeup of the Northern Neck. Only about 30 miles from the Chesapeake Bay, the Potomac River at this point is brackish. Because of the salinity, creatures you normally associate with bays or oceans are able to survive here. Blue and horseshoe crabs are often found on the sand. Note that horseshoe crabs are not really crabs but are more closely related to spiders and ticks. Despite its fearsome appearance, the horseshoe is harmless, mostly using its long, pointed tail to turn itself back over when flipped up onto the beach. Amid deer tracks in the sand you'll probably see lumps of clay that have broken off from the cliffs. The clay was a perfect pottery material for early Native Americans.

Return to, and turn left onto, the main trail and boardwalk, walking through the reed grass and rosehips of Yellow Swamp. If you didn't see them on the river, there is a good chance you will see a few buffleheads plying the stream in the swamp. A small duck, the male bufflehead is easy to identify—it has a nearly all-white body, a black back, and an almost perfectly round black head topped by a large patch of white. Buffleheads are also referred to as butterballs by duck hunters.

Passing arrowroot, a favorite food of muskrats, come to an intersection at 1.0 mile. The blue-blazed Turkey Neck Trail goes right; your route takes the trail's left branch, hugging the edge of Big Meadow, where park personnel often report seeing browsing deer and turkeys. At 1.2 miles you will rise to another intersection. Yellow-blazed Beaver Dam Trail is a shortcut and will rejoin your route at the 2.1-mile mark. Do not take that route. Keep left and continue following the blue-blazed trail, overlooking beaver dams and, maybe, lodges in the swampy meadow. As you walk along, look at the tops of the trunks of fallen trees; you may see that they are often used by woodland creatures as a table for feasting on nuts and pinecones. At around 1.6 miles you will pass some massive trees that have obviously been around for a long time. Stop for a few moments to pay your respects to these great-grandparents of the forest. Their branches are bigger around than most of the trunks of nearby trees. Ascend to swing away from Big Meadow and begin walking on an old road.

The other end of the Beaver Dam Trail comes in from the right at 2.1 miles; you want to stay left. Soon the other branch of Turkey Neck Trail comes in from the right; again, you want to stay left. At 2.4 miles the Turkey Neck Trail swings right—you could follow it back about a mile to the visitor center and your car. However, keep left on the old road to walk through campground C. Water and restrooms are available in the campground during the season.

Step across the paved Civilian Conservation Corps Trail and both lanes of the park road and turn right. In a few feet, turn left onto orange-blazed Laurel Point Trail, which descends into a holly- and laurel-crowded draw. At 3.1 miles, Rock Spring Pond shimmers emerald as it reflects the evergreen leaves of a laurel thicket. The pond was built in the 1930s by the CCC and now contains a variety of bass and other fish. Continue around the pond to 3.2 miles, where Laurel Point Trail bears left as a pathway to arrive at the boat dock in less than a mile. You, however, will keep right onto the woodlands roadway to follow green-blazed Rock Spring Pond Trail. If you are camped in the park, this wide, level road through the broad valley would make a great moonlight walk before retiring for the evening.

Arrive at the park road in 3.8 miles, cross the pavement, and turn left, soon coming to the conference center. Make a right and return to the visitor center at 4.1 miles.

There are two other short trails in the park. The 0.2-mile River Trail connects cabins 1–18 to the beach area; and the half-mile Beach Trail, which has scenic views of the river, descends from near the conference center to the swimming pool and beach.

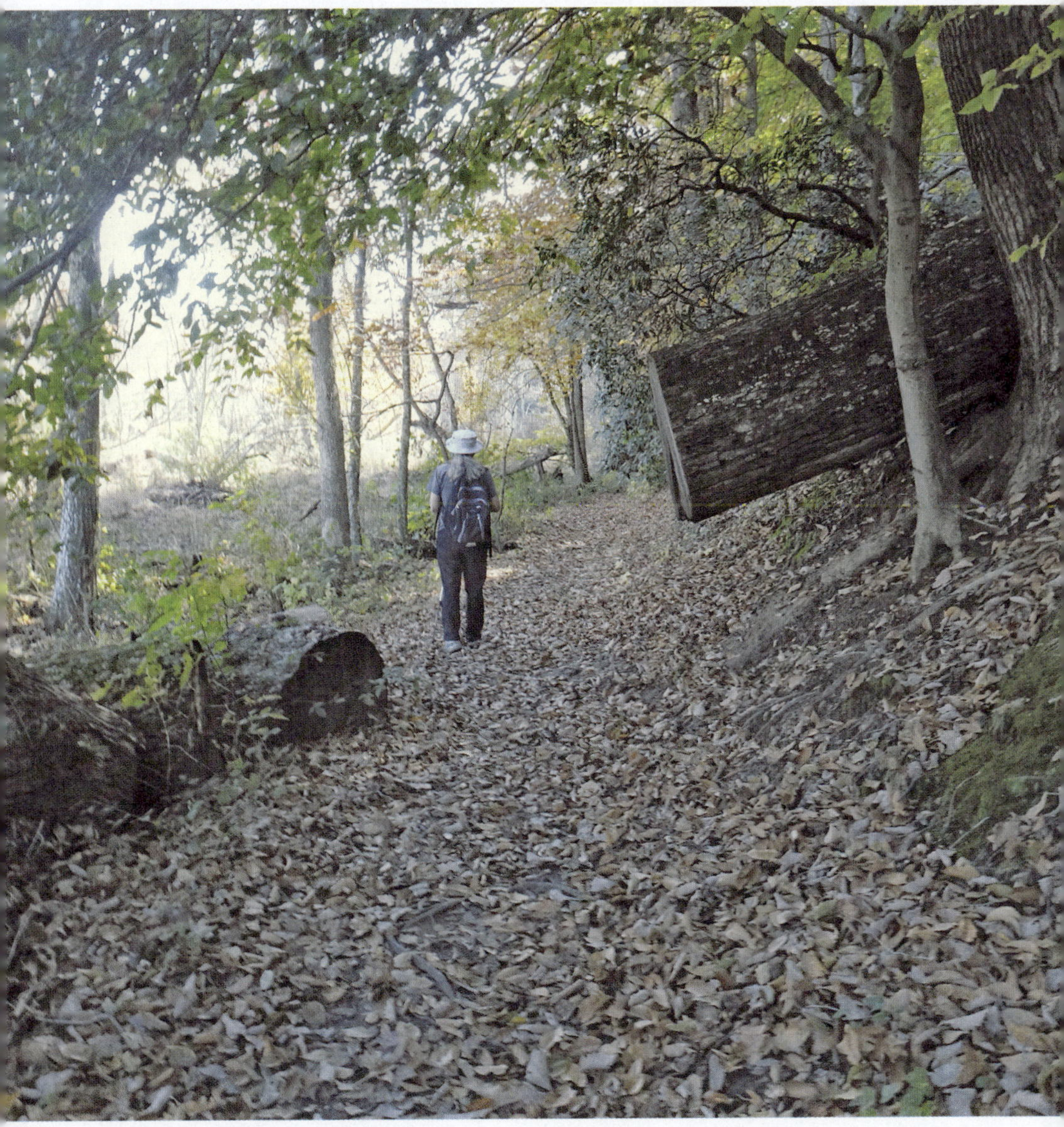

The trail hugs the edge of Big Meadow.

Central Virginia

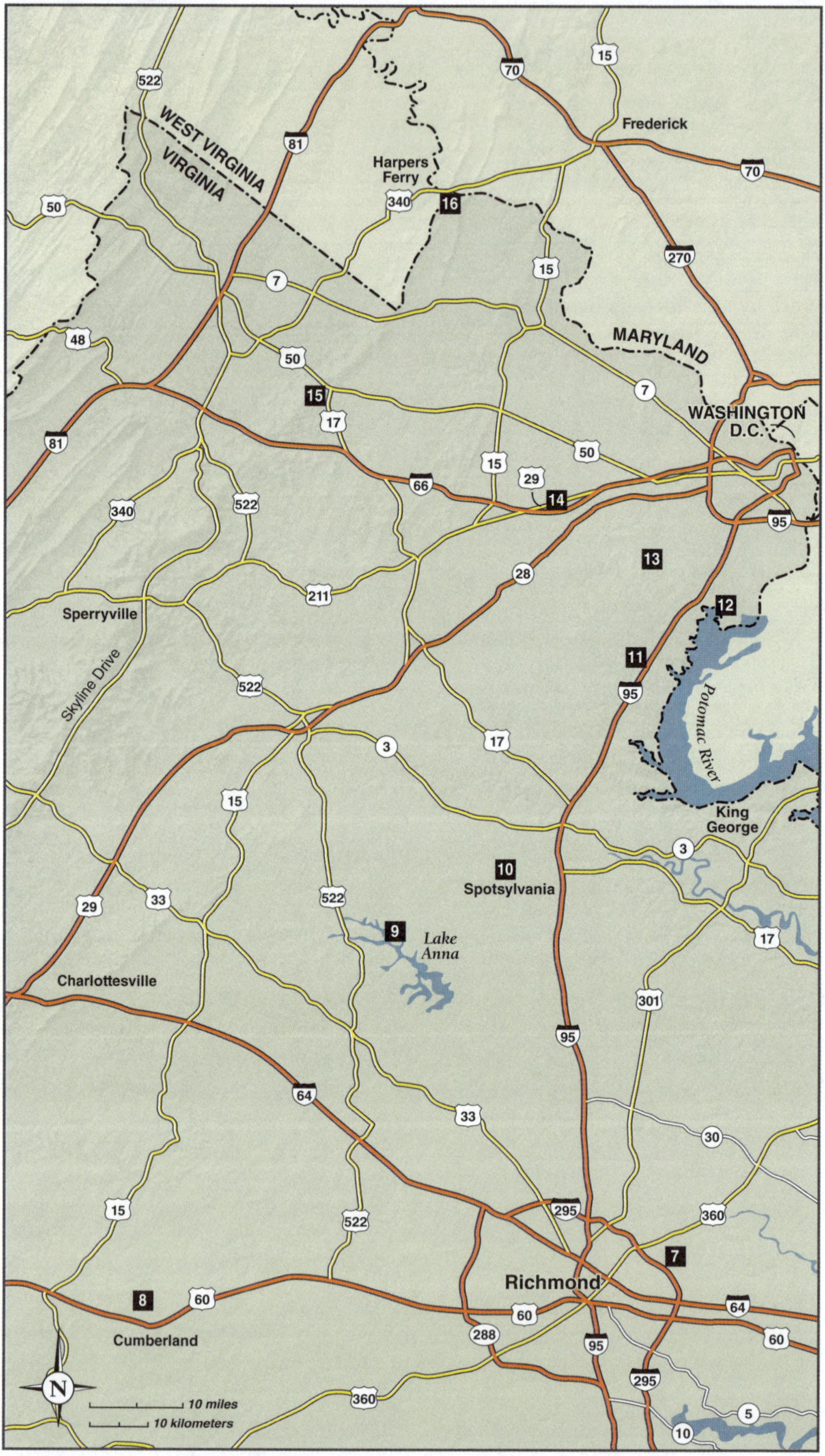

Central Virginia

Cold Harbor

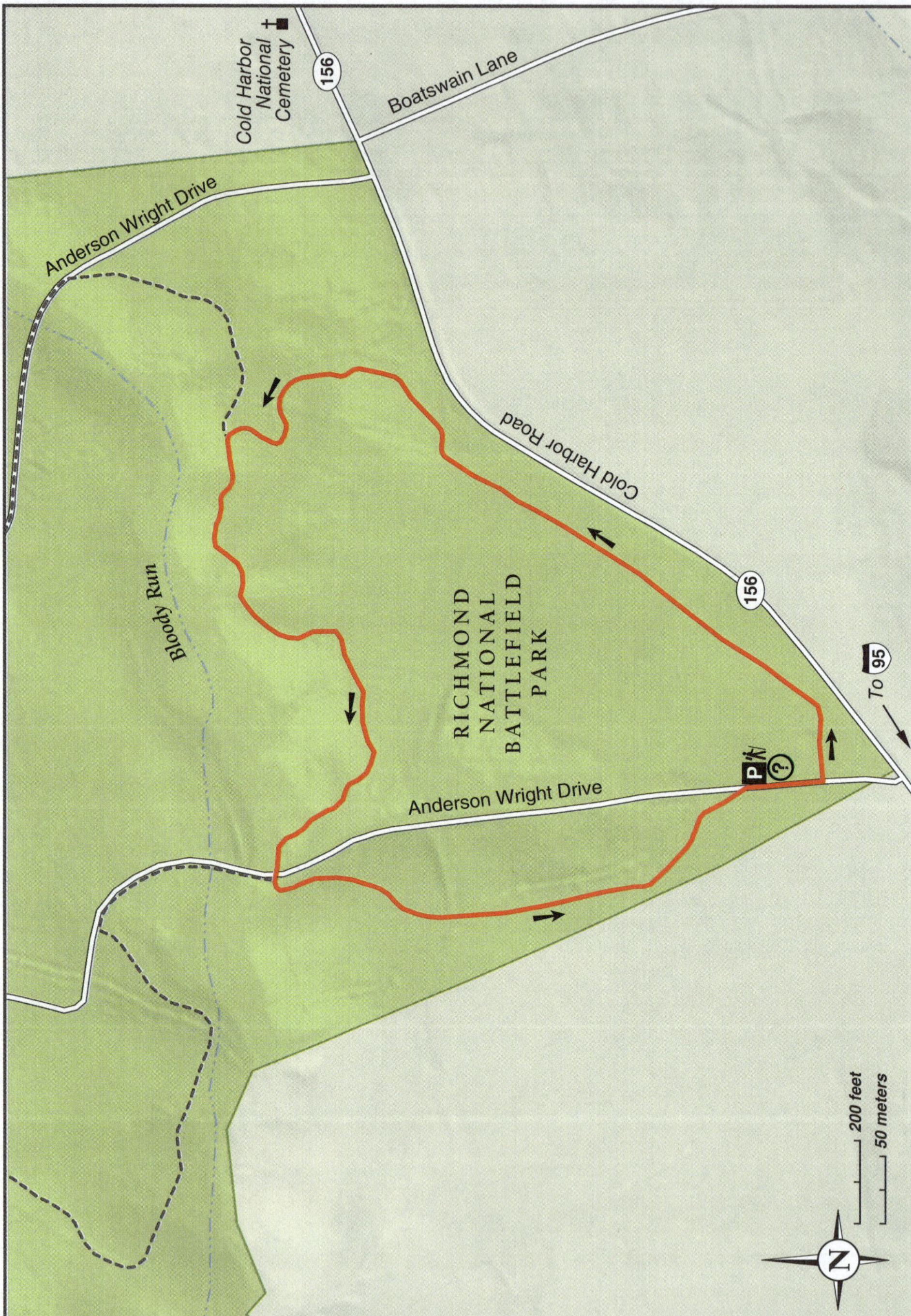

Cold Harbor National Cemetery
156
Boatswain Lane
Anderson Wright Drive
Cold Harbor Road
156
To 95
RICHMOND NATIONAL BATTLEFIELD PARK
Bloody Run
Anderson Wright Drive
200 feet
50 meters
N

7 Cold Harbor

- **GPS:** N37.5856309 W77.2871352
- **TOTAL DISTANCE (circuit):** 1.0 mile
- **HIKING TIME:** 30 minutes
- **VERTICAL RISE:** Less than 100 feet
- **MAPS:** USGS *Seven Pines;* National Park Service *Cold Harbor* map
- **CONTACT:**
Richmond National Battlefield Park
3215 E. Broad St.
Richmond, VA 23223
804-226-1981; nps.gov/rich

The Hike at a Glance

0.2 Swing away from VA 156

0.5 Bypass trail to right (that is an additional 2-mile-long loop option)

0.7 Cross paved park road (where the optional 2-mile loop rejoins this hike)

1.0 Return to visitor center

After May 21, 1864, and the somewhat stalemated battle of Spotsylvania (see Hike 10), Lieutenant General Ulysses S. Grant continued to move in a southward direction in his Overland Campaign to capture the Confederate capital, Richmond. In addition to several other skirmishes along the way, Grant's forces and General Robert E. Lee's Army of Northern Virginia clashed again near the crossroads of Old Cold Harbor. Union soldiers captured the crossroads on May 31, but fortifications, mostly in the form of extensive dirt breastworks built by the Southern army, turned the next three days of battle into a standoff.

The Union troops were never able to penetrate the fortifications, while the Confederate army just held its ground, unable to drive the invaders back. From June 4 through 12, the days were filled with minor attacks and occasional sniper fire. Unable to break through the Southern lines, Grant finally withdrew and turned his attention onto Petersburg. This successful defense of Richmond is considered Lee's last field victory of the war. Historians say the battle at Cold Harbor influenced the strategies of future wars by proving that well-selected defenses, supported by strong artillery power, are quite invulnerable to direct attack. It certainly turned the rest of the Civil War into a conflict where entrenchments and sieges took precedence over battles of direct assault.

From early 1862 to the city's surrender on April 3, 1865, Union forces engaged in numerous battles in attempts to capture Richmond. Many sites commemorating various conflicts and activities are scattered throughout the city and surrounding area and make up the National Park Service's Richmond National Battlefield Park.

DIRECTIONS In order to obtain a clear mental picture of Civil War events around Richmond, you should stop in at the visitor center at 500 Tredegar Street at the terminus of Fifth Street in Richmond, study the exhibits, and watch the audiovisual presentations. To reach Cold Harbor from the visitor center, follow Seventh Street to Broad Street to I-95 and take the interstate north to I-64. Take I-64 east to I-295 and follow that highway north to the VA 156 (North Airport Drive) exit. Continue on VA 156N for 5 miles, through several twists and turns, to the Cold Harbor park entrance, on the right. (The park service provides a pamphlet describing a circuitous driving tour of the sites of the Richmond National Battlefield Park. Following this tour will also eventually lead you to Cold Harbor.)

Route Description

In order to add even more background information to your hike, take a few moments to look in on the Cold Harbor Visitor Center. In addition to the usual ethical practices you should follow while on any hike, the park service requests that you refrain from removing any relics you may happen to find, park your automobile only in designated areas, and preserve the breastworks by not walking or climbing on them.

Start your hike by walking to the plaque behind the visitor center and continuing on the pathway along the edge of the meadow next to VA 156. You will be crossing the center of the Confederate main line of defense. On June 3, 1864, the Union army launched a massive attack but was soon pinned down by Confederate firepower, and in less than 30 minutes thousands of Union soldiers were killed or wounded. Remember that most of the land you will be walking upon throughout this hike was open farmland at the time of the Civil War; there were few trees or shrubs to hide behind or to use as shields against the showers of bullets filling the air.

Large oak and loblolly pine trees tower above, while sassafras and holly make up the understory as you swing away from the road at 0.2 mile. Holly is very shade tolerant and is often found flourishing, as it is here, under the canopy of an older and taller forest. Unlike many other trees, hollies are either male or female—thus, they must be in proximity to each other for the female to bear fruit. The berries, which turn bright red in the fall, are a favorite winter food for birds and deer. Wild turkeys are sometimes seen feeding high up in the trees as well as on berries that have fallen to the ground.

At 0.3 mile, cross a footbridge constructed to protect the breastworks. The fortifications here were made by Union soldiers, who, unable to advance or retreat, used bayonets, cups, canteen halves, and whatever other implements would work to dig the trenches in an attempt to escape the unrelenting Confederate artillery

Site of the main Confederate line of defense

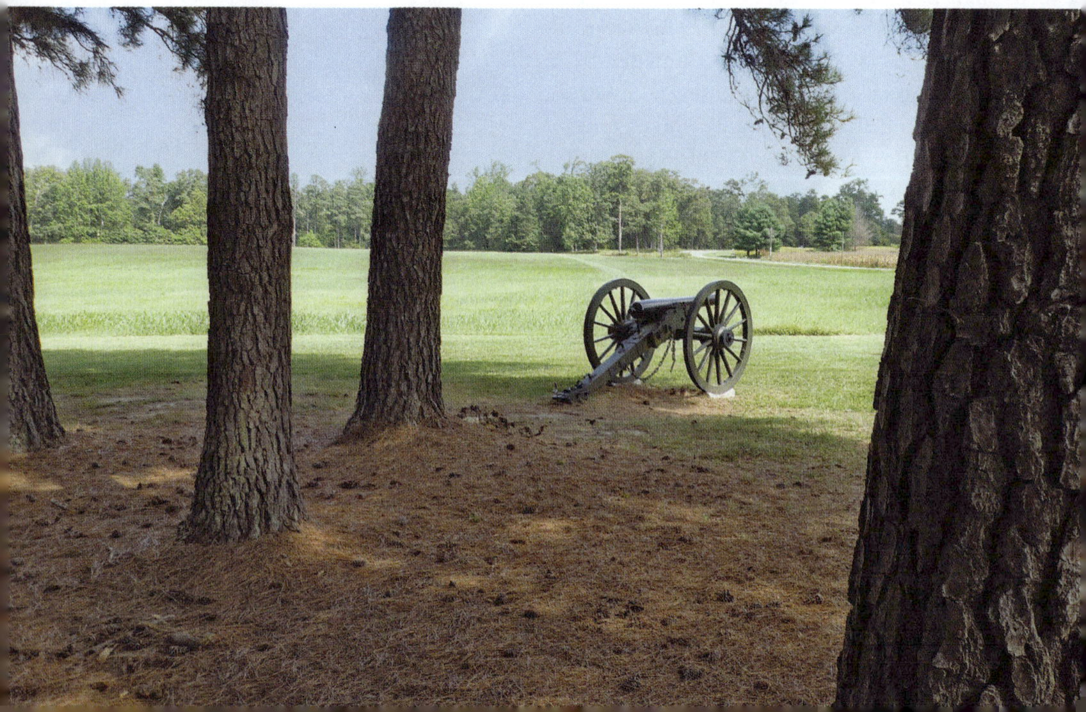

and musket fire. This area later became the main battle line for the Union forces.

The rifle pits you pass at 0.4 mile were dug so that guards could watch for enemy movement but be protected—more or less—from musket fire. Sweet pepper bush is now growing near the site, helping to heal the ground's wounds and obscure this little bit of history. In late July, the plant's wildly fragrant white flowers grow in spikes. Stop to smell one and discover how the "sweet" got into the name. The "pepper" portion was given to the plant, possibly, because the dried seedpods resemble small peppercorns. These remain on the plant through much of the year, making it a distinctive plant that is easy to identify.

If you wish to extend this hike by about 2 miles, you could follow the trail that takes off to the right at 0.5 mile to pass by more rifle pits and sites of the battle. However, this description continues on the main route to the left, crossing tiny Bloody Run and the paved park road at 0.7 mile, where those who have followed the longer route will rejoin the main trail. Ascend slightly and pass by a bit of Virginia creeper running along the ground and up some of the tree trunks.

You'll pass some of the best-preserved and deepest breastworks and trenches at 0.8 mile. If these trenches and mounds of dirt are still this obvious, just think how deep and tall they must have been more than a century and a half ago! Imagine what it was like to be a soldier engaged in this desperate attempt to stay alive. Although historians have not found any proof that it happened, a persistent tale maintains that men of the Union army wrote their names on bits of paper and attached them to their own clothing in the hope that their bodies could be identified after the battle. It's unfortunate that through the course of history, the human race seems to have expended more energy for hostile actions than for peaceful pursuits.

Swing to the left when you emerge into an open field. Due to the excellent forest-field mixture, foxes have adapted well to living in the rural Richmond area. Very likely the scat that you see on the trail is evidence that one of them has walked the same path you have. Take a stick and break open the scat to find out what the fox has been eating—perhaps there's fur and bones of a mouse, feathers from a bird, wild cherry and grape seeds, or remains of various insects.

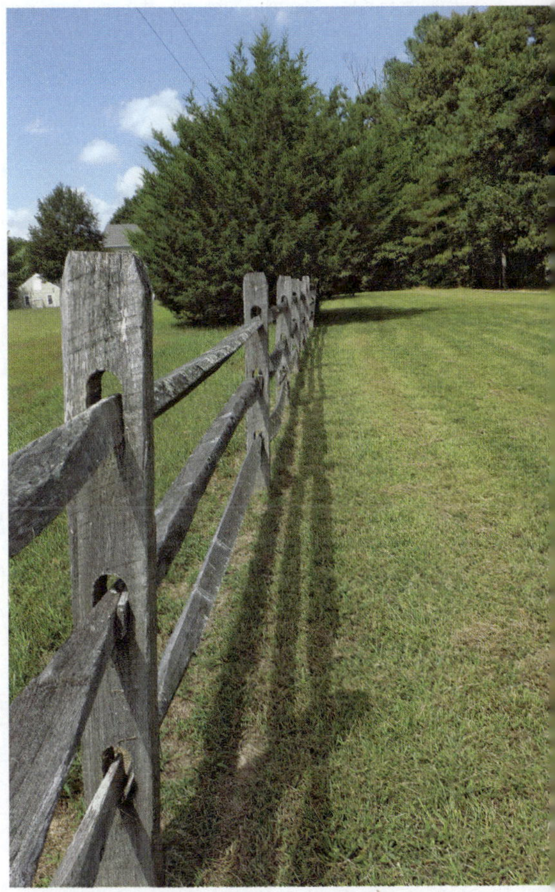

This fence marks the national battlefield park's boundary.

The hike comes to an end as you return to the visitor center at 1.0 mile. (See Hike 14 for information on additional Civil War sites in Virginia.)

Willis River Trail

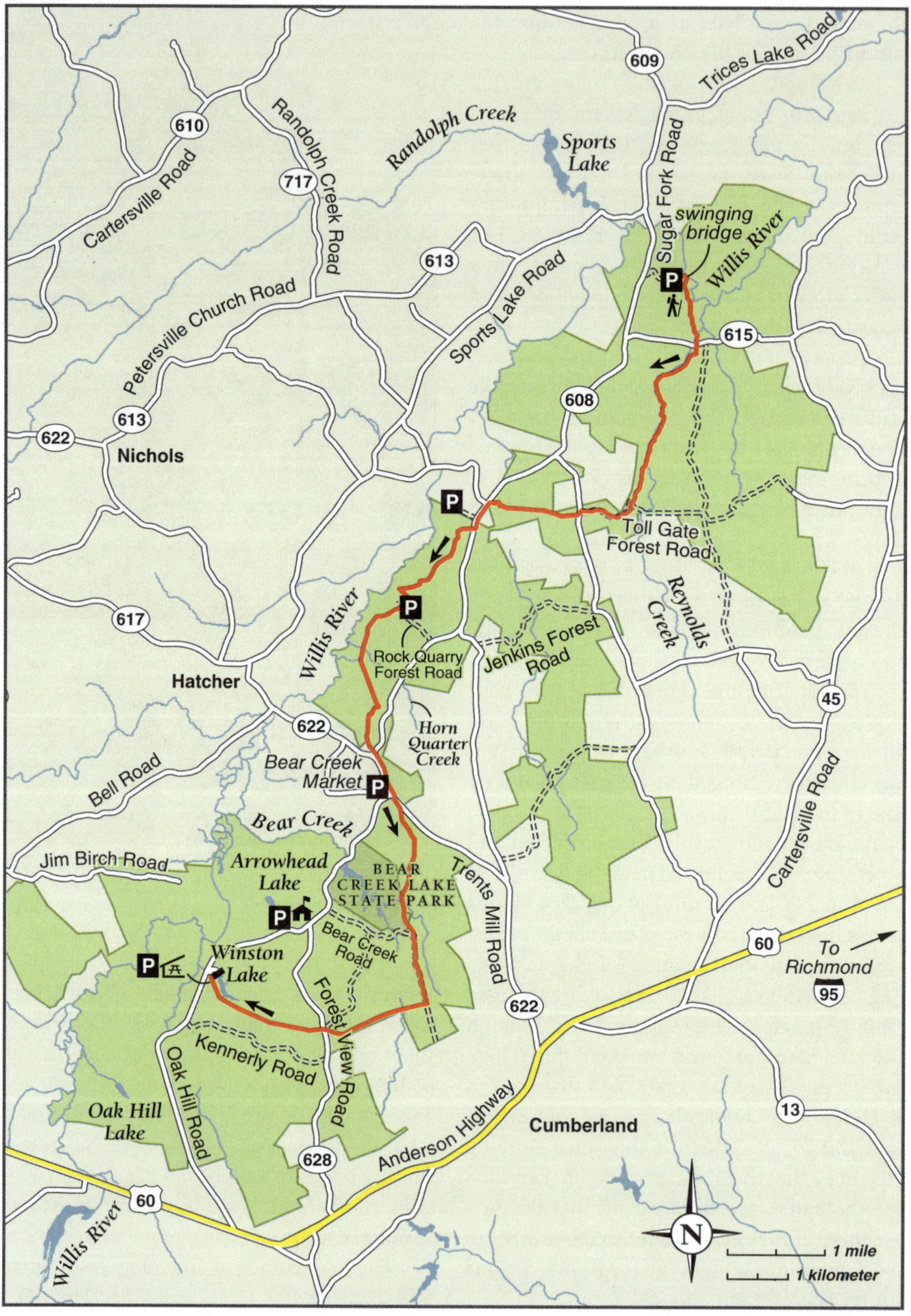

8 Willis River Trail

- **GPS:** N37.619646 W78.213735
- **TOTAL DISTANCE (one-way):** 15.3 miles
- **HIKING TIME:** 9.75 hours
- **VERTICAL RISE:** 700 feet
- **MAPS:** USGS *Gold Hill* and *Whiteville;* VA Department of Forestry *Cumberland State Forest/Willis River Trail* map
- **CONTACT:** Cumberland State Forest
751 Oak Hill Road
Cumberland, VA 23040; 804-492-4121
dof.virginia.gov/education-and-recreation/state-forests/virginia-state-forests/cumberland-state-forest

The Hike at a Glance

0.7 Cross Reynolds Creek on VA 615 bridge
1.8 Ford Reynolds Creek
2.9 Right onto Toll Gate Forest Road
4.8 Left onto VA 624
7.9 Ford Horn Quarter Creek
9.6 Bear Creek Market
10.3 Pass by Forest Trail 24
12.6 Ford Big Bear Creek
15.3 End of hike

After you have traversed several of the Tidewater's and Piedmont's easier and tamer hikes, you may be ready for a change of pace—a walk on the wilder side. The Willis River Trail is a cooperative venture of the Department of Forestry and volunteers from the area and courses its way for more than 15 miles through many of the lesser-visited regions of the Cumberland State Forest. While volunteers—who provide most of the labor for construction and maintenance of the route—do an admirable job, quick-growing summer vegetation and fallen trees rapidly overtake even the best-maintained sections. In addition, there are no bridges to get you across streams or aids to help you climb some of their high banks. There may be no discernible treadway on the ground in some places or the trail may be rerouted for short sections, so always follow the white blazes to make sure you on the correct route. Also be aware there are a few places where there may be short designated high-water routes; use these in times of wet weather. In addition, the forest has been logged in several places along the trail in recent years, sometimes making it even more difficult to discern the pathway.

You probably should not attempt this hike until you feel comfortable about being in such situations, but once you've gained that confidence, the Willis River Trail is a recommended adventure. Nowhere else in the Piedmont can you feel like you are one of the few explorers to pass through such a concealed countryside yet have the safety of trail blazes showing the way. Bring tackle to try your luck fishing the river for bluegill, crappie, largemouth bass, and pickerel.

Consider breaking this trip into two day hikes, as you'll sometimes need extra time to find your way. A number of options exist, but since the parking lot of the Bear Creek Market (see below) is a good place to leave one of your automobiles (after asking permission), splitting the trail into 9.6-mile (6.5-hour) and 5.7-mile (3.0-hour) segments is the most convenient. The store is also well stocked to provide you with ample lunch and munchies supplies. Water sources should not be considered potable, so carry plenty. With an abundance of ticks, flies, chiggers, and mosquitoes during the warmer months, plus ensnaring growths of briars, poison ivy, and other prickly vegetation, long pants and shirts should be your hiking garb here any time of the year. You will cross a well-developed multiuse trail, but it will be obvious that you want to continue to follow the lesser-used Willis River Trail. The only camping option is the developed campground in 326-acre Bear Creek Lake State Park a little more than 10 miles into the journey. In addition to its campground, the park has picnic facilities, a swimming area, concessions, fishing, and about 4 miles of trails.

DIRECTIONS To reach the hike, turn off US 60 onto VA 629, which soon becomes dirt. If coming from the west you will make this turn about 12 miles from the US 15–US 60 intersection in Sprouses Corner; coming from the east it will be about 1 mile from the VA 45–US 60 intersection west of Cumberland.

Three miles from US 60, a sign identifies Winston Lake, the Willis River Trail's southern trailhead. You can leave a car in the small parking area. Continuing the drive, come to a four-way intersection with the Cumberland State Forest headquarters to the left (obtain free maps of the trail here) and VA 628 coming in from the right. Continue straight on now-paved VA 629, passing the entrance to Bear Creek Lake State Park, 2.0 miles from Winston Lake. From the state park, it's 0.8 mile to a T-intersection and the Bear Creek Market, where you will turn left onto paved VA 622. Turn right onto dirt VA 623, 0.4 mile from the market, making a left onto paved VA 624 in 1.7 additional miles. From this intersection it is 2.2 miles to where you bear left onto paved VA 608, which almost immediately becomes dirt. When VA 615 comes in from the right, keep to the left for 0.4 mile to make the last right turn onto dirt Warner Forest Road. Park the car in another 0.5 mile in the small dead-end turnaround.

Route Description

Do not cross the swinging bridge over the Willis River; instead, look for double white blazes on the southern side of the parking area, which direct you into the woods along a pathway lined by Virginia creeper, mayapple, pawpaw, false Solomon's seal, running cedar, partridgeberry, and a host of entangling vegetation. The partridgeberry is an important ground cover; its roots are shallow but intertwining, forming a compact mat that helps stabilize the soil and keep it from washing away in times of high water. Look for deer tracks and other animal prints as you pass through the damp area just before emerging onto VA 615 at 0.7 mile.

Make a left to cross Reynolds Creek on the roadway's bridge, and in less than 300 feet look for double blazes that tell you to make a right onto a probably overgrown pathway beside a swampy area. At 0.9 mile, the trail bears right into the woods and then makes a left along a low ridge before it crosses and ascends out of a gully to the right. From here, it's important to keep a close watch on the blazes as the trail turns left to follow a water run uphill, crosses the run, climbs steeply to cross a ridge and descend, crosses an old trail at a right angle, and continues southward to return to Reynolds Creek at 1.8 miles. Go upstream a few feet and rock-hop the creek at its shallowest point. You may need to search for blazes before moving away from the stream. When you come back to Reynolds Creek at 2.1 miles, the trail can be hard to follow, but just stay between the creek on your left and the ditch (which looks almost like it could be an old railroad grade) on your right. Be very alert at 2.3 miles, where ironwood is spread throughout the forest, as the trail swings right to ascend and descend the hillside around a bend in the stream. Deep-red fire pinks dotting the woods in spring and summer, the rippling of little shoals, and reflections of large green cedars may be enticements to linger.

The trail crosses a very old road at 2.5 miles and swings to the right, ascending away from the creek to follow a grassy woods road below cedars and loblolly pine trees. At 2.9 miles, make a right onto the dirt Toll Gate Forest Road before going straight across dirt VA 624 and reentering the woods. That patch of wonderfully lush and green vegetation you walk through at 3.7 miles is poison ivy, so tread carefully as you gradually descend next to the small streambank punctuated by animal dens. Sycamores prosper in the wet bottomland you will be walking on once you begin to parallel Bonbrook Creek. The fording of the creek at 4.3 miles may be a little easier if you go upstream a bit. Be careful here if it has been raining hard; Bonbrook Creek has been known to have 10-foot-high flash floods.

At 4.8 miles, make a left onto paved VA 624, following it for 400 feet before turning right onto a gated forest road. Be alert because your route will take a left off this roadway in a short distance, descending along a small creek. Make a left to walk upstream next to the Willis River at 5.4 miles. Although the river is slightly murky, its cool, shallow waters would be nice to wade on those hot August days in the Piedmont. At 5.8 miles, make an abrupt turn to the left away from the river, soon entering the 27-acre Rock Quarry Natural Area. The Department of Forestry has reserved several of these natural areas in a number of the commonwealth's state forests. No recreational developments or logging are permitted in them, as these natural areas are intended to be used as laboratories to study the ecology of the areas they preserve.

After crossing a small stream at 6.2 miles, you will follow a defined footpath to a left turn onto a grassy woods road that will, in turn, bring you to a right onto Rock Quarry Forest Road (dirt VA 623 is 0.4 mile to the left). When the road ends in a forest of tall maple and poplar trees, enter the woods to the left, returning to walk along the river, though it is barely visible through the summer vegetation. It is hard for a camera to capture the colorful mixture of ground cover here—the green of running cedar and hundreds of ferns, the crimson red of fire pinks, and the vivid white and yellow of bloodroot. A bit later, rise from the waterway for a short distance before dropping to skirt a flat bottomland. The vegetation is so lush and quick growing that, even if it receives maintenance on a regular basis, the trail is likely to be quite overgrown and tricky to follow as it returns to the river through twists of honeysuckle vines. At 7.5 miles, once again you must be very alert when, for no apparent reason, the trail makes an abrupt left turn away from the river; be sure to keep a sharp eye out for the blazes (and try not to step on the jack-in-the-pulpits).

Horn Quarter Creek, at 7.8 miles, is quite different from the river. Its clear water and flat rocky bottom, combined with the quiet beauty of the surrounding forest, make this possibly the prettiest spot of the entire hike. Watch for giant snapping turtles when you cross the creek at 7.9 miles (and be careful crossing any stream around here). They can grow up to 18 inches in length and weigh more than 40 pounds. The one I nearly stepped on as I was fording the creek was well over a foot in size, and it was almost perfectly camouflaged with long fronds of river moss flowing from its back. The turtle's powerful jaw muscles (which it is not reluctant to use) and a belligerent disposition are what give it its name.

After making a left onto an old road, watch closely for blazes as the route continues south to VA 623, turns right, follows an old logging road, turns left, and then makes a junction with a creek.

You will soon come onto paved VA 622 (Trents Mill Road), which you should follow past dirt VA 623, the Bear Creek Market, and VA

Fire pink

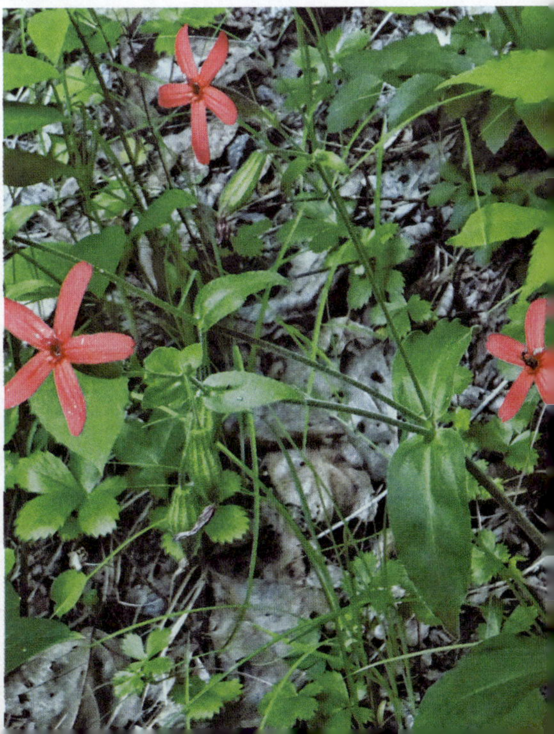

629 at 9.6 miles. Three hundred feet beyond the intersection, leave VA 622 (across the road from a utility box turnaround) by making a right into a grove of planted loblolly pines, soon following an old woods road, and continuing straight past several road junctions. When the woods road ends at 10.1 miles, take the pathway across a small water run. If you have walked the Willis River Trail from its beginning and have had a hard time following its route, you will be happy to know that it will make use of fairly well-defined pathways from here to the end of the hike.

The grassy road (Forest Trail 24) you cross at 10.3 miles goes right about 0.3 mile to the main road in Bear Creek Lake State Park. The forest is populated by birch, beech, and sycamore trees, some of them especially large along the scenic and winding stream you'll cross at 10.9 miles. Enjoy the walk next to clear-flowing Little Bear Creek, with its small ripples, 2-foot-high cascades, and sandy and rocky bottom. Cross over to the other side of the creek at 11.5 miles, continuing upstream amid a garden of mayapple on the ground and pawpaw leaves at eye level.

Pass by a flowing spring, rarer in the Piedmont than in the mountains, under giant grapevines hanging from the trees before crossing dirt Bear Creek Forest Road. After fording Big Bear Creek at 12.6 miles, bear left onto the grassy woods road, with wild rose blooming under the tall pines. After 150 feet, make a left turn, come to a power-line right-of-way, and cross paved VA 628 to enter a woods of dogwood and sweet gum.

Descend to cross a stream at 14.4 miles and pass by a walled-in spring (often dry) on your right just before crossing a larger creek; going upstream a bit may help you find a place to rock-hop across the water. You are now in the backwater area of Winston Lake, and there may be signs of beaver when the trail brings you close to the lake before veering away to ford another tributary. Again, go upstream to find the best place to cross. The ferns and running cedar are a plush carpet from where you look out to the lake and its dam. Descending, you'll make a right onto a hand-laid stone pathway, crossing the footbridge to arrive at the Winston Lake picnic shelter and the end of the hike at 15.3 miles.

After successfully facing the rigors and possible confusions of the Willis River Trail, you may reach the same conclusion I have: Sometimes it is more interesting and gratifying to hike a route that requires you to use a bit of your own navigational skills rather than one that coddles you with groomed treadways and manicured foliage.

Mayapple

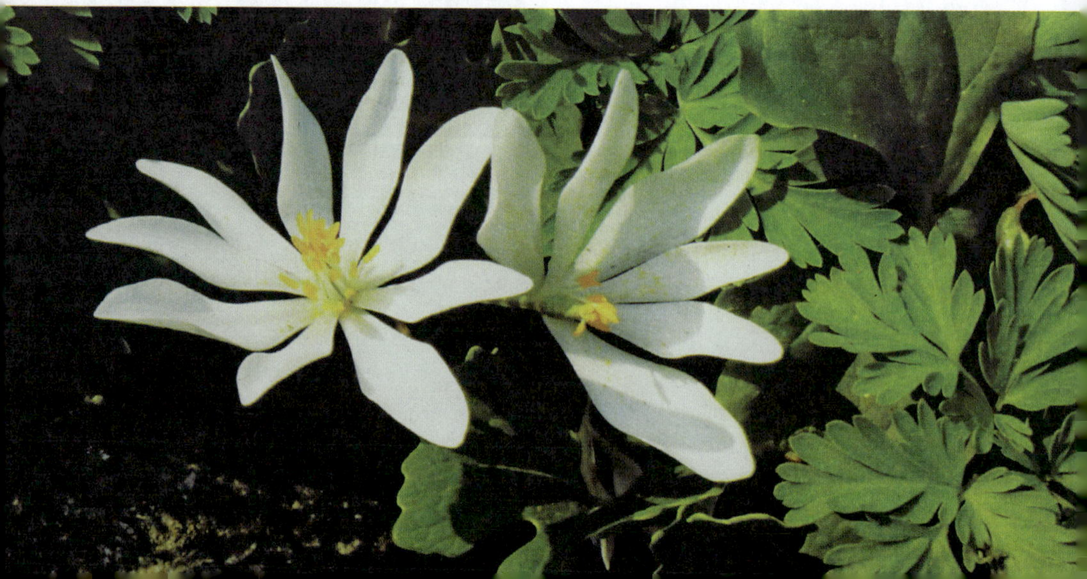

9 Lake Anna State Park

- **GPS:** N38.1166108 W77.8188920
- **TOTAL DISTANCE (circuit):** 12.9 miles
- **HIKING TIME:** 6.75 hours
- **VERTICAL RISE:** 660 feet
- **MAPS:** USGS *Lake Anna West; Lake Anna State Park* map
- **CONTACT:** Lake Anna State Park
6800 Lawyers Road
Spotsylvania, VA 22551
540-854-5503
dcr.virginia.gov/state-parks/lake-anna

The Hike at a Glance

- 0.7 Stay on Mill Pond Trail at intersection
- 0.9 Cove on Pigeon Run; retrace steps to intersection and turn right onto Pigeon Run Trail
- 2.1 Bear right on Gold Hill Trail
- 2.7 Swing right onto loop portion of Gold Hill Trail
- 3.6 Left at Y intersection
- 4.0 Left onto utility line right-of-way
- 5.5 Right onto Pigeon Run Trail
- 5.9 Left onto Sawtooth Trail
- 6.8 Left onto park road
- 7.0 Return to car; take spur of Sawtooth Trail to continue hike
- 7.1 Left onto Sawtooth Trail
- 8.0 Left onto Glenora Trail
- 8.6 Bypass Big Woods Trail and arrive at Glenora Plantation site; retrace steps and turn right onto Big Woods Trail
- 10.0 Bypass Cedar Run Trail for the moment and turn right to arrive at Taylor homesite; retrace steps
- 11.5 Turn right onto Cedar Run Trail
- 12.3 Right onto Turkey Run Trail
- 12.9 Return to car

Nearly every bit of land on Earth has gone through countless changes in its topography, geology, natural history, and uses by the human race. A walk through Lake Anna State Park can provide physical evidence of how past events have shaped the present-day makeup of Virginia's central Piedmont.

Long before humans set foot on this continent, a fault formed in the crust of the earth near what is now Lake Anna State Park. Molten lava poured through this north–south fracture and, as the general lay of the land sloped toward the Atlantic Ocean, the liquid rock spread eastward. Unimpeded, the leading edge of the flow fanned out widely, eventually cooling into a large area rich in iron ore, while behind it the flow was compressed into a narrow band now called the Gold-Pyrite Belt of Virginia.

The Mannahoacks, an eastern tribe of the far-flung Sioux Nation, lived in the area at the time settlers from the Old World began to arrive. Being hunters, food gatherers, and small-plot farmers, the native tribe had little use for the mineral riches below their domain, and the land remained more or less unchanged throughout their occupancy. Within 100 years of the newcomers' arrival, though, the Mannahoacks had been forced off their ancestral territories, and use of the land began to shift.

Virginia's colonists needed a steady supply of nails, farm implements, and other tools to establish their farms and settlements, and the early 1700s saw the rise of numerous iron furnaces making use of the rich ore deposits in what is now Spotsylvania County. Iron mines pockmarked the countryside, and logging roads crisscrossed the landscape to enable harvesting of what was known as the Big Woods. The lumber was made into charcoal to fire the furnaces, one of which was on Douglas Run, just east of the present-day parklands. By the end of the 18th century, however, most of these furnaces had closed, replaced by other furnaces on the more easily navigable James, Potomac, and Rappahannock Rivers.

Agriculture became the region's primary means of livelihood, yet many farmers found

Lake Anna State Park

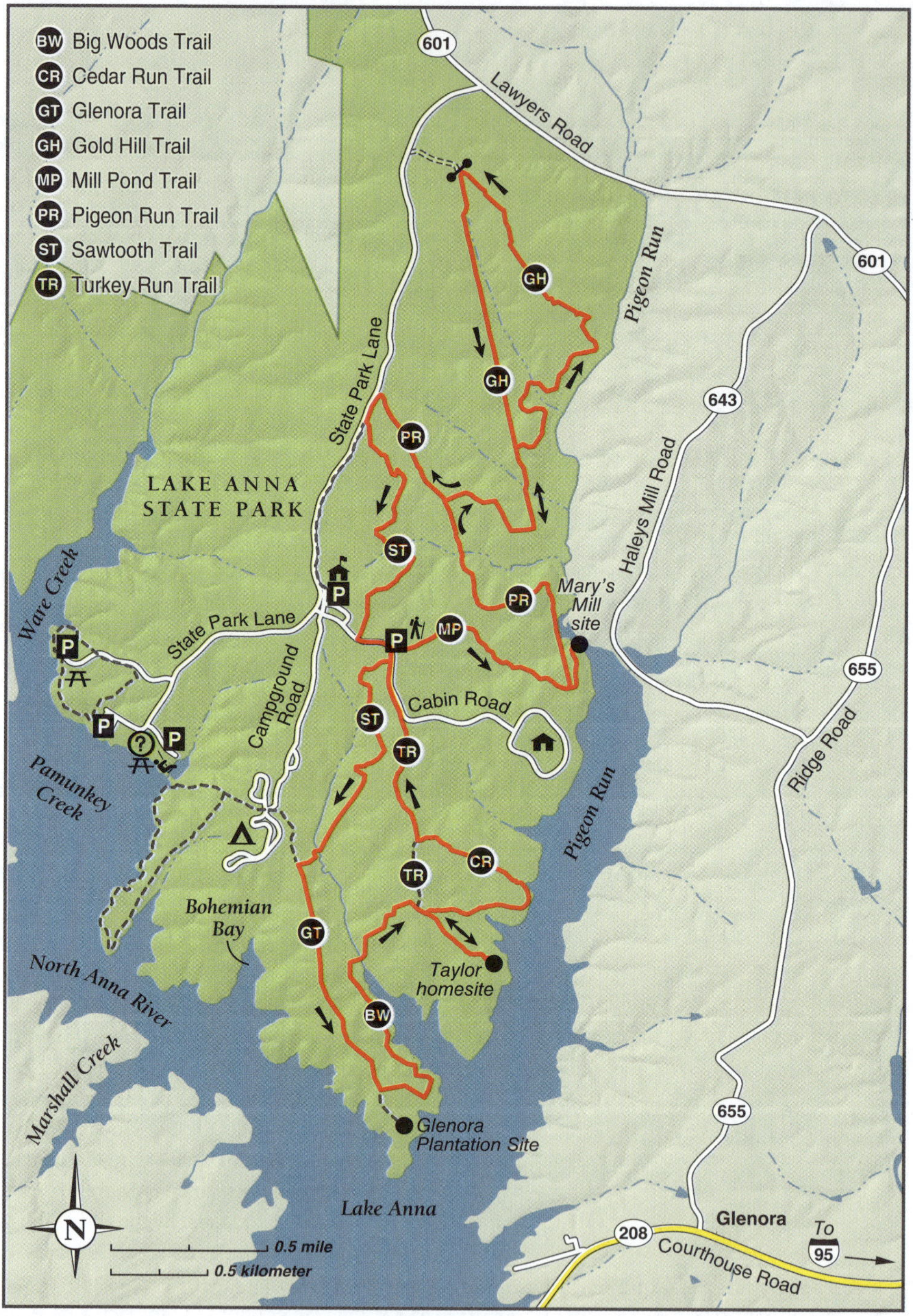

that "panning" their water runs resulted in small but profitable rewards. The first recorded gold mine in Virginia was in western Spotsylvania County in 1806, and the Goodwin Mine opened on Pigeon Run in the 1830s. At one time there were at least 23 mines operating in the county, helping make Virginia the nation's third largest gold producer from 1830 to 1850. The California gold rush of 1849 diverted attention from Virginia, and the population around North Anna River once again adopted an agrarian way of life supplemented with a bit of mineral mining.

Lake Anna was created to fulfill the water needs of the cooling system of Virginia Power Company's North Anna Nuclear Power Station, a short 3 miles from the state park. When the dam across the North Anna River was completed in 1971, the power company gave the lake to the Commonwealth of Virginia. With 8 miles of shoreline, the state park opened to the public in 1983 and offers picnic areas, rental cabins, a campground, a boat ramp, excellent nature and history exhibits in the visitor center, swimming in the lake from Memorial Day to Labor Day, a bathhouse, interpretive programs (one program will teach you how to pan for gold), and concessions. A network of trails allows you to roam the park's more than 2,400 acres to discover natural secrets and beauties and find reminders of all the human activity that has taken place in the past and continues into the present. This hike consists of two loops, with your parked car being in the middle, so you could decide to do the loops on two separate occasions if you don't have the time or inclination to do the entire outing all at once.

DIRECTIONS To reach the trailhead, take I-95 Exit 118 at Thornburg (a few miles south of Fredericksburg). Turn onto Mudd Tavern Road (VA 606), following it westward (as it becomes VA 208) for 7.9 miles, where you will keep left to stay on VA 208. Turn right onto Lawyers Road (VA 601) in an additional 8.2 miles, turn left into the park in another 3.4 miles, and go 1.8 more miles to turn left onto the road marked as leading to the hiking trails. Parking is on the right in another 0.4 mile.

Route Description

Cross the road and enter a forest of sweet gum, sassafras, and hickory on the Mill Pond Trail. Partridgeberry grows abundantly along this old woods road. At 0.7 mile, come to an intersection with the Pigeon Run Trail in the cleared swath of a utility line right-of-way. Continue straight on the Mill Pond Trail and descend to a cove on Pigeon Run at 0.9 mile, where Hailey's gristmill ground locally grown corn from 1857 to 1889. Some of the huge stones that made up the dam for the mill are still visible in the water. If it hasn't rained hard for a few days, the water is usually very clear and you are likely to see dozens of tiny clamshells just below the surface. Anglers may be interested to know that the lake contains bluegill, black crappie, channel catfish, walleye, several kinds of bass, and other fish. Check at the visitor center for fishing regulations.

Although private homes are located on the other side of the cove, this is one of the quietest spots you will have on this hike, so take a break at the water's edge and maybe observe a heron or two trolling the shallow water in search of a meal, a muskrat taking an early morning swim, or a broad-winged hawk surveying its domain. If you are lucky enough to catch a couple of beavers at work, you will see some heavy-duty industry in action. Two adult beavers can bring a 3-inch sapling down in about three minutes and are able to construct a 12-foot-long, 2-foot-high dam with only two nights of labor.

Return to the utility line and turn right onto the Pigeon Run Trail as it follows the arrow-straight right-of-way across the small ups and downs of the landscape. However, be alert at 1.4 miles! The trail swings to the left, away from the utility line, and enters a woods where holly trees are quite prominent and running cedar covers much of the ground as

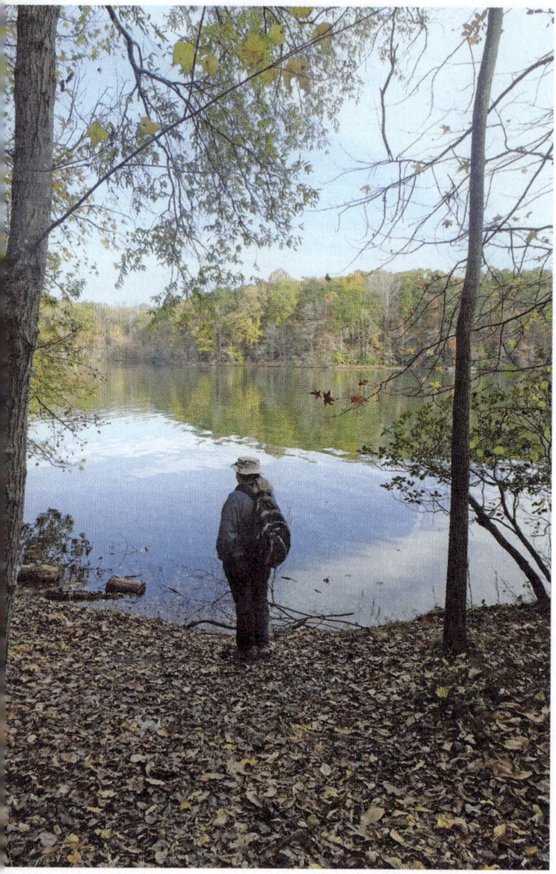

Lake Anna

you swing around a ravine. Bear right onto the Gold Hill Trail at 2.1 miles. (If you are becoming tired or are running out of time, you could shorten the trip by 3.4 miles by continuing straight and following the hike description from the 5.5-mile point.)

Turn left and resume walking along the utility line at 2.5 miles, but pay close attention because you need to swing right into the woods on a footpath at 2.7 miles to begin following a loop portion of the Gold Hill Trail. Cross a stream at 3.0 miles and rise slightly into a forest where the floor is covered with so much running cedar that it looks green even in the middle of winter.

Pay attention so that you don't miss the trail's sharp left turn close to some buildings at 3.3 miles and another left when you come to a Y-intersection at 3.6 miles. It seems as though you have returned to an old, familiar friend when you make one more left at 4.0 miles and resume walking along the utility line right-of-way. Expect to get wet and muddy feet along this portion if it has rained recently. However, you are compensated for this when you observe the multitude of deer tracks in the muck.

When frightened, white-tailed deer will flee at speeds of up to 35 miles per hour, all the while flashing the white of their tails to alert other deer of the danger. This white "flag" also helps the young to follow their mothers through the thick forest vegetation. Fawns are born in the spring after a gestation of seven months—one fawn to a doe bred for the first time, and twins, or sometimes triplets, thereafter. White-tailed deer are not as polygamous as other members of their family, and it's not uncommon for a male to mate with only one doe throughout his life.

Having returned to the intersection with the beginning of the loop portion of the Gold Hill Trail at 4.9 miles, stay straight and retrace your steps to make a right turn into the woods at 5.2 miles. At 5.5 miles, turn right onto the Pigeon Run Trail, which comes to an end at 5.9 miles, where you need to bear left and parallel the main park road on the Sawtooth Trail. Cross a couple of small water runs and turn left onto the paved road at 6.8 miles, and return to your car at 7.0 miles.

If this is all the time you have, drive away with plans to do the rest of this outing another day. If not, take a short break and enjoy the snacks and drinks you stashed in the car.

When ready to resume, enter the woods from the parking area on a spur of the Sawtooth Trail, soon passing the site of an old well that once supplied water for a nearby steam-powered sawmill. At 7.1 miles, turn left onto the main route of the Sawtooth Trail, lined by a large number of holly trees. Unlike the leaves of the holly tree, which remain green throughout the year, the leaves on the beech trees next to the water run you cross at 7.8 miles turn brown yet remain on the tree through most of the winter.

Turn left onto the Glenora Trail at 8.0 miles and follow this old country lane through a mixed forest of sweet gum, hickory, oak, holly, maple, sassafras, and cedar. Hornets' nests are spotted regularly on this trail, so be attentive. In the mountains of Virginia, blueberries usually slow hikers down in August. Here in the Piedmont you will probably enjoy them by no later than mid-July.

Big Woods Trail comes in from the left at 8.6 miles. Continue straight for a short distance to the renovated smokehouse building. This is the only structure still standing from the Glenora Plantation; most of what was once the plantation is now under the waters of Lake Anna. Standing guard over this silent scene is a large, venerable sycamore. Sycamores are generally acknowledged as attaining the most massive proportions of any American hardwood tree. A sycamore's leaves also have the distinction of being the largest single-bladed leaves (4–10 inches in length and breadth) native to the US. Even in a dense mixed forest you can easily spot sycamores by the gleaming white bark of their upper portions.

Retrace your steps back to, and turn right onto, the Big Woods Trail, an old logging road. Walking next to the lake, you will gradually ascend to where the Big Woods Trail ends and meets the Turkey Run Trail at 10.0 miles. Turkey Run Trail goes left 1.0 mile to the trailhead parking; you should turn right onto it and bypass the Cedar Run Trail for the moment to come to a chimney marking the old Taylor homesite (look for the nearby cemetery) close to the shore of the lake.

Return to the intersection with Cedar Run Trail at 11.5 miles. Turn right onto it and descend on this old country road, walking through fields of running cedar. You will soon cross a wooden bridge (the lake is visible through the vegetation) before swinging around an old homesite on a point of land next to the lake, where planted daffodils still bloom in the spring.

Cedar Run Trail ends to meet back with Turkey Run Trail at 12.3 miles. Turn right onto Turkey Run Trail and bring this outing to a close when you return to your automobile at 12.9 miles.

The renovated smokehouse is all that remains of the Glenora Plantation.

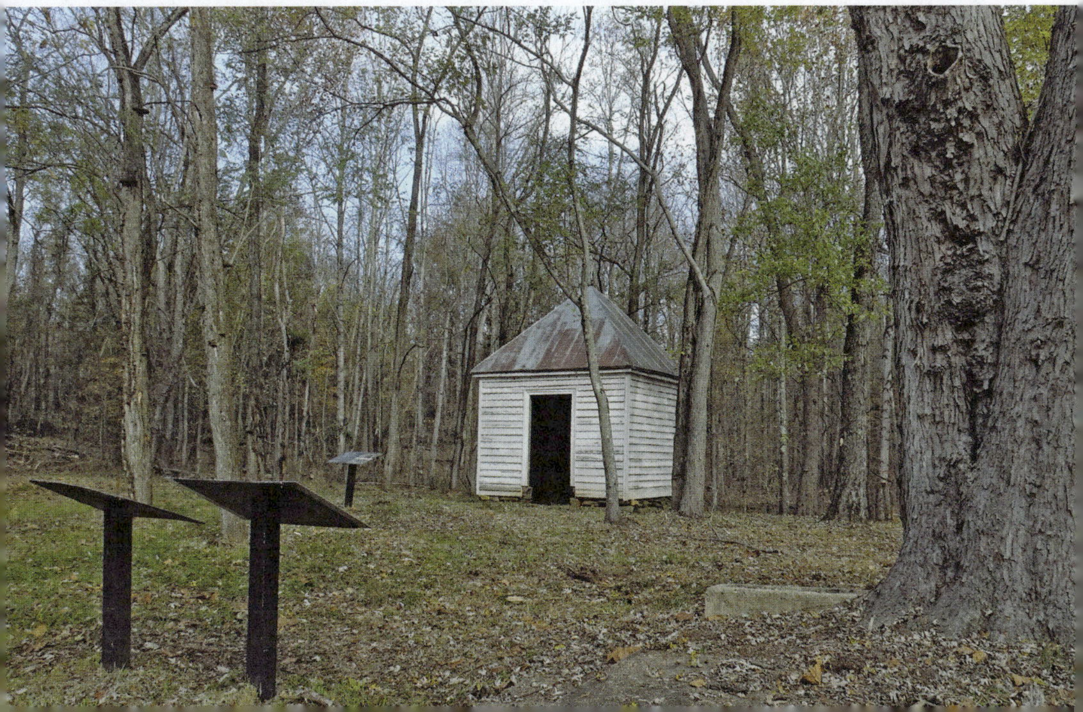

Spotsylvania

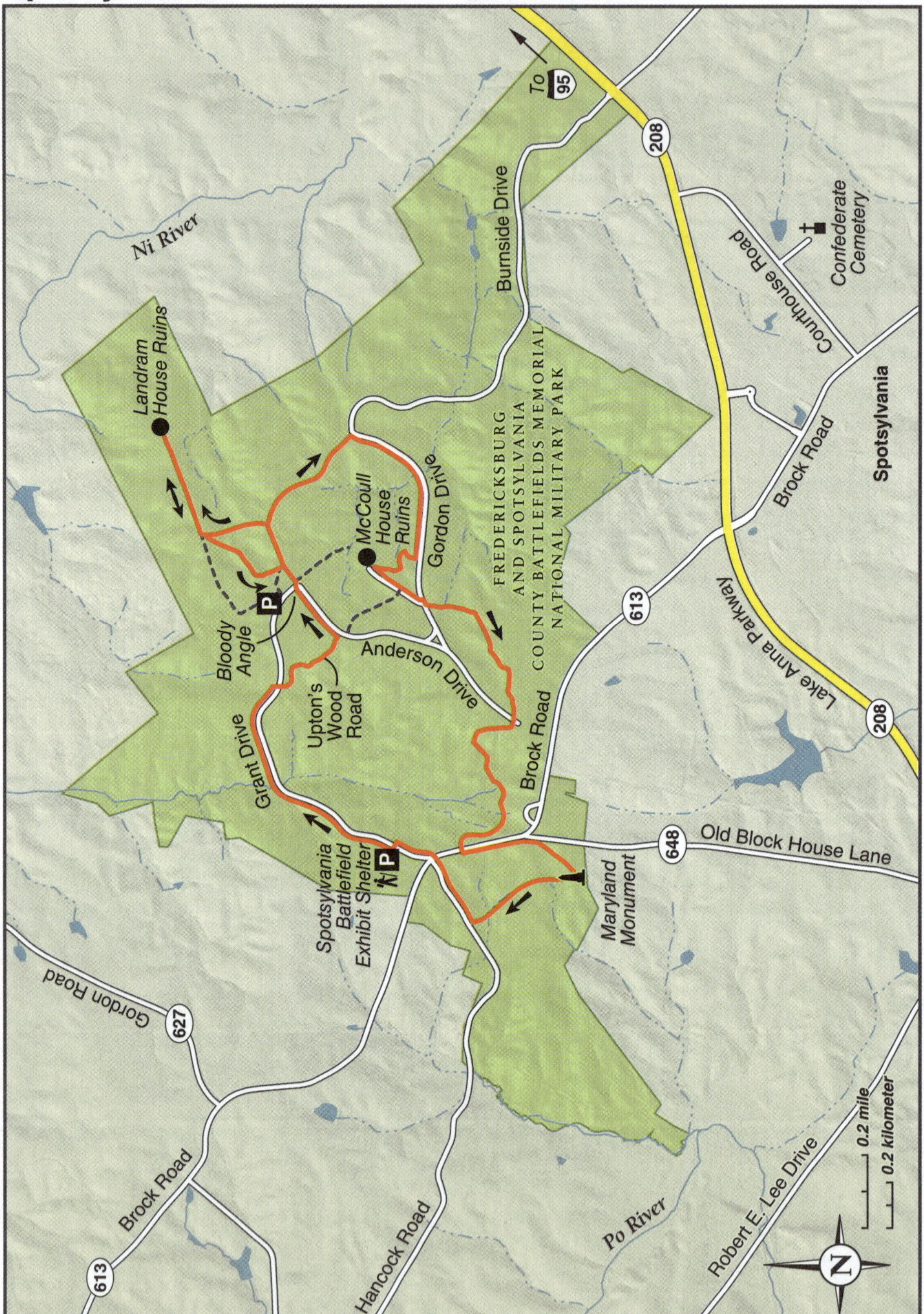

10 Spotsylvania

- **GPS:** N38.2191288 W77.6140721
- **TOTAL DISTANCE (circuit):** 5.3 miles
- **HIKING TIME:** 3.0 hours
- **VERTICAL RISE:** 240 feet
- **MAPS:** USGS *Spotsylvania; Spotsylvania History Trail* map
- **CONTACT:** Fredericksburg and Spotsylvania National Military Park
120 Chatham Lane
Fredericksburg, VA 22405
540-693-3200; nps.gov/frsp

The Hike at a Glance

0.6 Cross paved roadway
1.1 Bloody Angle
1.4 Right onto gravel road, arrive at Landram House site; retrace steps to make right onto mowed pathway
2.3 Recross Boody Angle salient
2.8 Right onto Gordon Drive
3.2 Make right into woods
4.4 Use caution crossing VA 613
5.0 Right onto Hancock Road and, again, cross VA 613
5.3 End of outing

During the course of the Civil War, four major battles—those at Fredericksburg, Chancellorsville, Wilderness, and Spotsylvania Court House—were fought in Fredericksburg and Spotsylvania County, and today the National Park Service preserves some of the lands on which these conflicts occurred. The four sites are a short drive apart, each one offering a variety of hiking opportunities.

The battle of Fredericksburg, December 11–13, 1862, gave Robert E. Lee what many consider to be his most one-sided victory. The Sunken Road and National Cemetery walks and the 5.0-mile Lee Drive Trail are within the city limits of Fredericksburg. General Thomas J. "Stonewall" Jackson was fatally wounded by his own men a few miles west of Fredericksburg during the battle of Chancellorsville (April 27–May 6, 1863). The 3.5-mile Chancellorsville History and 1.0-mile Hazel Grove Trails lead hikers past important points of that battle.

After his encounter on May 5–6, 1864, with the resolute Confederate forces of General Lee at the Battle of the Wilderness, southwest of Chancellorsville (the 0.5-mile Tapp Farm and 2.0-mile Gordon Flank trails help put this conflict into perspective), the general-in-chief of all Union armies, Ulysses S. Grant, marched his forces southward in hopes of seizing the village of Spotsylvania Court House. If the crossroads could be put in Union hands, the Union would control the shortest route to Richmond. Determined to prevent the North's forces from eventually moving on to the capture of the Confederate capital, Lee rushed his troops to the outskirts of Spotsylvania and hurriedly constructed an intricate network of earthen fortifications. The ensuing battle lasted from May 8 to May 21 and included a 20-hour struggle so horrendous that the location came to be known as Bloody Angle.

While all four of the national park sites are worth hiking, I'm going to direct you to the Spotsylvania battlefield because it has one of the longest possible walks through some of the most serene and bucolic scenery. The lay of this land in the Piedmont makes the hike a moderately easy one, alternating between open fields of green grass, sunny meadows crowded with wildflowers, and shaded forests of hardwoods and pine.

DIRECTIONS Before going to the Spotsylvania battlefield, though, stop at the Fredericksburg Battlefield Visitor Center (take I-95 Exit 130A at Fredericksburg, follow VA 3 eastward, turn left onto Lafayette Boulevard, and go 0.5 mile to the visitor center) to gain an overview of all the battles by watching a short film, visiting the excellent museum, and talking to park personnel. You can also pick up free pamphlets about the trails, so be sure to obtain the ones for Spotsylvania and Bloody Angle (dispenser boxes at the trailheads are sometimes empty).

From the visitor center parking lot, make a right onto Lafayette Boulevard/ Business US 1. Stay on the same roadway when the route number changes to VA 208, bringing you to a T-intersection in Spotsylvania Court House. Turning right onto Brock Road (VA 613) and continuing for 1.5 miles brings you to the battlefield entrance, on the right.

Route Description

After studying the exhibits in the shelter, begin the hike by following blue blazes on the left side of Grant Drive past the picnic area. Dogwoods blossom along the road in early spring; their deep crimson joins other leaves in the mixed deciduous forest to make this an exceptionally colorful excursion in the fall. At 0.6 mile, after walking beside fortifications built by Union soldiers, cross the paved roadway and enter the woods on partridgeberry-lined Upton's Road. During the afternoon hours of May 10, 1864, Union colonel Emory Upton brought 12 regiments down this farm road, a move unanticipated by a Georgia brigade entrenched behind the fortifications that you'll cross just before reaching the paved road at 0.9 mile. The element of surprise enabled Upton to take nearly 1,000 prisoners, but because he was unsupported by other Union troops, he was forced to retreat in the face of a Confederate counterattack, losing 1,000 of his own men in the process. Yet immediately after the fighting, Grant promoted Upton to the rank of brigadier general "for gallant and meritorious services."

After studying the old fortifications, known as Doles' Salient, turn left onto paved Anderson Drive, soon crossing over to the right side of the road. At 1.1 miles, pass through a fence stile to where signs mark the site of Bloody Angle. In the present day, the entrenchments may not look like they would have provided much protection, but you must remember that when General Edward Johnson's Confederate division built them on May 8, 1864, the trench was deep enough and the mound high enough that the men could fire their muskets and still be protected. Also, to make it more difficult for an attacking army to overrun them, trees were felled in front of the works, their sharp branches pointing toward the attackers.

Passing by the first footbridge over the salient, make a left to cross the ditch on the second bridge and continue walking on a mowed pathway. This peaceful field of wildflowers was in use as a cultivated field on May 12, 1864, but it should be easy to use your imagination to picture the scene when Union forces burst from the woods to quickly capture General Johnson and 3,000 of his men.

At 1.4 miles, turn right onto the gravel road; Union forces built the trenches along this road after the early morning attack. Come to the site of the Landram House (destroyed by fire in 1905). It was from here that General Winfield S. Hancock's Second Corps swept across the open ground toward the Confederate lines. Retrace your steps along the gravel road, returning to take the right-hand pathway mowed through the meadow, and pass several monuments before recrossing the salient of the Bloody Angle at 2.3 miles. Union general Louis A. Grant's firsthand account may best describe the melee and carnage of Bloody Angle: "Nothing but the piled up logs of breastworks separated the combatants. Our men would reach over the logs and fire into the faces of the enemy, would stab over with their bayonets; many were shot and stabbed through the crevices and holes between the logs; men mounted the works and with muskets rapidly handed them kept up a continuous fire until they were shot down, when others would take their place."

Turn left after crossing the footbridge to come to the parking lot behind East Angle.

Follow the paved roadway with breastworks to the left, bearing right onto Gordon Drive at the intersection at 2.8 miles. As you come to the edge of a field on your left at 3.2 miles, pay attention because the route suddenly leaves the road to enter the woods on the right. Running cedar next to the trail fades as the pathway quits the forest to arrive at the McCoull House site, which was located within the center of the Confederate salient and served as headquarters for General Johnson. From here, take the mowed trail marked with a sign back in the direction of the paved road. This trail will lead you to the Harrison House site, where Confederate general Richard S. Ewell was headquartered and Robert E. Lee pitched his tent. At 3.7 miles, you'll enter the woods, passing an incredibly large and intricate maze of winding trenches—Lee's last line of defense, constructed on May 12. Cross the paved roadway, reentering the forest on a blue-blazed pathway. In May, look for large tulip tree flowers blooming beside tall and straight loblolly pines.

Take care in crossing busy VA 613 at 4.4 miles to follow the mowed route to the Maryland Monument, marking the spot of the first assault on Southern forces on May 8. Swing right from the monument to gain the high point on Laurel Hill. Having arrived on the run from the Battle of the Wilderness, the Confederate army had barely enough time to set up defenses before Union soldiers came swarming toward them.

The smell of honeysuckle permeates the air on the edge of the field at 5.0 miles as you enter the woods and make a right onto dirt Hancock Road. Once again, use caution crossing VA 613. Pass by the monument to Major General "Uncle" John Sedgwick, commander of the Union Sixth Corps of the Army of the Potomac, struck down by a sharpshooter's bullet on May 9. The exhibit shelter and end of this 5.3-mile hike are just a few feet away.

As in the case of the Battle of the Wilderness, both the Union and Confederate armies sustained tremendous casualties at Spotsylvania—a combined estimated loss of more than 25,000 men. Many historians say the Wilderness conflict ended in a stalemate and that because Grant was unable to capture the crossroads town, he failed to win a decisive victory in Spotsylvania. Yet these were certainly victories of a sort. When Grant pulled his forces away, it was not in retreat. Rather, he continued his relentless drive southward that, in less than a year, ended with Lee's surrender at Appomattox.

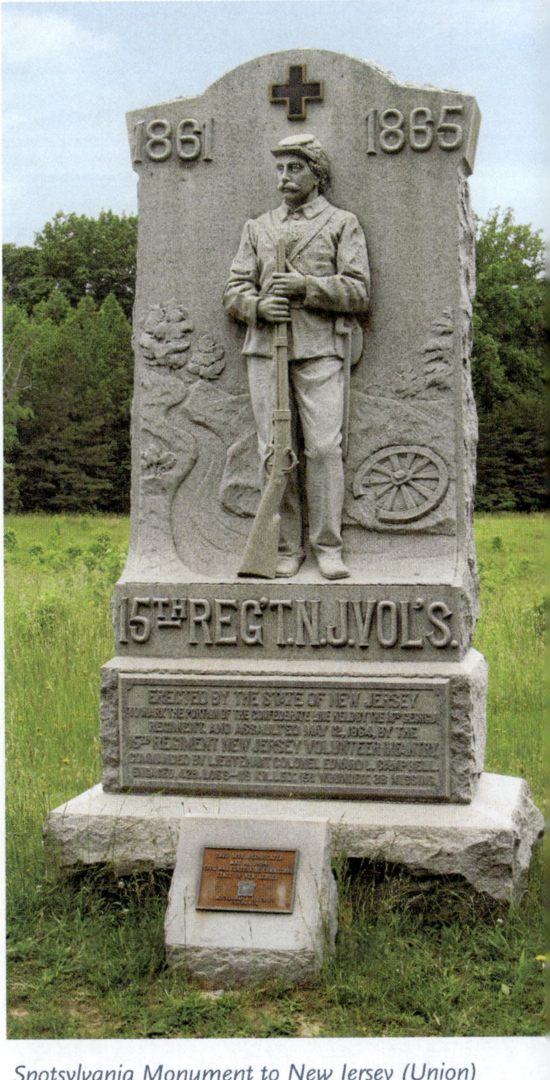

Spotsylvania Monument to New Jersey (Union) volunteers who fought and died in this place

photo: Johnny Molloy

Prince William Forest Park

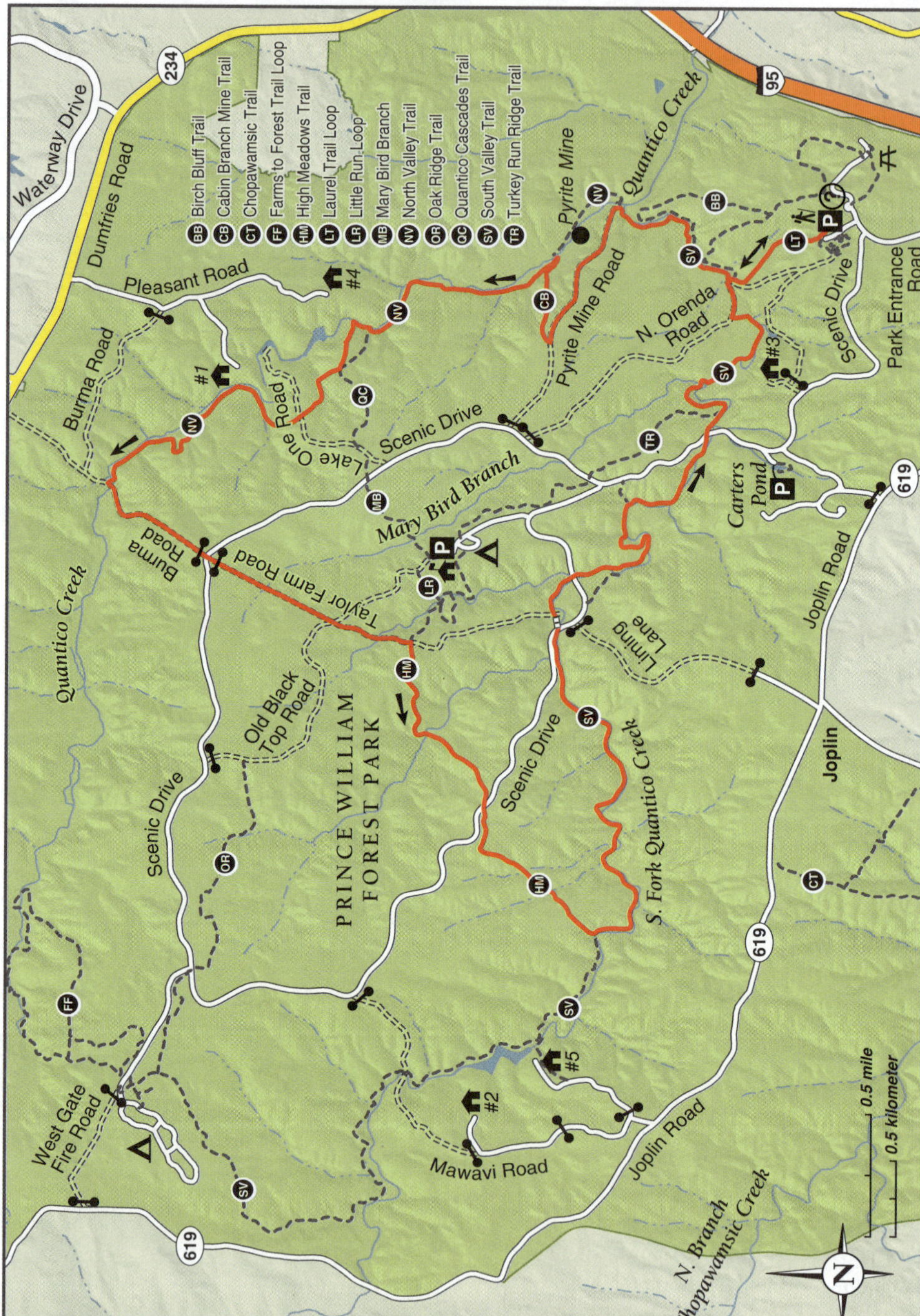

11 Prince William Forest Park

- **GPS:** N38.5598234 W77.3479762
- **TOTAL DISTANCE (circuit):** 13.5 miles
- **HIKING TIME:** 7.75 hours
- **VERTICAL RISE:** 400 feet
- **MAPS:** USGS *Joplin* and *Quantico (VA and MD); Prince William Forest Park* map
- **CONTACT:** Prince William Forest Park
  18100 Park Headquarters Road
  Triangle, VA 22172
  703-221-7181
  nps.gov/prwi

The Hike at a Glance

- 0.4 Cross footbridge; turn right onto South Valley Trail
- 1.3 Left onto Pyrite Mine Road
- 1.9 Right onto Cabin Branch Mine Trail
- 2.2 Left onto North Valley Trail
- 3.3 Rise above small cascades, soon turn right onto Quantico Cascades Trail
- 3.8 Right onto North Valley Trail
- 4.1 Keep right on North Valley Trail
- 5.3 Left onto Burma Road
- 6.0 Cross paved Scenic Road and walk onto gravel Taylor Farm Road
- 6.8 Right onto High Meadows Trail
- 8.5 Left onto South Valley Trail
- 13.1 South Valley Trail continues left; this hike makes a right, crosses a bridge, and makes a right onto Laurel Trail Loop
- 13.5 End of hike

Just as the mountains to the west in Shenandoah National Park were, in places, farmed by unsound practices during the 19th and 20th centuries, so, too, was the acreage around Quantico Creek. This area, however, was subjected to that form of abuse from the mid-1700s. Two hundred years later, when the federal government acquired much of the land fed by Quantico Creek, the soil had become so nutrient-deficient that farming was quickly becoming impractical. Tons of topsoil had washed downstream, turning the harbor at Dumfries into a marsh. For nearly a decade, the Great Depression–era Civilian Conservation Corps (CCC) labored to reclaim the area. Their work, and good stewardship by the National Park Service, has borne fruit. A hike through the park reveals a healthy and green hardwood forest bisected by clear-flowing streams filled with aquatic life and providing sustenance for beavers, muskrats, raccoons, deer, turkeys, and more. Herons, kingfishers, and egrets fish the waters; several different kinds of hawks may be observed year-round; and at least 140 other species of birds have been seen flying by flowering mountain laurel and into pine boughs.

DIRECTIONS The quiet beauty of the park is made all the more remarkable by the fact that it is less than an hour's drive from heavily populated Washington, D.C. The park, which charges an entrance fee, is located on VA 619, only a few hundred feet from the I-95 Exit 150 at Triangle (just south of Dumfries).

Route Description

In addition to nearly 40 miles of trails, the park provides picnic grounds, fishing, individual and group camping cabins, ranger-led programs, tent and RV campgrounds, and a backcountry camping area reachable only by foot (required permits and detailed information on current conditions are available from the visitor center). The short Piedmont Forest Trail is covered with rubber mulch, making it more accessible. Because of these amenities and its close proximity to the D.C. metro area, the park attracts many visitors, yet I've always found the trails to be wonderfully underused. In fact, I did this 13.5-mile hike on a Labor Day weekend and saw only five other people, and four of them were within 10 minutes of a picnic area!

Before undertaking the hike, consider walking the Farms to Forest Trail, located next to the Oak Ridge Campground. This short loop provides a vividly clear example and explanation of forest succession from farmland to woodlands.

Your extended exploration of the park begins in the Pine Grove Picnic Area, where there are two different trailheads of the yellow-blazed Laurel Trail Loop. You want to begin on the western end of the trail, heading northward out of the picnic area. (Be sure to make use of the visitor center—where you should pick up a trail map as a supplement to this guide—or the picnic area's amenities to fill up your water bottles before embarking, as this is your last chance to obtain potable liquids until you return here at the end of your journey.) Enter a hardwood forest with an understory of mountain laurel and azalea.

Continuing on gently sloping terrain, you'll come to the intersection of Laurel Trail Loop and South Orenda Road where, at 0.4 mile, a footbridge enables you to cross over the South Fork of Quantico Creek. Turning right onto white-blazed South Valley Trail, the route is a pleasant downhill walk next to the stream. Be sure to pay attention at 1.3 miles, where you'll make a left turn onto Pyrite Mine Road.

The road receives its name from an operation that existed along the creek from 1889 to 1920. The mine extracted and processed pyrite, which was valued for its high content of sulfur—used to make soap, fertilizer, glass, gunpowder, and a host of other products. Miners were lowered and raised into three main shafts in buckets suspended by 80-foot cables attached to the mine's ceiling. The ore, called fool's gold for its resemblance to that coveted commodity, was raised from the depths and deposited into railroad cars by this same cable system. Due to the great demand for sulfur during World War I, the mine flourished, and the 200- to 300-man crew was exempted from active duty in the armed forces. But with the discovery of pyrite in places of the world where it could be more easily recovered, the mine

Azaleas

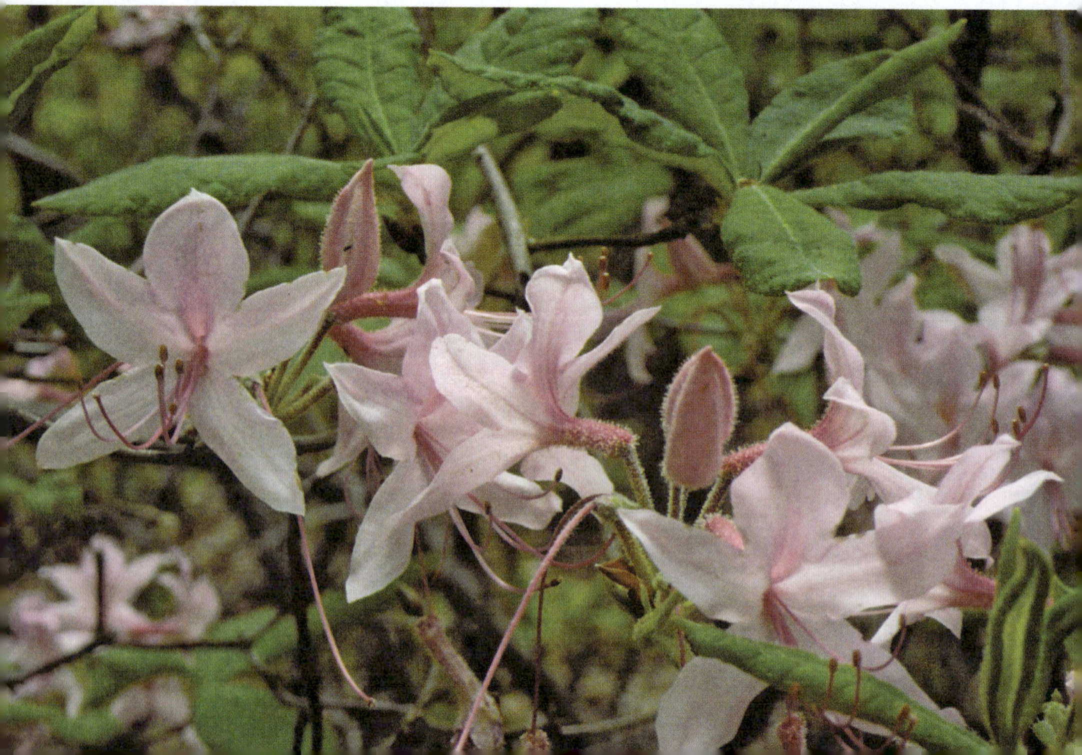

closed in 1920, amid the throes of a miners' strike. The CCC dismantled the vacant buildings and used the material to construct many of the cabins, roads, and other developments still in use in the park. When the mine was in full operation, there were more than 70 structures along the banks of the North Branch of Quantico Creek. As part of the process of reclaiming the mine lands, the park service capped the mine shafts and covered the area with topsoil, grasses, and trees.

Continue rising on Pyrite Mine Road to 1.9 miles. At this point you need to make a right and descend along orange-blazed Cabin Branch Mine Trail. At 2.2 miles, turn left onto blue-blazed North Valley Trail, where beavers may have been gnawing on trees. After you rise above some small cascades at 3.3 miles and drop into a laurel thicket, keep right on yellow-blazed Quantico Cascades Trail, forsaking the North Valley Trail for a while.

Quantico Creek's small cascades, which you passed just a short while ago, are at the fall line, the place where the Piedmont drops onto the coastal plain. While it may not look like much here, the fall line is a major geological feature and, in several places, determined the location of some of Virginia's largest cities. Fredericksburg, Richmond, and Petersburg were all established as transshipment centers on the fall line because their respective rivers became unnavigable beyond those points for large ships bringing cargo upstream from Chesapeake Bay.

The trail makes an abrupt left from Quantico Cascades to ascend past tulip poplars to the four-way intersection at 3.8 miles. Going straight would bring you to parking lot E in 0.6 mile; left goes back to the pyrite mine via the North Valley Trail. You want to make a right onto blue-blazed North Valley Trail, crossing a water run and coming to another intersection at 4.1 miles. Bearing left on blue-blazed Lake One Road would take you to parking lot E in 0.7 mile; keep to the right on the North Valley Trail, soon following a level route upstream along the North Branch of Quantico Creek. The ironwood in this forest of pines and ferns receives its name from its trunk's resemblance to bulging, sinewy muscles. It is in this wide, isolated valley that you are finally away from the constant dull roar of traffic on I-95. The trail negotiates two low ridges before crossing the creek, where beeches are one of the more dominant trees and evidence of beavers may be seen. At 5.3 miles, Burma Road goes right toward the RV campground on the park's northern boundary. You should make a left to rise on Burma Road and cross the paved main park road, Scenic Drive, at 6.0 miles, continuing on the gravel Taylor Farm Road. Gradually descend, accompanied by mountain laurel blossoms in spring and an abundance of blueberries later in summer. Continuing straight, cross Old Blacktop Road—actually made of dirt and a bit of gravel—which runs to the left 0.5 mile to the Turkey Run Ridge Group Campground and to the right 1.0 mile to parking lot F.

Arrive at a four-way intersection at 6.8 miles. To the left it's 0.4 mile to the group campground; you want to turn right onto orange-blazed High Meadows Trail. Before leaving the area, do a little exploring around the old orchards, fields, and cemetery of the Taylor Farm site. (If you want to cut the length of this hike by about 3 miles, you should continue straight from the four-way intersection on blue-blazed Taylor Farm Road for 0.6 mile to intersect the white-blazed South Valley Trail at the 10.4-mile point of this description.)

From the farm site, your route, the High Meadows Trail, ascends just a bit before dropping to cross a tributary of the South Branch of Quantico Creek—another good place to possibly see a beaver or two. At one time, trapping had decimated the beaver population, but their reintroduction in the 1950s has been successful. Having come to parking lot H at 7.7 miles, cross the paved park road, Scenic Drive, then continue to follow orange-blazed High Meadows Trail, with oaks towering above and running cedar hugging the ground. Footbridges bring you across several water runs to the junction with white-blazed South Valley Trail at 8.5 miles.

To the right, this trail takes a winding route of several miles to the Oak Ridge Campground. You, however, make a left onto it, headed down Quantico Creek's South Branch. It can be hard to believe you're only 20-some miles from downtown Washington, D.C., as you walk through this wide, broad, and quiet valley. Like the beavers that use the creek as part of their home and the deer that use it to quench summer thirsts, you might want to make use of the creek's many little pools to cool your feet or take a quick wade. Be careful about wading if there has just been a heavy rain; sand on the pathway shows that the stream can become pretty wild in times of high water. Cross a side stream (the same one you crossed while on the High Meadows Trail) on a footbridge, step across the paved park road, and keep right when Taylor Farm Road comes in from the left at 10.4 miles. Cross under the main park road on a most interesting wooden footbridge and come to a large pool just above the fall line of this branch of Quantico Creek. During the warmer months you may see a snowy egret swishing the water with its feet—its hopes are to stir up some prey to stab with its sharp bill. Switchbacks bring you past three short side trails to the left, successively leading to parking lots C, B, and A.

Cross the paved park road one last time at 12.0 miles and keep right when blue-blazed Turkey Run Ridge Trail comes in from the left. Look for deer tracks in the soft sand when your trail bears right to continue following white blazes of the South Valley Trail on a woods road. (The roadway to the left is North Orenda Fire Road, leading 1.6 miles to parking lot D.) When you come to the next intersection at 13.1 miles, it is time to leave white-blazed South Valley Trail, as it continues straight toward the pyrite mine site. Make a right, cross the bridge, and make an immediate right onto yellow-blazed Laurel Trail Loop, following it back to the picnic area at 13.5 miles.

12 Mason Neck State Park

- **GPS:** N38.6441501 W77.1984970
- **TOTAL DISTANCE (circuit):** 2.7 miles
- **HIKING TIME:** 1.5 hours
- **VERTICAL RISE:** 50 feet
- **MAPS:** USGS *Fort Belvoir; Mason Neck State Park* map
- **CONTACT:** Mason Neck State Park
  7301 High Point Road
  Lorton, VA 22079; 703-339-2385
  dcr.virginia.gov/state-parks/mason-neck

The Hike at a Glance

0.15 Right onto Bay View Trail

0.55 Make a hard right at intersection; continue past observation platform

0.7 Keep right onto Bay View Trail

0.8 Right onto Wilson Spring Trail

1.4 Cross paved park road

1.6 Right onto Kane's Creek Trail; stay left on Kane's Creek Trail at next intersection, but go right at following intersection

2.7 Return to parking area

Mason Neck, a narrow stretch of land rimmed by Belmont, Pohick, and Occoquan Bays and Gunston Cove, juts out into the wide Potomac River about 20 miles south of Washington, D.C. The first recorded mention of the area was by Captain John Smith as he traveled up the Potomac during his exploration of the Chesapeake Bay and its tributaries in 1608. In about 1755, on the northeastern side of the neck, George Mason constructed Gunston Hall, his plantation home, which is still considered one of Virginia's most attractive Colonial homes.

In the 1776 Declaration of Rights of Virginia, Mason stated, "All men are by nature equally free and independent and have certain inherent rights . . . namely, the enjoyment of life and liberty, with the means of acquiring and possessing property, and pursuing and obtaining happiness and safety." He refused to sign the US Constitution because it did not oppose slavery or protect individual rights, but many of his ideas were later incorporated into the Constitution's first 10 amendments (the Bill of Rights); they were also used as inspiration for the French Rights of Man and even the United Nations' Universal Declaration of Human Rights.

It seems somewhat fitting that an area named after the author of a bill of rights for human beings is now largely a preserve for birds, plants, animals, and aquatic life, granting them the most basic of rights, that of survival.

In the 1960s, the Conservation Committee for Mason Neck was formed to save the region from encroaching urbanization. Through that organization's zealous labors—and with help from the Nature Conservancy—the Pohick Bay Regional Park, Gunston Hall Plantation, Mason Neck National Wildlife Refuge (later dedicated to Elizabeth Hartwell, who helped spearhead these efforts), and Mason Neck State Park now protect more than half of the neck's approximately 10,000 acres. All of these areas provide good recreational and walking opportunities and will be passed on your way to your hike in the state park.

DIRECTIONS Take the Lorton I-95 Exit 161 and head eastward for a short distance on Lorton Road to US 1. Turn northward onto US 1, following it to a left turn onto Gunston Road (VA 242). In 3.3 miles, the entrance to Pohick Bay Regional Park is on the left. In addition to a 150-site campground, one of the largest swimming pools on the east coast, a picnic area, an 18-hole golf course, and boat-launching facilities, the park has several marked trails (totaling more than 4 miles) that twist and turn through stands of holly and laurel, passing small inlets covered with water lilies.

Mason Neck State Park

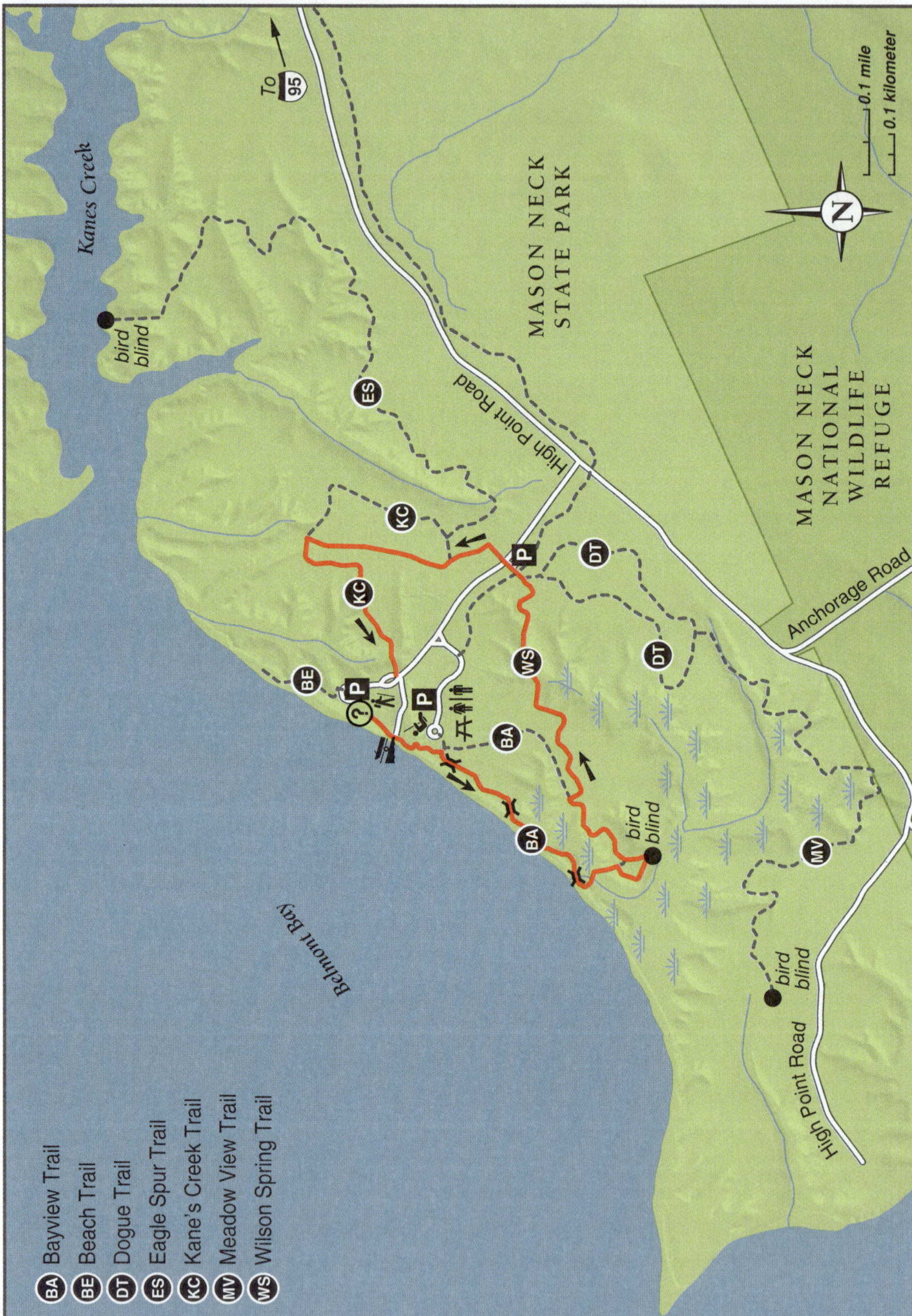

To reach Gunston Hall, continue on VA 242 a short distance past the regional park. A 2-mile trail shows off the natural beauties of Mason's homestead. Beyond Gunston Hall, the roadway becomes VA 600, which you should follow to a sign pointing you to Mason Neck State Park and a right turn onto High Point Road (VA 5733). High Point Road cuts through the Elizabeth Hartwell Mason Neck National Wildlife Refuge, established in 1969 as the country's first national sanctuary for the endangered bald eagle. A parking area on the left is the access point for the approximately 3-mile Woodmarsh Trail. A brochure (sometimes available at the trailhead) provides information on places such as Eagle Point, which overlooks the 250-plus-acre Great Marsh. It is estimated that more than 30 eagles nest or roost in the refuge and state park over the winter and spring to mate and raise their young.

Continue on High Point Road to enter Mason Neck State Park. Continue another 1.9 miles to arrive at the parking area for the visitor center. As you should always do when a visitor center offers interpretive displays, spend a few moments here to learn a little bit of the human and natural history of the area you are about to tour.

Route Description

Even though it is far north of the mouth of the Chesapeake Bay, the state park's shoreline is still subject to the rise and ebb of the Atlantic Ocean's tides. This means that the area's marshlands provide the right habitat for saltwater creatures, such as an occasional blue crab, and attract a wide variety of birds and waterfowl. Despite its proximity to large population centers, this hike can present the opportunity to see, or at least observe signs of, an amazingly diverse array of wildlife. Because of this, and the ease of walking, Mason Neck is the perfect spot to bring city-bound children who have never been delighted by the sprinting leaps of a white-tailed deer, the cry of an osprey flying overhead with a fish grasped in its talons, the gobble of a wild turkey (Ben Franklin's choice for our national bird), or the bark of a red fox calling out to its young. There are copperheads in the park's more remote areas; exercise common-sense precautions. However, don't be alarmed—sightings are almost nonexistent, whereas eagle sightings are quite common.

Begin the hike behind the visitor center by enjoying the sunshine sparkling on Belmont Bay. Turn to your left, walking toward trailheads and picnic areas and passing sweet gums, eastern hemlocks, black walnuts, and red cedars. Drop to a small canoe- and sailboard-launching beach. Cross a bridge over the pond outlet and switchback uphill through pawpaws to the picnic area. The pawpaw's 4- to 5-inch fruit, which resembles a short, fat banana, is at first green but ripens to a purplish-brown. Its meat, with the consistency of an overripe banana, was a food source for rural families up to the mid-20th century and is still considered somewhat of a delicacy by many people.

Come to the Bay View trailhead at 0.15 mile; avoid the trail to the left and take the one to the right that goes along the edge of the bay. Cross a wet area on a wooden footbridge and begin walking on a high bank above the bay. The sound of small waves lapping along the shore is bound to have a calming effect on those willing to listen. Staying quiet will increase your chances of seeing a bald eagle or two, but don't be disappointed if you fail to see any. Keep a sharp eye out for other creatures—great blue herons, Canada geese, wood ducks, and an occasional raccoon hoping to catch a frog or dig up some shellfish to include in its omnivorous diet. Muskrats and beavers are often spotted, usually in early morning or early evening, making ripples on the surface of the water when swimming to or from their burrows on the shoreline.

Use a boardwalk at 0.45 mile to cross a creek that contains northern largemouth bass, black crappie, and bluegill. Take a last glance at the bay as the route swings to the left, using another boardwalk to cross a wide, swampy area of the creek. Here, turtles often bask in the sun atop logs floating in the water.

Leave the boardwalk and follow a pathway lined with laurel as it enters the woods. Look at these woods and reflect back to the time of Captain Smith's ventures in the 17th century. In his journal he noted that, at some places where he set ashore, the virgin forest canopy was so thick that direct sunlight almost never penetrated it. Deprived of this nourishment, very little, if any, vegetation grew on the forest floor, and Smith claimed he could peer a mile or more through the trees!

Come to an intersection at 0.55 mile and make a hard right. Blueberry bushes abound here. In a few hundred feet you'll arrive at an observation platform overlooking a cattail-lined marsh. Surprisingly, marshes are one of the most important areas, ecologically, in the world. They produce more organic material than any other area on Earth—almost 10 tons per acre per year. The marshes are dominated by grasses, which decay and, along with other material, are washed out to the rivers and bays. This decayed material, known as detritus, is the first link in a food chain that reaches far out into the ocean.

Continue past the observation platform to come back to the Bay View Trail at 0.7 mile and keep right. Leave that pathway at 0.8 mile and turn right onto the Wilson Spring Trail. Undergrowth is not quite as thick here, making it easier to spot some of the park's resident deer or gray squirrels. Walk into a darker forest of beech and holly at 1.2 miles, passing small, wet-weather marshlike ponds. Walk over and take a rest break next to one. Many people see eastern painted turtles, one of the most common turtles in the United States, but never know it because they don't look for the reptile's special markings. You'll know if one slides into the pond in front of you because you'll be looking for red markings on the side of its shell and red and yellow stripes on its head, legs, and tail.

Just after bypassing the Dogue Trail, stepping over the paved High Point Trail, and crossing the paved park road at 1.4 miles (the visitor center is about 0.5 mile to the left), continue to follow the trail through another open area of the forest. In 1.6 miles you will come to the end of the Wilson Spring Trail. The visitor center is to the left; your route goes right onto Kane's Creek Trail through a typical Potomac lowland forest of mature oak, hickory, and poplar above an understory of holly and laurel. Stay left on the Kane's Creek Trail at the next intersection; the Eagle Spur Trail to the right goes 1.3 miles to an overlook of Kane's Creek.

Stay right at the next intersection to follow the trail marked as leading to the visitor center, and return to your parked car at 2.7 miles.

Gaze across Belmont Bay from near the visitor center.

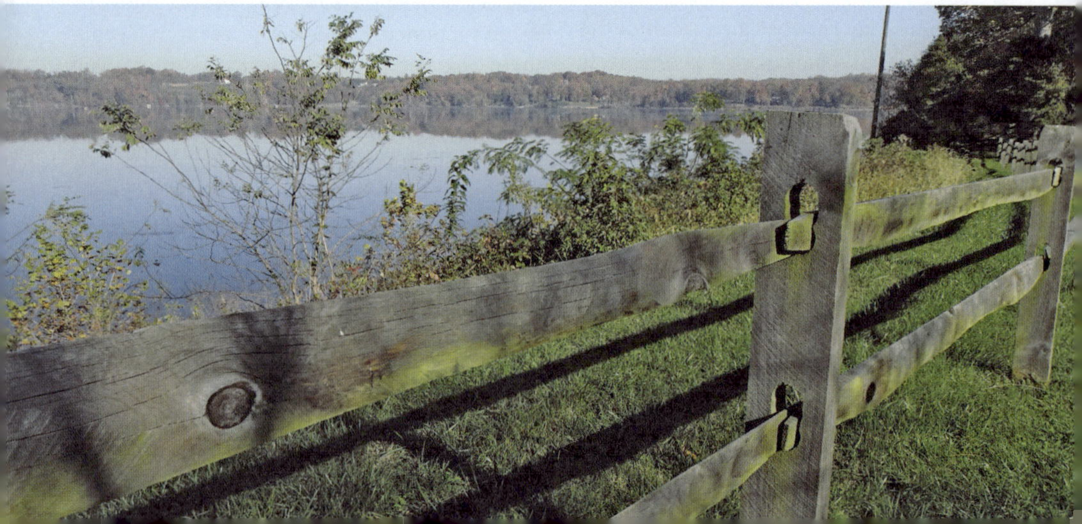

13 Bull Run–Occoquan River

- **GPS:** N38.766341 W77.406927
- **TOTAL DISTANCE (one-way):** 11.0 miles
- **HIKING TIME:** 7.5 hours
- **VERTICAL RISE:** 3,180 feet
- **MAPS:** USGS *Manassas, Independent Hill,* and *Occoquan*
- **CONTACT:** NOVA Parks
  5400 Ox Road
  Fairfax Station, VA 22039; 703-352-5900
  novaparks.com/parks/bull-run-occoquan-trail

The Hike at a Glance

- 0.5 Turn left onto BROT
- 3.0 Walk near soccer field
- 4.4 Bull Run Marina; soon cross Old Yates Ford Road
- 8.0 View of Occoquan River; soon cross Wolf Run Shoals Road and pass cemetery
- 9.4 Utility line right-of-way
- 9.8 Utility line right-of-way
- 11.0 End of hike

Concerned about urban sprawl in the northern Virginia region, a group of farsighted citizens banded together in the late 1950s and, along with several local governments, formed the Northern Virginia Regional Park Authority (now known as NOVA Parks). More than 12,800 acres are now preserved under the auspices of the authority.

Five of the regional parks—Bull Run, Hemlock Overlook, Bull Run Marina, Fountainhead, and Sandy Run—contain 5,000 of these acres along the shore of the Bull Run–Occoquan stream valley. This continuous strip of parkland is a valuable conservation area, preserving marshes and forests and protecting the shoreline of the Occoquan Reservoir, the source of water for a large percentage of northern Virginia's population.

Following the winding course of Bull Run and the Occoquan River through four of the five parks, the Bull Run Occoquan Trail (BROT) makes it possible—despite continued, rapid development of the region—to walk nearly 20 miles in basically one direction and still be almost continuously on public lands. The shoreline is a nesting place for ducks, geese, osprey, and other bird life. Chipmunks, squirrels, wild turkeys, snakes, turtles, raccoons, foxes, and a large population of deer inhabit lands along the trail. Numerous gnawed trees, especially near and in Hemlock Overlook Regional Park, are evidence of an active beaver community.

The northern section of the BROT begins in Centreville in Bull Run Regional Park and runs to Hemlock Overlook Regional Park. That portion is quite wet and marshy. Therefore, this hike takes in the more pleasurable southern 11 miles of the trail, from Hemlock Overlook Regional Park to Fountainhead Regional Park. Camping is not permitted along the BROT. Like all trails, the BROT is sometimes relocated for short distances, so be sure to follow blue blazes in case the trail on the ground differs from this description.

DIRECTIONS For this long, one-way hike, you will need two cars in order to do a shuttle. To reach Fountainhead Regional Park, which is south of Washington, D.C., take I-95 Exit 163 at Lorton. Go westward on Lorton Road (VA 642) to make a right turn onto Ox Road (VA 123) and then a left onto Hampton Road (VA 647). Turn left onto VA 727 to enter Fountainhead Regional Park. Leave one car at the trailhead parking lot, then go back and turn left onto Hampton Road (VA 647). Intersect and turn left onto Henderson Road (VA 643). Continue to the right where Old Yates Ford Road (VA 612) goes off to the left to Bull Run Marina. Bear left onto Clifton Road (VA 645) and watch for the left turn onto Yates Ford Road (VA 615).

Bull Run–Occoquan River

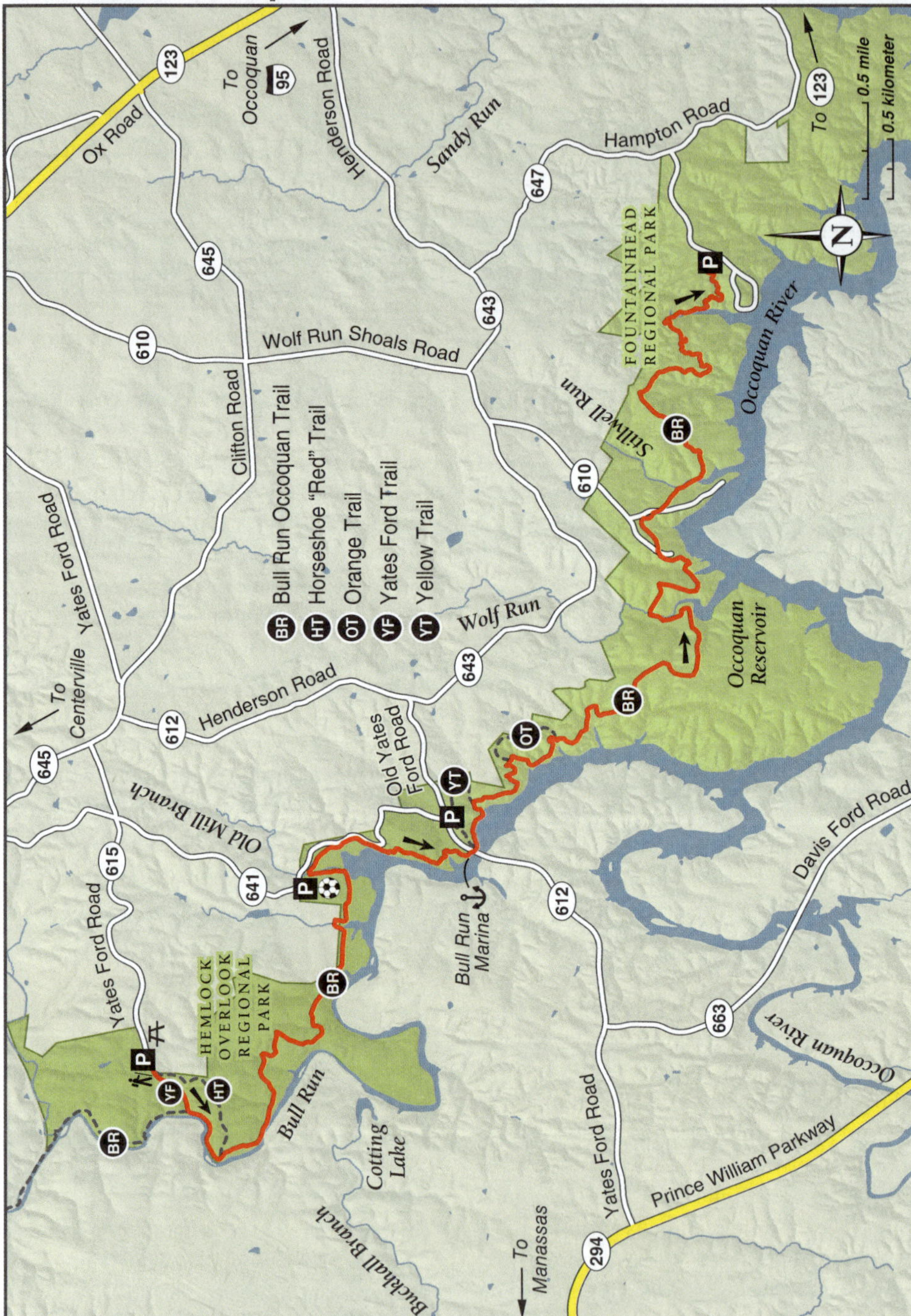

Cross Kincheloe Road and continue on Yates Ford Road. Turn into the small trailhead parking area directly across the road from Hemlock Overlook's mailbox (marked 13220 Yates Ford Road).

Route Description

From the trailhead parking lot, walk along the pavement toward the park's gated entrance, but in 0.1 mile do not follow the road as it swings to the right through the gate; rather, continue by entering a hardwood forest directly ahead on an old dirt road that used to be the carriage road leading to Yates Ford on Bull Run.

At 0.2 mile, the Horseshoe Trail on the left intersects with the old road. It is possible to take this trail and rejoin your route at the 0.9-mile point of this description. However, you should continue to descend along the road, passing a plaque to Sol M. Edinin (1920–1981) placed by the Clifton Horse Society Ltd. At 0.45 mile, notice the small rows of circular holes drilled into the inner bark layer of nearby trees. Yellow-bellied sapsuckers drill the holes; sap rises into them, and, true to their name, these woodpeckers feed by sucking the liquid out with long, bristly tongues. Often ants and other insects are attracted by the trees' sweet juices, and the sapsuckers can get both "dinner" and "dessert" from just one hole. Pileated woodpeckers also inhabit Hemlock Overlook—the holes they make are large, deep, and almost rectangular.

Arrive at Bull Run at 0.5 mile and turn left through laurel to begin walking on the BROT and paralleling the stream. Several small rock overhangs are located at 0.7 mile and would make great emergency shelters in case of a sudden spring shower.

In a large open area, the Horseshoe Trail joins the BROT at 0.9 mile. Spring flowers such as mayapple, spring beauties, violets, bluebells, and bloodroot are found in profusion here. Dogtooth violet is also abundant later in the spring. Sycamores grow well along this bottomland, reflecting their preference for moist soil as opposed to the rockier, drier ground of the hillsides.

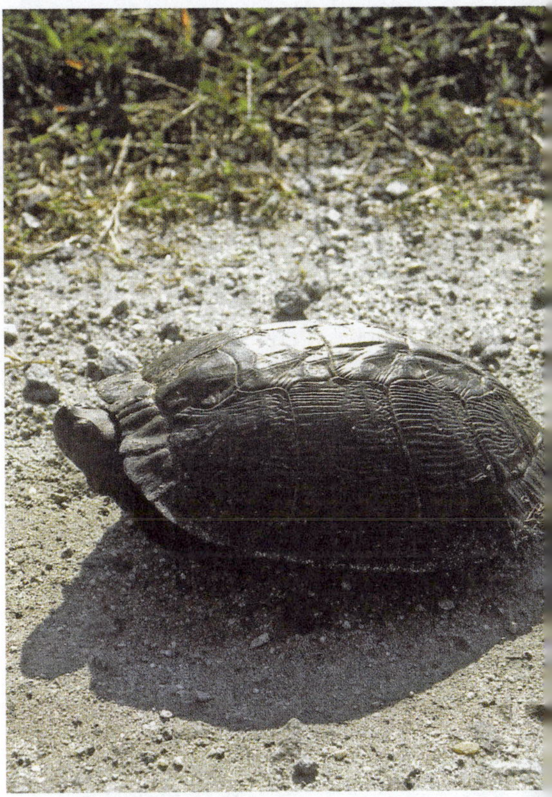

Box turtle

At 1.4 miles, the sounds of a firing range may be evident as the trail swings away from the stream to enter a newer forest of cedar and pine. Running cedar spreads itself across the ground, helping to stabilize the soil. Reenter the older-growth forest at 1.6 miles, cross a small creek, and ascend along an old woods road. At the top of the rise, at 1.8 miles, you must be alert and take the woods road to the right, not the one to the left. Again, at 2.1 miles, watch for the spot where your route leaves the road. Descend on a pathway to the left. Soon you will ascend to follow another old road through laurel, only to descend steeply and begin walking along a creek and another dirt road at 2.4 miles.

The trail leaves the road at 2.6 miles, turns left, crosses a creek, and enters a field. Ducks,

Canada geese, and great blue herons are frequent visitors to the backwater area on your right. You may see great blue herons standing motionless in the shallow water, waiting for a dinner of fish, snakes, mice, frogs, or small birds to come close enough to be quickly grabbed and consumed. The field is a good place to catch a glimpse of rabbits or deer in the early morning or early evening.

Swing around another backwater area, cross an inlet stream, and at 3.0 miles walk along the edge of a soccer field, heading toward a parking lot. Just before the lot, turn right, cross a stream, and walk through a field, aiming for the place where the trail reenters a wooded area of pines and cedars.

You must be alert again at 3.9 miles, as the trail makes an abrupt change to the left to steeply climb the hillside. It drops steeply down and climbs again to begin a series of short ups, downs, and meanderings through a wonderful older forest. Enter Bull Run Marina at 4.2 miles, passing a yellow-blazed trail to the left. That trail is a circuit hike of about 1 mile that rejoins the BROT. Continue to your right, crossing a backwater stream on a footbridge at 4.35 miles, where the yellow-blazed trail rejoins your route from the left. Again, continue to the right; ascend to pass restrooms, picnic tables, and the boat-launching area in Bull Run Marina at 4.4 miles.

Take care in crossing busy Old Yates Ford Road. Follow a paved trail a short distance into the woods, but do not follow it back uphill. Continue on a dirt pathway next to Bull Run, which gets wider as you work your way downstream toward the reservoir. Honeysuckle and grapevines wind their way over the trees and across the trail. Watch where you step, as the vines, especially the honeysuckle, could cause

A deer strikes an elegant pose in the field.

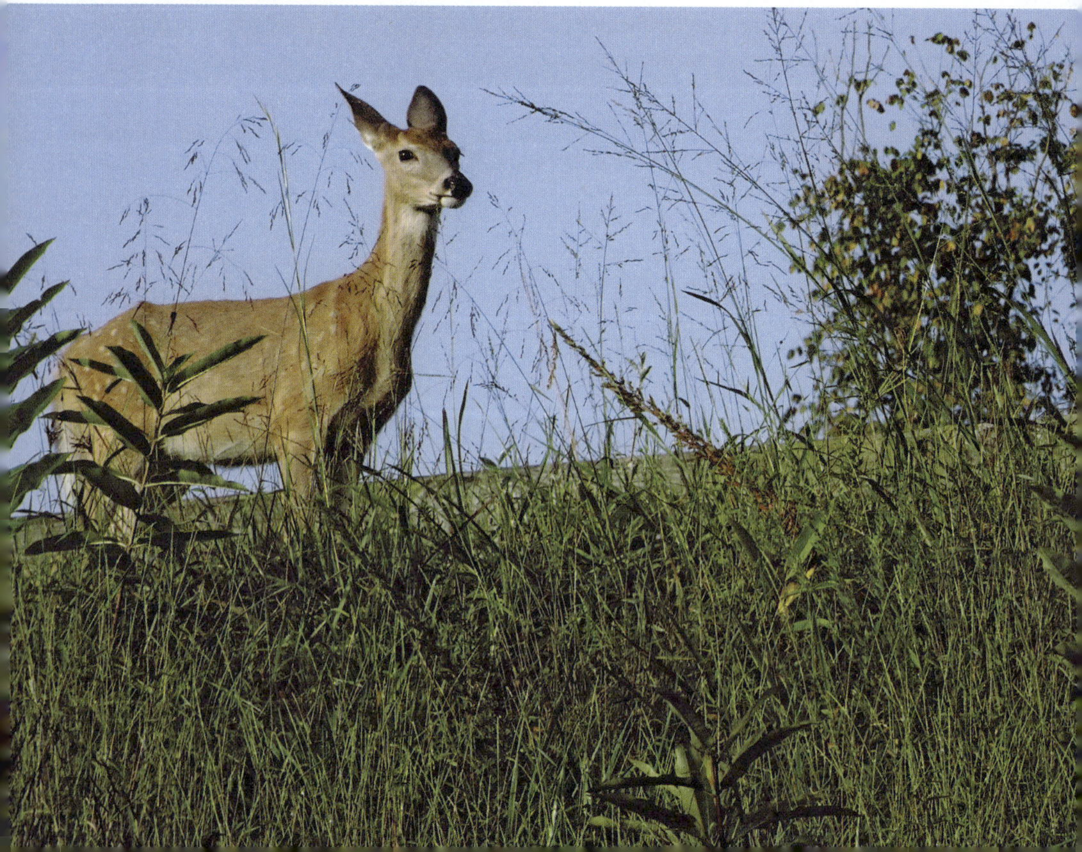

you to trip. However, the forest will become more open once you swing around a backwater area. As you walk this upland pathway away from Bull Run, it, unseen by you, is intersected by, and becomes, the Occoquan River.

An orange-blazed trail comes in from the left at 4.9 miles. It, too, is a circular trail of a little more than a mile. The orange-blazed trail rejoins the BROT at 5.1 miles. Begin a series of ups and downs as you meander through the woods close to a housing development. Turn right onto an old road to swing away from the houses and, amazingly, after just having been so close to civilization, enter a wonderfully isolated valley at 5.9 miles.

At 6.0 miles, ascend out of the valley, cross a low knob, and descend into another small valley, only to rise again. Songbirds are especially active here in the early morning as they flitter among the exceptionally large beech trees. You will walk by a few upscale homes as you turn right onto a dirt road at 6.5 miles. There is a T-intersection at 7.5 miles, where you need to make a left turn to descend, leaving behind the houses and road noise. At 7.6 miles, make a left turn onto a trail following a water run upstream. The creek is deep, murky, and slow moving, giving the area an almost swampy feeling. Skunk cabbage is one of the earliest plants to bloom here after the first of the year, and, if you are hiking in late winter, look for its purple-and-brown flowers surrounded by broad green leaves. Touch one of the leaves to learn how it received its name.

Cross a stream at 7.8 miles. After ascending to a T-intersection at 8.0 miles, turn right and gradually descend to come to your only view of the Occoquan River. This valley was originally inhabited by Native Americans of the Powhatan confederacy, and *occoquan* can be translated to mean "at the end of the water." The name presumably refers to where the Occoquan empties a few miles downstream into Belmont and Occoquan Bays. Arrive at a four-way intersection at 8.2 miles and turn left to swing around a backwater area and ascend to cross a small creek. Look backward for a few moments to enjoy your last glimpse of the river.

Come onto paved Wolf Run Shoals Road, walking by a cemetery with quite a number of gravestones identifying 1918 as the year of death. Could all of these people have passed away because of the great flu pandemic? A thousand feet beyond the cemetery, you must be alert, as your route makes an abrupt turn to the right off the paved roadway to follow a cedar-lined, dirt-and-gravel driveway. Soon bear right and descend on an old dirt road.

Cross a creek at 9.1 miles and ascend in a mixed hardwood and evergreen forest. The trail comes to a utility-line right-of-way at 9.4 miles and turns left uphill. Just 0.2 mile beyond, turn left, away from the utility line. You will cross under another line at 9.8 miles, where you need to make an abrupt turn to the right, soon making another right turn onto a dirt road.

Be alert at 10.1 miles, as your route leaves the dirt road, enters the woods to the left, and descends. At 10.4 miles, you come to a right turn onto a woods road, where you parallel a small stream. Rock-hop a creek at 10.5 miles and ascend steeply, entering Fountainhead Regional Park and soon passing a horse trail that heads off to the right.

A white-blazed trail comes in from the left at 10.6 miles. On the right, the horse trail rejoins the BROT at 10.8 miles. Stop to look through the late-1800s cemetery.

Reach the trailhead parking at 11.0 miles. Restrooms are to your right. The park offers nature trails, a picnic area, and a boat-launching ramp. A snack shop and visitor center are a short distance down the road, to the right.

Manassas National Battlefield Park

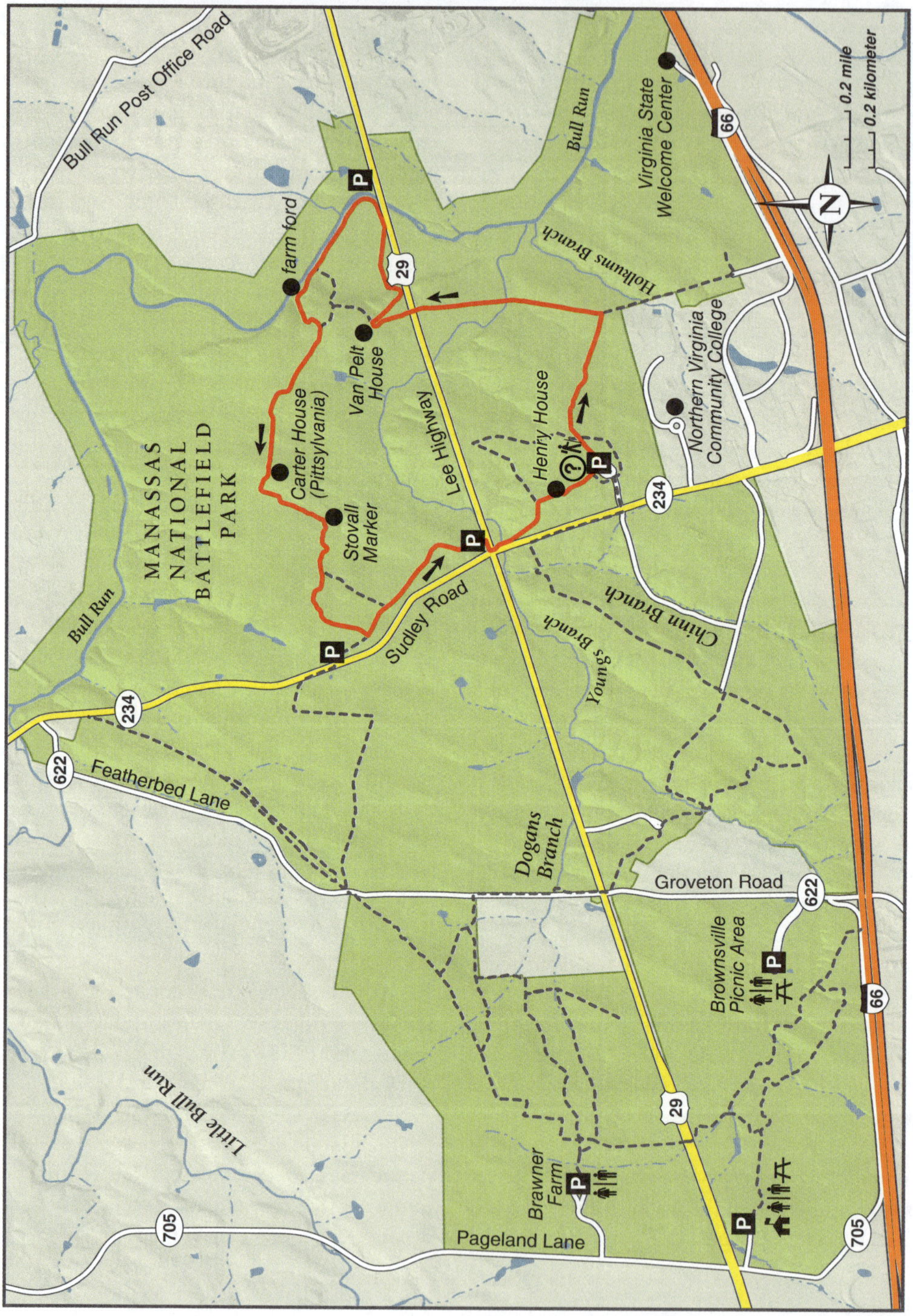

14 Manassas National Battlefield Park

- **GPS:** N38.8130539 W77.5212668
- **TOTAL DISTANCE (circuit):** 5.5 miles
- **HIKING TIME:** 2.5 hours
- **VERTICAL RISE:** 390 feet
- **MAPS:** USGS *Gainesville; Manassas Battlefield Walking Tours* map
- **CONTACT:**
  Manassas National Battlefield Park
  1251 Lee Hwy.
  Manassas, VA 20109-2005
  703-361-1339
  nps.gov/mana

The Hike at a Glance

- **0.6** Left onto Rock Road
- **0.9** Cross Youngs Branch
- **1.25** Follow pathway to left and soon cross US 29
- **1.4** Van Pelt House site
- **2.5** Keep right at intersection and arrive at Farm Ford
- **3.3** Trail levels out and soon comes to Landan Carter home site
- **4.2** Trail breaks out in open; soon bear left to descend and cross US 29
- **5.3** Henry House
- **5.5** Return to Visitor Center

The peaceful, rolling hills of the broad Manassas plateau were the site of two intense, bloody, and significant battles of the Civil War. On July 16, 1861, General Irvin McDowell marched 35,000 Union troops out of Washington, D.C., in an effort to capture an important railroad junction at Manassas. Most of the Union forces were 90-day, poorly trained volunteers who had answered President Abraham Lincoln's call to arms after the April 1861 attack on Fort Sumter. Most of the volunteers, the Union commanders, and even Lincoln felt this would surely be a short war.

On the morning of July 21, 1861, McDowell opened fire near Stone Bridge, which spans Bull Run. At first the battle appeared to be going in favor of the Union forces, but as General Thomas J. Jackson held his ground on Henry Hill and fresh units were rushed to his aid, the Confederates eventually forced the Union into a chaotic retreat to Washington. This first major clash in the War Between the States set the stage for four more years of bitter conflict.

In August 1862, the two forces met once again at Manassas. General Robert E. Lee, now in command of the Army of Northern Virginia, divided his army, sending Stonewall Jackson's wing behind Major General John Pope's Union line. In this way, he caused Pope's army to flee across Bull Run and back to Washington. This opened the way for Lee's first drive into Northern territory and a possible recognition of the Confederate States of America by major European powers.

DIRECTIONS Leave I-66 at Manassas Exit 47 and follow Business VA 234 north. In a little more than 0.5 mile, turn right into the park to arrive at the visitor center.

Route Description

To add to your enjoyment of the hike, you should devote at least some time to the exhibits and multimedia programs presented in the center. Several brochures describe the battles, the physical features of the 5,000-plus-acre park, and itineraries for a number of different hiking opportunities.

The circuit hike described here follows a route that touches upon a number of sites relevant to the first battle of Manassas. In addition, it offers a quiet and moderate walk across open meadows, through heavily wooded forests, and along the meandering and shallow Bull Run. The quiet and peace of this hike are made even more enjoyable when you realize you are only

26 miles from the hustle and bustle of downtown Washington, D.C., and within a couple of miles of its sprawling suburbs.

Begin by walking through the open field from the visitor center to the statue of General Thomas J. Jackson. The Henry House is visible to your left. Ignore it for now; your return route will bring you past it. Follow the pathway to the cannons. These guns mark Jackson's line of defense on the afternoon of July 21, 1861. It was here that Jackson earned his famous nickname. His troops held their ground while other Confederate soldiers dropped back in disarray. Hoping to stop the rout and inspire the brigade under his command, Brigadier General Barnard E. Bee pointed out Jackson's resolute troops and shouted, "There stands Jackson like a stone wall! Rally behind the Virginians, boys!" Although the Confederate forces did rally behind Jackson, Bee was fatally wounded during the battle.

Near the cannons, take the pathway heading into the woods. At 0.3 mile enter the woods where an old road veers off to the left. You should bear right and follow the marked pathway. The dogwood's pink-and-white leaf bracts color the springtime forest; its red berries dot the woods in the fall, providing food for passing birds.

Descend through a mixed hardwood forest and, at 0.5 mile, cross a small, sometimes dry, water run. At 0.6 mile from the visitor center turn left onto old Rock Road, a route used by Confederate troops coming from the south. Honeysuckle, greenbrier, and poison ivy hang copiously from tree branches. Arrive at a four-way intersection at 0.8 mile. Continue along Rock Road, now lined by cedars and other evergreens.

To save you from having to ford Youngs Branch, be alert at 0.9 mile, where a pathway bears left from the road and makes an almost immediate right to cross the stream on a footbridge. This shaded place, where the shallow, slow-moving waters reflect the trees and sunlight, is a nice spot for a rest break. Within a few hundred feet the trail breaks out into the open and your route turns left to rejoin Rock Road.

At 1.25 miles, leave the gravel road, follow the pathway to the left, and in 200 feet take care in crossing busy US 29 (Warrenton Turnpike). Pass through a gate and ascend along the right side of an open field. At 1.4 miles you must make an abrupt turn to the right to arrive at a sign marking what was once the site of the Van Pelt House, Avon. Confederates stationed here had a clear view of Stone Bridge and watched as Union forces approached along Warrenton Turnpike.

There is a large intersection of trails at the Van Pelt House site. Trails ahead and to the right would eventually bring you to the Farm Ford. However, to continue following this description, make a hard right, heading southeast, in the direction of US 29.

Descend the knoll at 1.6 miles and continue on a boardwalk through a moist bottomland forest dominated by oaks to arrive at Stone Bridge. Early in the morning of July 21, 1861, the opening shots of the first battle of Manassas were fired nearby. To prevent any further use by Union forces, the Confederates destroyed the bridge in March of 1862. It was rebuilt in 1884.

Do not cross the bridge. Instead, look for the trail going off to the left to begin paralleling Bull Run. The hike now becomes quieter and more relaxed as you move into the woods and away from US 29. Come to an intersection at 2.5 miles and keep right, soon coming to the Farm Ford, where Colonel William T. Sherman's troops crossed Bull Run to join other Union soldiers already engaged in the battle on Matthews Hill.

Just beyond the ford, the trail swings away from Bull Run and stays to the right at an intersection (the trail to the left leads back to the Van Pelt House site). Continue along the edge of the woods, cross a gravel road at 3.0 miles, enter woods, and ascend along the pathway.

The trail levels out at 3.3 miles, and soon you will reach a small clearing. Here the curious may wish to do some off-trail explorations. To the left of the pathway you can search for the foundation and remains of the two-story mansion home, known as Pittsylvania, of the Landon Carter family. The family cemetery, hidden by trees and underbrush, is a little farther into the woods. Now is the time to contemplate the reclamation powers of nature. Note how tall the trees are and how full the forest is. Yet, at the time of the battle, Pittsylvania could be seen easily from the surrounding countryside. The land around the house was open farmland, clear of trees.

Return to the main route and continue following blue blazes along the old woods road. Join up with, and follow, the Matthews Hill Loop Trail. Sixty feet to the left is a marble stone marking the spot close to where Private George T. Stovall of the Eighth Georgia Infantry was killed. There are a number of park service interpretive signs along this heavily wooded section of trail. They contain quotes from battle participants and other bits of information. Although it may slow your hiking pace, taking the time to read the signs will add greatly to your understanding and appreciation of your surroundings.

Proceed straight as your route crosses a horse trail. At 4.2 miles the trail breaks out into the open and continues across the field; a line of cannons on your left marks the Union position. Enjoy the clear view across to Henry Hill. In 200 feet you have the option of extending the hike to a full length of about 11 miles by following the trail to the right, crossing Sudley Road (VA 234), and continuing along the second battle of Manassas itinerary. Consult the visitor center for information on this option.

To continue following this description, do not cross VA 234, but instead turn left in the field to parallel the roadway. Keen observers may note a number of piles of scat, indicating that raccoons, opossums, and foxes frequent this meadow on a regular basis.

A bench provides a resting place to enjoy commanding views of Matthews Hill and other points to the west and south. Major General John Pope headquartered his Union forces here on August 29 and 30, 1862, during the second battle of Manassas. Walk downhill a few hundred feet to the Stone House, built around 1848. The Union army used the structure as an aid station during both battles. The house is sometimes open to the public; check with the visitor center for dates and times.

Cross US 29 at the stoplight, follow a pathway to the footbridge over Youngs Branch, and continue to the top of Henry Hill. Bear right on the Henry Hill Loop Trail to arrive at the postwar Henry House at 5.3 miles. Captain James B. Ricketts's forces deployed guns here, but as the battle progressed, Confederate troops drew ever closer and the Union army began its withdrawal from the first battle of Manassas. Follow the line of cannons to return to the visitor center at 5.5 miles.

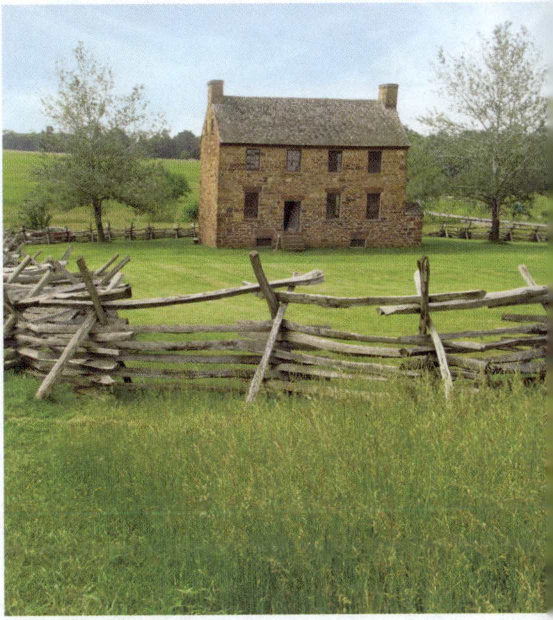

The Stone House

photo: Johnny Molloy

Other nearby hiking opportunities are at Bull Run Regional Park (a sign on US 29 points the way to the park, a few miles to the east of the Manassas National Battlefield Park) and the Bull Run Occoquan Trail (see Hike 13), which follows Bull Run for a little less than 20 miles. For hikers desiring to learn more about the Civil War in the state, Virginia contains other Civil War parks with walking opportunities. Among them are Fredericksburg-Spotsylvania National Military Park (see Hike 10), Richmond National Battlefield Park (see Hike 7, Cold Harbor), Appomattox Court House National Historical Park, and Petersburg National Battlefield (consult *Hike Virginia South of US 60* for the latter two).

Sky Meadows State Park

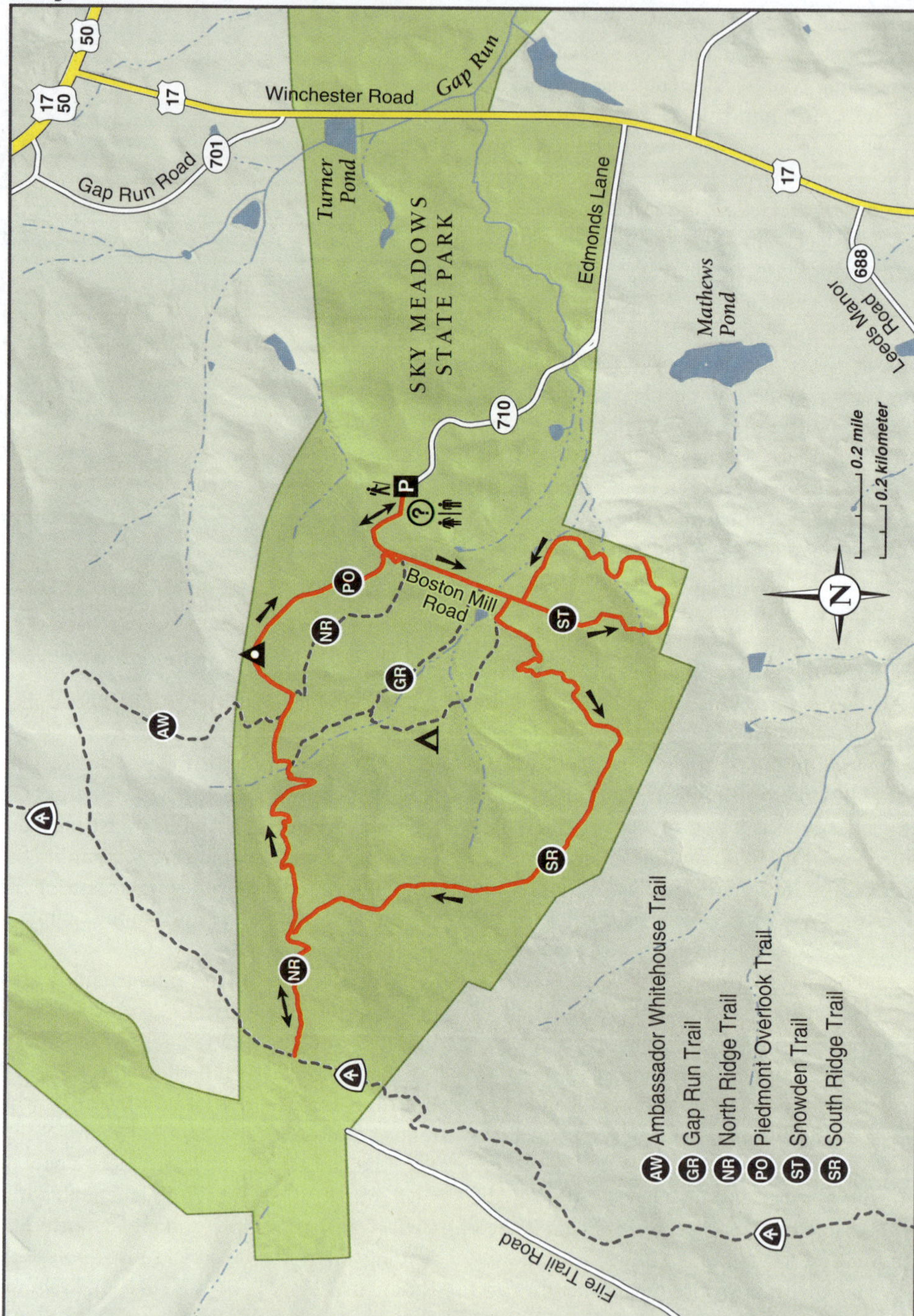

15 Sky Meadows State Park

- **GPS:** N38.9917351 W77.9661228
- **TOTAL DISTANCE (circuit):** 5.4 miles
- **HIKING TIME:** 3.5 hours
- **VERTICAL RISE:** 1,460 feet
- **MAPS:** USGS *Upperville; Sky Meadows State Park* map
- **CONTACT:** Sky Meadows State Park
11012 Edmonds Lane
Delaplane, VA 20144
540-592-3556
dcr.virginia.gov/state-parks/sky-meadows

The Hike at a Glance

- 0.1 Left onto Boston Mill Road
- 0.4 Left at loop trail intersection onto Snowden Trail
- 1.5 Return to loop tail intersection, bear right, turn left into meadow, and soon turn left onto South Ridge Trail
- 3.2 Left onto North Ridge Trail
- 3.5 Arrive at AT; retrace steps to intersect of South Ridge and North Ridge trails; keep left on North Ridge Trail
- 4.6 Left onto Piedmont Overlook Trail
- 5.2 Rejoin North Ridge Trail; go a few steps and turn left onto Boston Mill Road
- 5.4 End of hike

I had always thought that it was obvious how Sky Meadows State Park received its name. For, even from miles away, it's possible to spot the large, open, richly green fields that dapple vast areas of the hillside as the topography sweeps upward from the rolling piedmont to the eastern slope of the Blue Ridge Mountains. However, the name comes from former owner Robert Hadow calling his rural landholdings *Skye Farm*, for an island in Scotland. Yet, the story of the origin of the name does not detract from the park's stunning scenery.

From the 1700s, most of what is now park property passed through a number of owners. In the early 1840s, farmer and general merchant Abner Settle bought acreage from a neighboring farm, built a fieldstone structure, and called it "Mount Bleak." By the 1850s, the owners were successfully raising hogs, chickens, turkeys, oxen, and horses and harvesting fields of wheat and corn. Other structures include a carriage barn, ice cellar, and log kitchen.

DIRECTIONS Sky Meadows State Park is about an hour's drive from Washington, D.C. You can leave US 50 near Paris and follow US 17 south for a little more than a mile.

Route Description

The park has a picnic area, a visitor center, the Mount Bleak House, a bridle trail, restrooms, water, and a hike-in campground (with primitive sites and water). Reservations and payment of a fee are required to camp. Camping anywhere else in the park is prohibited. You may fish in the pond close to US 17 if you have a valid Virginia fishing license.

Sky Meadows has one of the best and most active interpretive programs I have ever come across in a state or national park. Among other things, you may find yourself gazing at the stars with an astronomer, making a rag doll, identifying birdcalls while on a morning stroll, or listening to tall tales around an evening campfire. The Mount Bleak House is open for tours. The visitor center can provide dates and times of activities and a park map.

One of the main attractions of hiking in the 1,860-acre state park is that it contains a wide array of plant life, both wild and cultivated. Trees around the Mount Bleak House include crabapple, plum, Chinese chestnut, walnut, Norway maple, green ash, sugar maple, forsythia, pecan, dogwood, lilac, and Kentucky coffee tree. The contrast of open meadows and deep forests, coupled with an elevation difference of

1,840 feet as a high point and 640 feet as the low, ensures that wildflower lovers are in for a treat from late winter to mid-autumn. Skunk cabbage could be blooming in moist, wooded areas by mid-February. Cutleaf toothwort and rue anemone begin appearing on the forest floor about the beginning of April. Shortly thereafter, purple and yellow violets, spring beauties, and star chickweed begin to bloom in the woods. By late April and early May, the wooded areas are at their most colorful—tall wild geranium, with its pink blossoms, grows above the tiny yellow trumpets of corydalis, while green and purplish jack-in-the-pulpits stick out of moist ground on singular, strong stems.

Sun-tolerant plants line the roadways during the hot summer months. White or violet trumpet-shaped flowers of jimsonweed grow from the poor soil of the road banks. Thriving in the pastures are white oxeye daisies and tall, yellow crown-beard. Both of these plants are members of the daisy family, which, according to Roger Tory Peterson, is the largest family of flowering plants and possibly the newest one to evolve on Earth.

Spotted touch-me-not will still be blooming in wet areas in the woods in September, and moth mullein adds a bit of yellow to roadsides as late as October. Animals inhabiting the park include fox squirrels, chipmunks, gray squirrels, skunks, opossums, red foxes, coyotes, eastern cottontails, deer, and raccoons.

A system of trails wanders through the fields, into the woods, and along small streams; the following hike touches upon most of the highlights to be discovered. It also comes into contact with the Appalachian Trail, furnishing additional hiking opportunities (and primitive camping for those who take it south out of the park).

Begin by following the trail signs from the far end of the parking lot of the Mount Bleak House. In 0.1 mile turn left onto gravel Boston Mill Road. At 0.15 mile you should bypass the turnoff to the North Ridge, Piedmont Overlook, and Appalachian Trails and continue on the road, enjoying the views of open farmlands above and below you. In the 1800s this old roadway stretched for about 3 miles, connecting Paris, Virginia, with gristmills on Crooked Run.

At 0.4 mile, bear left onto the Snowden Trail. You could shorten the overall length of this hike by 1.0 mile by turning right and following the Gap Run Trail. However, the Snowden Trail is an easy walk and will help you further appreciate what you will see and experience on the rest of the hike. Proceed through a mature oak forest along the old roadway built in the 1820s. Bear right at an intersection; you will be returning on the road coming in from the left. Holes in trees mark this as a favorite woodpecker feeding site.

At 0.6 mile, the trail turns left off the old road. At 0.75 mile, ascend via switchbacks next to a fenceline and open field. Deer apparently are quite fond of this section of the park; I counted more than 15 running through the woods, their white tails raised and flashing a warning of my encroachment upon their forest home. At 1.0 mile descend into an open woods.

The undergrowth becomes fuller and thicker at 1.2 miles as you begin to parallel a small stream that provides nourishment to this lusher vegetation. Turn right onto an old woods road at 1.3 miles. At 1.4 miles you should turn left onto Edmonds Lane, another 1800s roadway. The builders of the stone wall must have known what they were doing, for even after all these years, it still lines the road, a testament to their skill and hard work.

At 1.5 miles, return to the loop-trail intersection, bear right, and in 200 feet turn left and enter a meadow. At 1.6 miles, you'll reach an intersection. The Gap Run Trail goes right for 0.2 mile to the campground and 0.7 mile to the North Ridge Trail, but you should bear left onto the South Ridge Trail.

At 1.7 miles, follow an old road ascending through a wooded area. Pay attention as the trail breaks out into the open—it does not ascend to the bench overlooking the farmland but makes an abrupt turn left and back into the woods. Pass by the site of Snowden Manor. Only the foundation, chimney, and a few stone walls mark where this large, white, frame-columned house stood from the mid-1800s to when it burned in 1937.

At 2.0 miles, bear right and then swing left along the edge of the meadow. Continue ascending and enter the woods. Abundant grapevines drape themselves over the trees as you ascend along a nicely graded woods road. If you are the first person to come this way in several days, be ready to run into scores of spiderwebs spanning the width of the road. The webs are even more numerous in the fall, when the spiders work furiously to catch as much prey as possible before the insects disappear with the coming of cold winter weather.

The South Ridge Trail comes to an end as it intersects the North Ridge Trail at 3.2 miles. A descent to the right would lead 0.9 mile to the campground, but you want to bear left and ascend as the route becomes steeper and rockier, passing through large patches of poison ivy.

At 3.5 miles, arrive at the junction with the Appalachian Trail (AT). The AT runs to the right 2.9 miles to US 50 in Ashby Gap and 7.0 miles to the left to Manassas Gap Shelter. Use this spot to take a well-deserved break in this quiet and isolated place. I have experienced something new and wonderful every time I've visited this spot. I've heard the staccato sounds of a woodpecker to the right of me answered by another on my left, then by one behind me and again by one in front of me, permitting me to enjoy nature's version of "surround-sound stereo." Other times, in late winter, bloodroot has begun to force its way through the hoarfrost-frozen ground, while spring walks about 3 miles south on the AT have been rewarded with one of the most profuse arrays of trillium ever seen in one area.

Sky Meadows State Park has many great viewpoints.

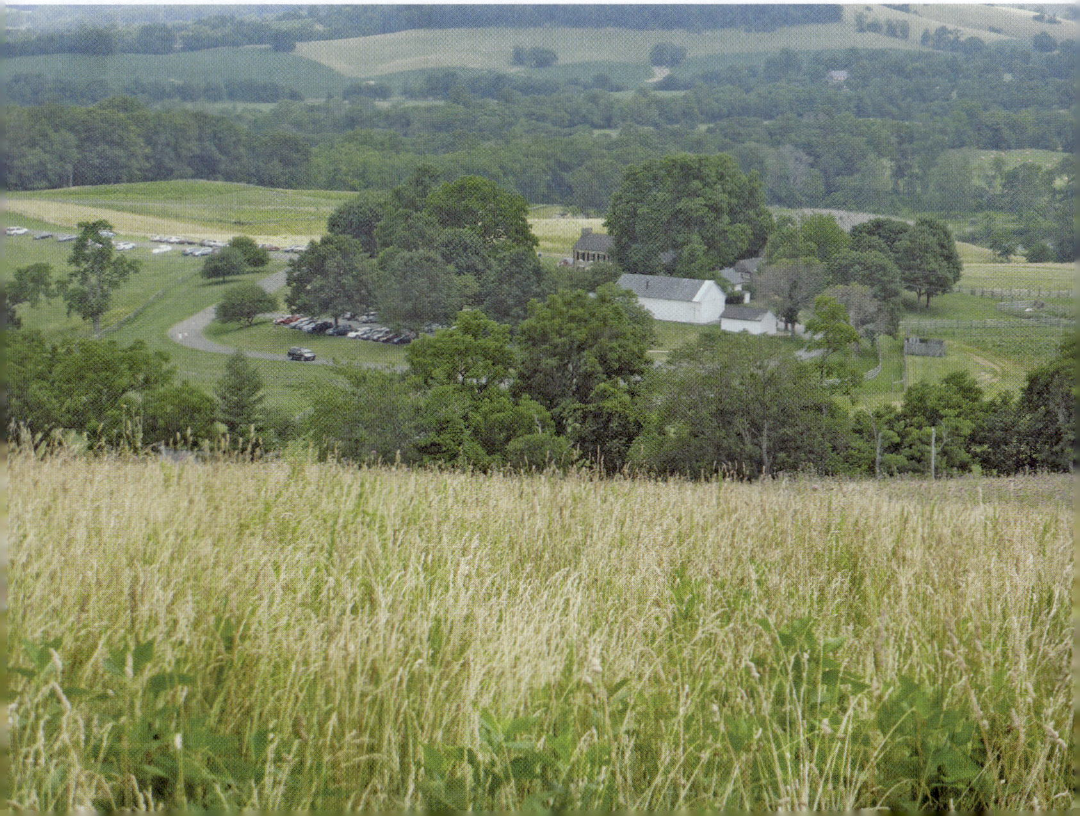

From the intersection, descend to retrace your steps to the intersection with the South Ridge Trail. This time bear left to continue descending and following the North Ridge Trail. The going is rough and rocky as you pass by several crumbling stone walls, evidence that the mountainside was used at one time for the grazing of stock. At 4.0 miles, pass through an area that was infested by spongy moths (*Lymantria dispar dispar)* in the mid-1980s. Many of the oldest and largest trees are dead and decaying. It's interesting to see, however, that nature is going through the long, slow process of eventually returning the area to a climax forest.

Cross Gap Run. At 4.4 miles is the intersection with the orange-blazed Gap Run Trail. The campground is 0.5 mile and the parking lot 1.3 miles along this trail to the right. Bear left to ascend switchbacks on the North Ridge Trail and bypass the Ambassador Whitehouse Trail that comes in from the left. At 4.6 miles, come to an intersection. The North Ridge Trail now goes right, descending to the parking lot in 0.6 mile. You, however, should turn left uphill to begin following the Piedmont Overlook Trail.

At 4.7 miles, break out into the open for what I consider to be one of the best grandstand views in the northern part of Virginia. From your perch on the eastern edge of the Blue Ridge Mountains, the rolling and flatter lands of the Piedmont stretch out before you. The meadows directly below slope down to a pond shimmering in the sunlight. Rectangular fields of nearby farms alternate with strips of woodland, turning the landscape into a patchwork quilt of greens, browns, and golds. Vultures soar on rising thermals as clouds float by, leading your eyes to focus on the distance where, on clear days, the high-rise buildings of the Dulles-Fairfax area can be seen poking above the horizon.

Descend through the meadow on a mown route, soon descending to the right at 5.2 miles to walk past an old cowshed. In a few steps rejoin the North Ridge Trail and turn left onto gravel Boston Mill Road. Follow the route back to the parking lot at 5.4 miles.

Boston Mill Road

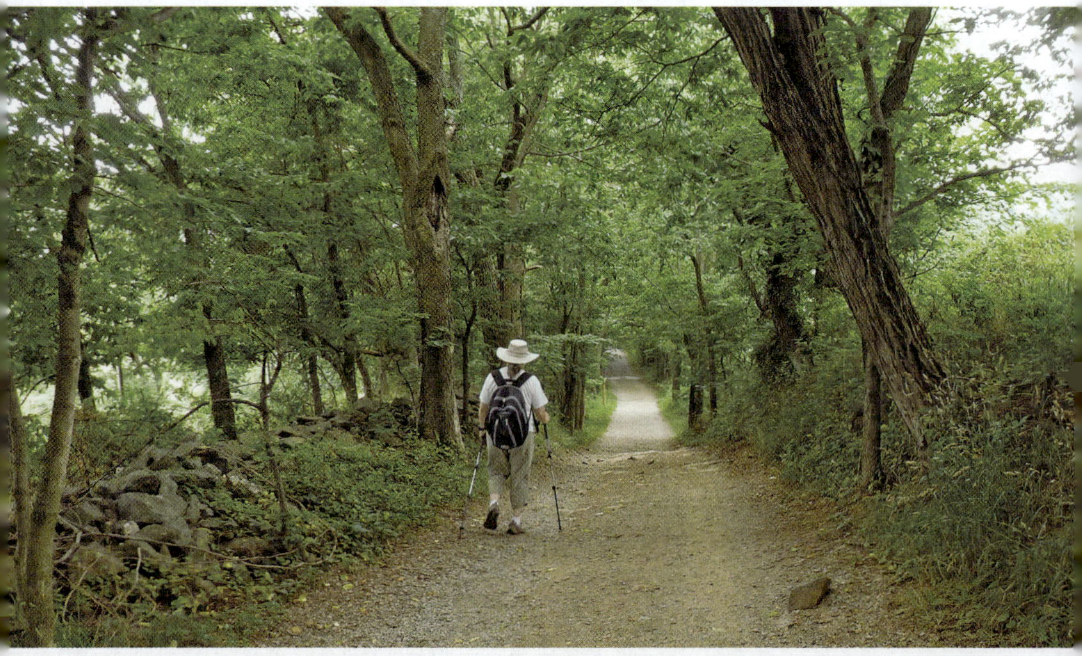

16 Split Rock

- **GPS:** N39.315549 W77.755790
- **TOTAL DISTANCE (round-trip):** 5.2 miles
- **HIKING TIME:** 3.0 hours
- **VERTICAL RISE:** 950 feet
- **MAPS:** USGS *Harpers Ferry (VA, MD, and WV); Harpers Ferry National Historical Park* map
- **CONTACT:** Harpers Ferry National Historical Park
PO Box 65
Harpers Ferry, WV 25425
304-535-6029
nps.gov/hafe

The Hike at a Glance

1.0 Left onto blue-blazed trail
1.6 Left onto ridgeline
1.9 Side trail to first view
2.1 Side trail to second view
2.6 Split Rock; retrace steps
5.2 End of hike

When hiking the Appalachian Trail (AT) for the first time, I was so impressed by the view from Split Rock in Virginia that I spent more than half a day there, etching the scene in my mind. Below the rocks is the Potomac River, punching its way eastward through the Allegheny and Blue Ridge Mountains and meeting up with the waters of the Shenandoah River in front of historic Harpers Ferry. Walking the trail again several years later, I was disappointed to find the AT had been rerouted into Harpers Ferry and away from the viewpoint. I felt compensated, though, when the trail delivered me to Jefferson's Rock in West Virginia, with its different perspective of the same scene.

However, a part of the old route of the AT had been maintained and a circuit hike through three different states afforded the opportunity to visit both of these splendid viewpoints. It also provided a chance to explore Harpers Ferry and walk a distance on the 184-mile towpath of the C&O Canal. Unfortunately, that circuit hike, too, is now no longer possible because of a landowner who began prohibiting hikers from passing through just a short section of private property near the turn of the 21st century.

Thankfully, though, it is still possible to hike to Split Rock on a round-trip path that begins in Harpers Ferry and uses the AT and a blue-blazed trail to reach the overlook. Be aware that camping is prohibited on the route of this entire hike because it is all on national park property. A commercial campground is located on US 340 between Harpers Ferry and Charles Town, West Virginia.

DIRECTIONS The hike begins in Harpers Ferry, West Virginia, from the small park service parking lot located immediately after US 340 crosses the Shenandoah River from Virginia into West Virginia. However, you will probably not be able to park here, as the lot is usually full. So, drive 1.0 mile southward on US 340 to the park's visitor center, where shuttle buses will bring you back to the historic town.

Route Description

Start the hike by walking back toward US 340 from the historic part of town and turning left on US 340 to follow the AT's white blazes. Take the bridge over the Shenandoah River, crossing to the other side when there is a break in the heavy traffic speeding by you. Be careful!

Follow the AT as it ascends stone steps and into a forest so full of vegetation that it soon begins to somewhat muffle the sounds of the roadway below. Continue the ascent into an attractive forest of hardy oaks and maples

Split Rock

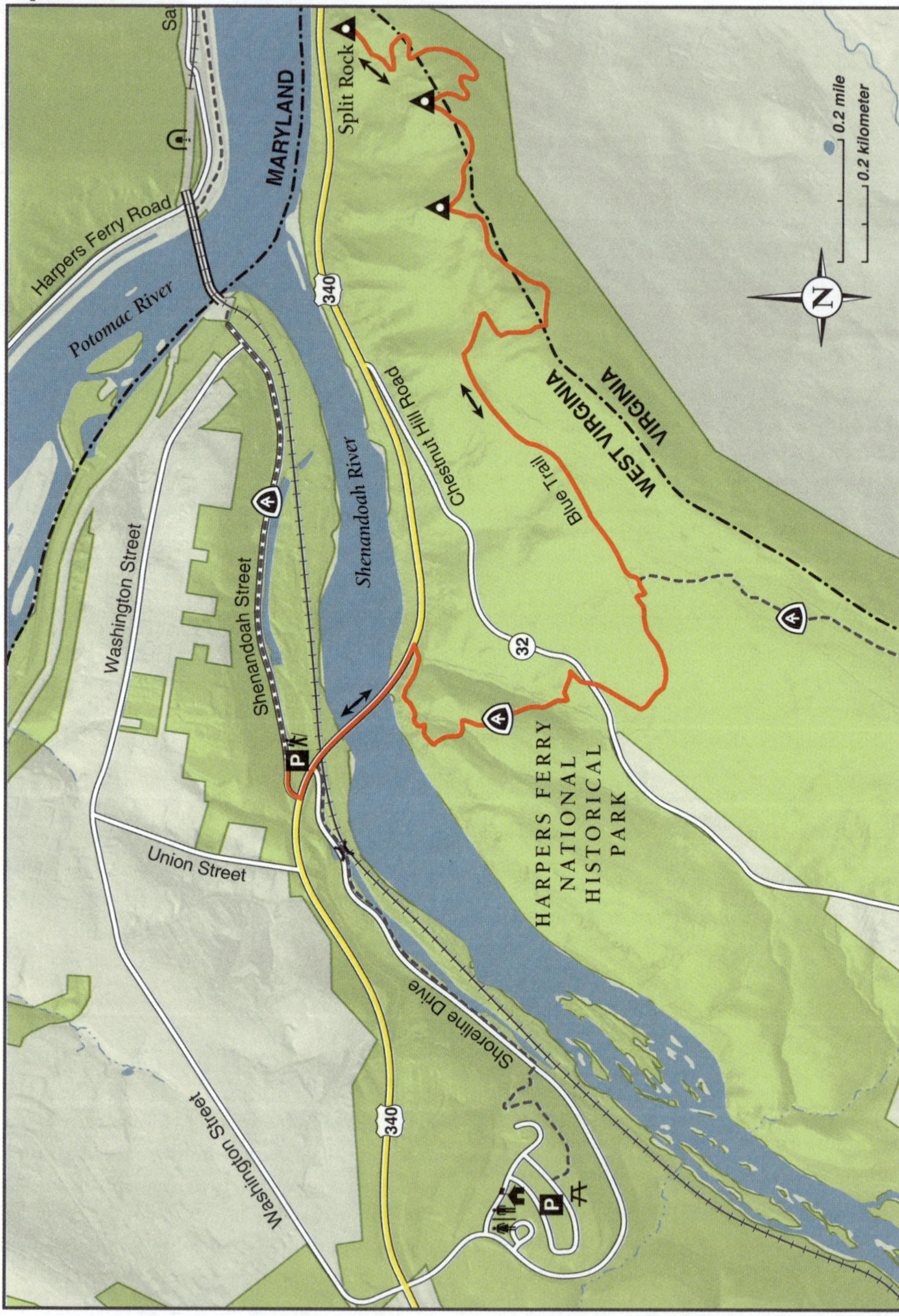

above an understory of dogwood, soon passing through an area of planted periwinkle that marks the site of a former homestead. In 0.6 mile, cross paved Chestnut Hill Road with the route becoming a bit steeper; a few switchbacks help ease the climb. The songbirds are especially active in the morning in the newer-growth forest on this side of the road, while the call of the pileated woodpecker is heard just about any time of day.

At 1.0 mile, the AT keeps to the right on its way to Georgia; you want to turn left onto the blue-blazed pathway. The ascent is a little more gradual for a short while, but you will eventually have to make the final push to attain the ridgeline to follow it to the left at 1.6 miles. Turn left onto a side trail at 1.9 miles that leads, in just a few yards, to a view of Harpers Ferry and the confluence of the Shenandoah and Potomac Rivers. A second short side trail at 2.1 miles goes to another view, this one with an increased range of where the AT ascends Weverton Cliffs in Maryland and onto the ridgeline of South Mountain.

The objective of the day is reached when you swing left to arrive at Split Rock, at 2.6 miles. Far below the rocks, shimmering ripples and bits of whitewater in the Shenandoah and Potomac Rivers reflect the light of bright sunny days. Spanning the Potomac River upstream from where the two rivers meet is the B&O Railroad bridge. The attached footbridge is the route of the AT. All of Harpers Ferry is spread out before you. Saint Peter's Catholic Church, with its prominent steeple, sits on the cliffs overlooking the Shenandoah, while Hilltop House Hotel (closed as this book went to press), high above the Potomac, towers over the historic district. Almost directly north of you are the cliffs of Maryland Heights. (A historical trail makes a circuit route around Maryland Heights, and it is an extremely scenic hike that you should consider doing while in the area. Check at the park service visitor center or in *50 Hikes in Maryland* for more information.) While lingering here, take time to think about the scene you are looking down upon. The small town has been the site of many major events throughout the country's history.

On his way to the Continental Congress in 1783, Thomas Jefferson proclaimed the confluence of the Potomac and Shenandoah Rivers a "stupendous" scene and "worth a voyage across the Atlantic." In 1794, George Washington

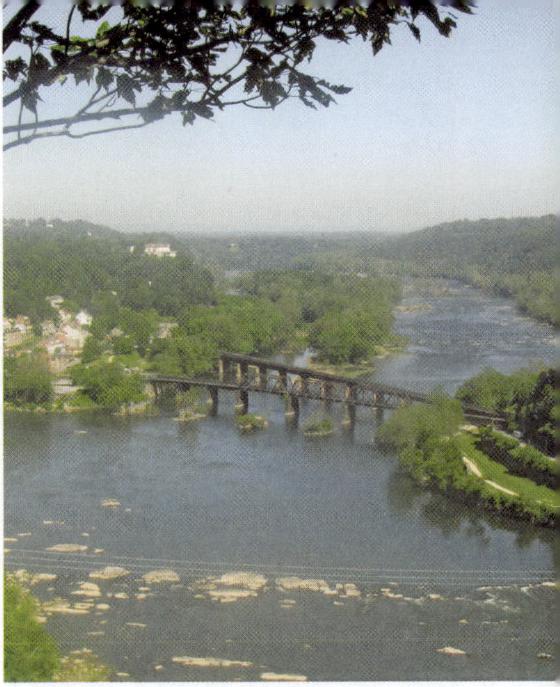

Harpers Ferry stands at the confluence of the Shenandoah and Potomac Rivers.

photo: Johnny Molloy

convinced the US Congress to establish a federal arsenal and armory on the site; Meriwether Lewis was so impressed with the arsenal's quality munitions that he obtained its rifles for his upcoming expedition into the newly purchased Louisiana Territory. And it is said that John Brown's failed raid on the arsenal to obtain arms for a slave insurrection in 1859 was the Civil War's opening act.

Strategically situated as it is near the border between North and South, the town changed hands eight times during the war. By the time the hostilities ended, much of the town and most of the factories had been burned and the railroad bridge destroyed. Massive floods in 1870 and 1889 damaged almost everything that the war had not. Floods in the 20th century completed the job, and by 1936, manufacturing in the town had ceased. Harpers Ferry National Historical Park was created in 1963.

When you decide it is time to leave, retrace your steps back to the right turn onto the descending route of the AT at 4.2 miles. Continue the descent by retracing your steps along that white-blazed pathway and return to the hike's starting point at 5.2 miles.

Blue Ridge and Massanutten Mountains

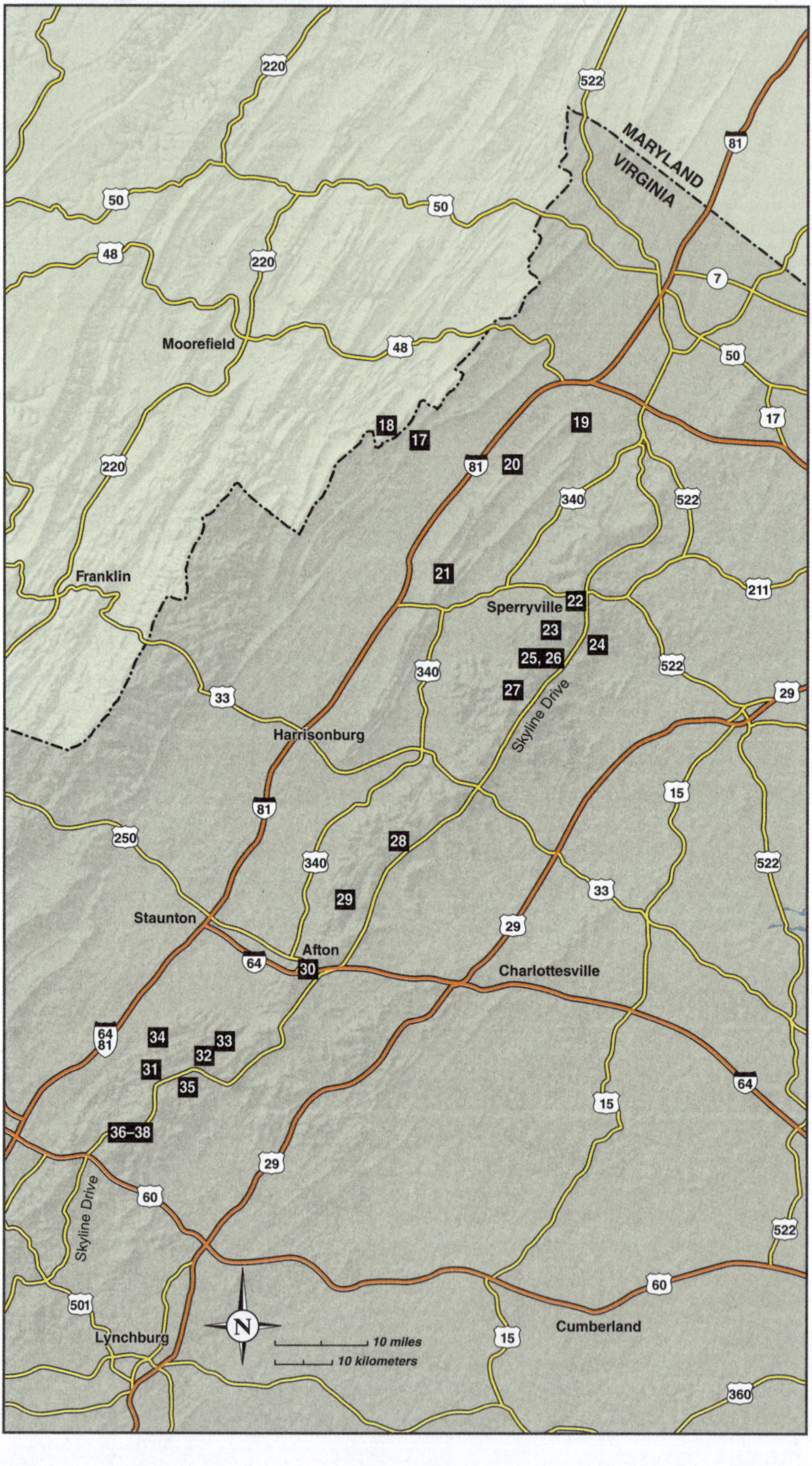

Blue Ridge and Massanutten Mountains

Little Sluice Mountain and Cedar Creek

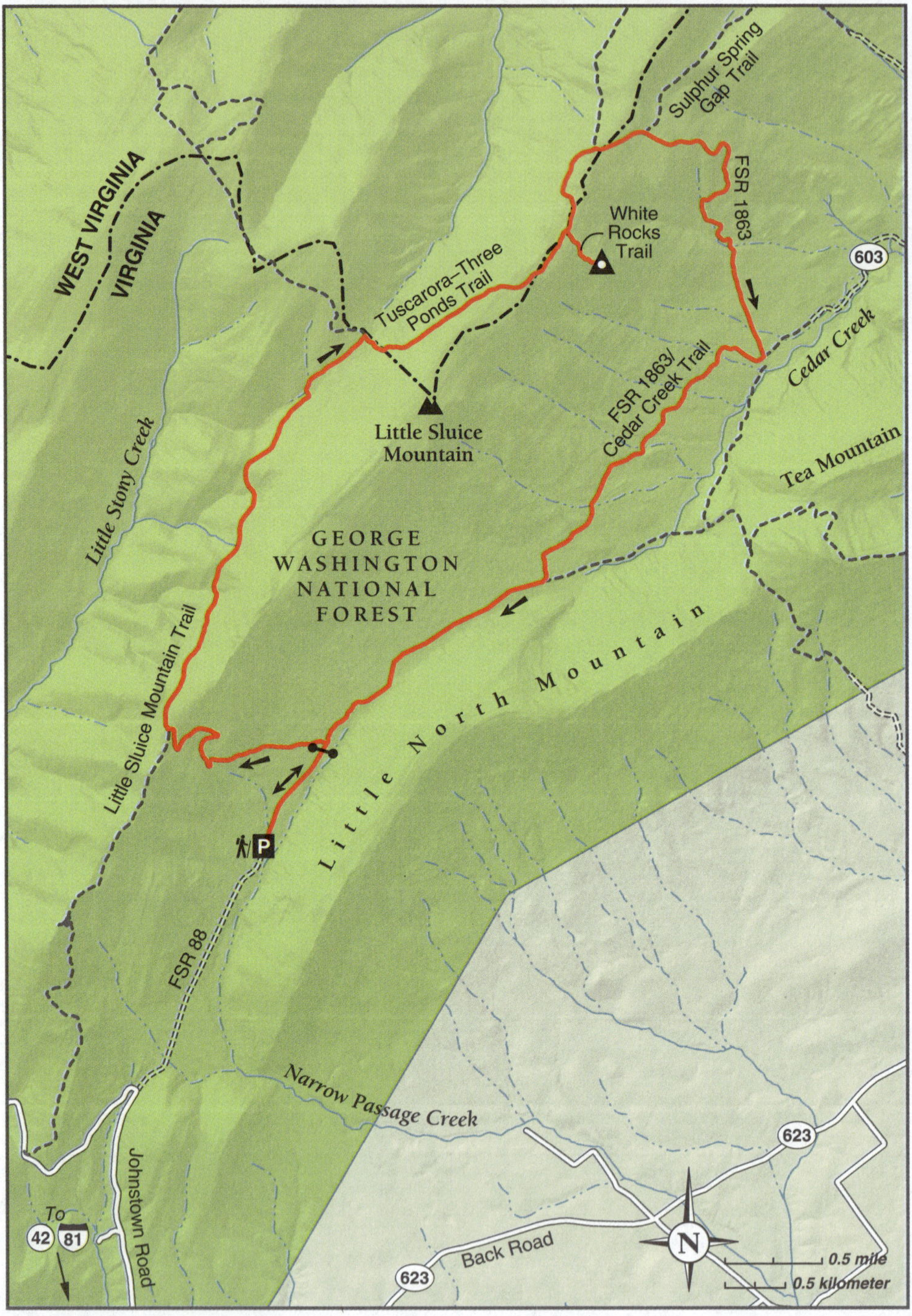

17 Little Sluice Mountain and Cedar Creek

- **GPS:** N38.932374 W78.617481
- **TOTAL DISTANCE (circuit):** 12.7 miles
- **HIKING TIME:** 8.0 hours
- **VERTICAL RISE:** 2,080 feet
- **MAPS:** USGS *Wolf Gap (WV and VA)* and *Woodstock (VA and WV); National Geographic Trails Illustrated Map #792 Massanutten and Great North Mountain*
- **CONTACT:** Lee Ranger District
  95 Railroad Ave.
  Edinburg, VA 22824; 540-984-4101
  fs.usda.gov/gwj

The Hike at a Glance

0.5 Left onto rising dirt road

1.6 Attain ridgeline; soon turn right onto Little Sluice Mountain Trail

2.3 Dirt road to right leads 60 feet to spring

3.8 Hard right to begin following Tuscarora/Three Ponds Trail

5.1 Right onto White Rocks Trail; descend steeply to viewpoint; retrace steps to Tuscarora/Three Ponds Trail and turn right

6.5 Bear right, bypassing Sulphur Spring Trail coming in from left

9.2 Begin following FSR 1863/Cedar Creek Trail

12.7 Return to automobile

A look at the Virginia–West Virginia border on a highway map shows large blank spaces between paved roadways. A topography characterized by long, high ridgelines and steeply sloping hillsides permits most modern highways to cross only in the few naturally occurring gaps in the mountains' rugged profiles. At one time, however, dirt logging, mining, and carriage roads carried a bustling variety of vehicles and people up creek valleys and over mountain summits. Those days are gone, but this hike makes use of many of these old roads, most now little more than footpaths, to explore environs that are once again isolated from outside influences. In addition to the seclusion, highlights include possible abundant wildlife, a strong-flowing high-elevation spring, and a grandstand viewpoint

As this is a long walk of more than 12 miles over rugged terrain, it would be best to do this hike when the daylight hours are many, or as a two-day, overnight backpack.

DIRECTIONS Take I-81 Exit 283 at Woodstock and follow VA 42 westward for 5.6 miles to Columbia Furnace, where you turn onto VA 675 for close to 0.7 mile. Make a right onto VA 608, which soon becomes Forest Service Road (FSR) 88. Keep right on FSR 88 where FSR 92 comes in from the left, pass by the Little Sluice Mountain trailhead 0.5 mile from this junction, and continue another 2.5 miles to the large parking area, on the left.

Route Description

Walk around the gate and ascend. When the first few editions of this guidebook were published, readers were directed to look to the left for the very indistinct Bread Road Trail {FS 411} (named in the early 1800s when wagons used it to haul food to charcoal makers cutting timber and producing fuel for nearby furnaces). Since that time, a newer and very distinct road at 0.5 mile into the hike goes off to the left. The old route had ascended at more than a 30% grade in places, so it's nice to follow this gradually rising road to arrive on the ridgeline at 1.6 miles (however, it is sad a bit of local history had been wiped out). A small clearing provides a limited view into Stoney Creek Valley and across to Big Schloss (see Hike 18) on the Virginia–West Virginia border. Turn right and gradually descend along the sparsely purple-blazed dirt road (it's open to motor vehicles, well used, and busy during hunting season, so take proper precautions), which is Little Sluice Mountain Trail {FS 398}. (To the left the road drops down the mountain to FSR 88 in about 2 miles.)

A low point is reached at 2.0 miles, where you begin a gentle ascent of about 500 feet to cross a spur ridge; its flat knob would provide a pleasant campsite. A very reliable piped spring is about 60 feet up the dirt road that comes from the right at 2.3 miles. Continue on the main route, passing what may be a somewhat indistinct hunter's camp. The quality of this spot as a campsite varies widely from year to year, depending on the amount of use or care—or both—that it receives.

Wild turkeys need great expanses of undeveloped, wooded country in order to prosper, and the extensive landholdings of the George Washington and Jefferson National Forests in this part of Appalachia support a large population of these birds. Wild turkeys seem to prefer walking through the forest rather than flying among the trees, and chances are good during the summer that you'll see a family flock making use of the same road you're using; the sexes tend to separate during the winter months. Ranging from 2.5 to 4 feet in size, turkeys are almost constantly hunting for food. Scratchings along the edge of the road may mark where they have been digging for beetles and other insects; searches for their favorite nuts, such as acorns, leave large areas of the forest floor cleared of decaying leaves and other small deadfall. In Virginia, poison ivy makes up about 5% of turkeys' diets.

Ignore the old road coming in from the right at 2.8 miles; ascend and descend another spur ridge. Begin nearly level walking at 3.4 miles, passing a small (maybe dry) water run and several good campsites. A riot of ferns adds to the beauty and color of this moist, hidden mountain valley located miles from the nearest paved highway. Be alert at 3.8 miles, where the road you have been following makes an apparent swing to the left; your route makes a hard right to begin following the Tuscarora/Three Ponds Trail {FS 1013.1}. (Some maps may show this to be FS 405.4.)

White Rock Cliff offers a spot for rest and contemplation.

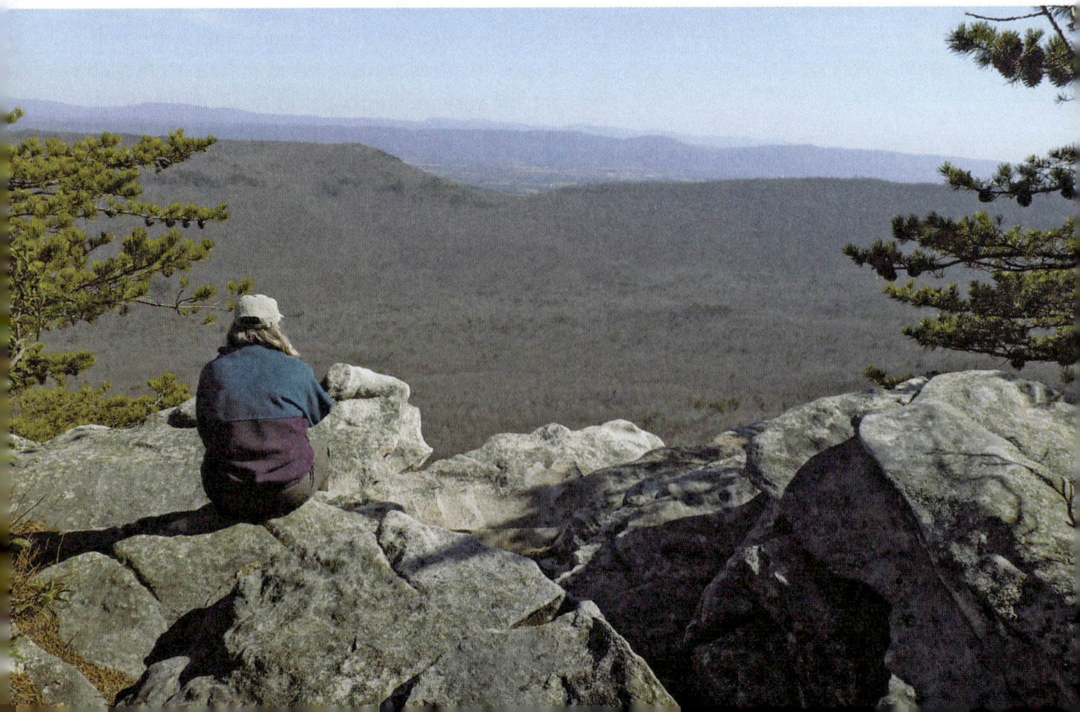

You have crossed into West Virginia. Just before you crest the ridgeline at 4.5 miles, a small outcrop to the left furnishes a view of Mill and North Mountains and Racer Camp Hollow.

Begin gradually descending, looking for a white-blazed trail (White Rocks Trail {FS 514}) coming in from the right at 5.1 miles. Take this rough, rocky, steep (53% grade!), downhill, 0.35-mile path for the best view you'll have on this hike. From your perch high atop White Rock Cliff, the Cedar Creek watershed is below you. Directly ahead, on the Little North Mountain ridgeline, is the obvious depression of Sheffer Gap. The Shenandoah Valley is visible through the gap, while Massanutten Mountain and the ridges of Shenandoah National Park can be seen far to the east.

Return to the main trail, turn right, and continue descending the mountain. Avoid the trail coming in from the left at 6.2 miles, keeping to the right as the treadway becomes softer and grassier. This would be a nice spot for a high mountain campsite. You must be alert again at 6.5 miles; purple-blazed Sulphur Spring Trail {FS 414} is more or less straight ahead, but you need to bear right onto the route that now looks more like a pathway instead of an old road. You have returned to Virginia, as you enter a large stand of pines for the first time on this hike. Emerge from the pines at 6.9 miles to descend steeply, soon passing a large outcrop with trees growing out of the rock.

Once again, be alert at 7.8 miles. Avoid the trail to the left; instead, bear right, cross a small water run, and continue to follow blue blazes, stepping onto FSR 1863 at 9.2 miles. In order to avoid the often-wet land near the creek, Cedar Creek Trail {FS 573} was rerouted onto the higher ground of FSR 1863 a number of years ago. So, follow the yellow-blazed road (which soon becomes a dirt woods road and then a footpath) through the gate and past a few old mine sites. Although it was designed to be a dryer route, this can still be a quite wet walk along the lower portion of the mountain during the spring or after heavy rains.

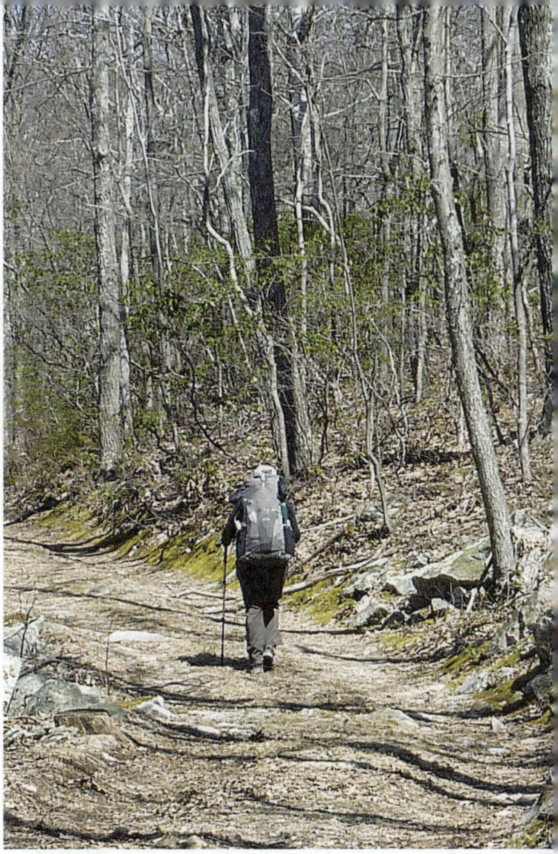

Little Sluice Mountain Trail

Looking down so that you can see where to place your feet on the uneven treadway, you will probably see numerous deer tracks in the soil of this moist bottomland. A close examination of these tracks can tell you what the deer were doing when they passed this way. If the points (which point in the direction the deer was going) of the two sections of the hoof are nearly touching each other, then the deer was probably on a "leisurely stroll." When the print shows the two halves splayed, the deer was on the run.

The footpath eventually reconnects you with FSR 88, which returns you to your automobile at 12.7 miles. If you arrive at your car toward the end of the day, consider spending the twilight hours here. This is the time of day when many forest creatures become active, and you just might see some deer, a raccoon, a skunk, an opossum, or, if you're lucky, a bobcat. You are almost guaranteed to hear at least one owl hoot, if not many, as night overtakes day.

Big Schloss

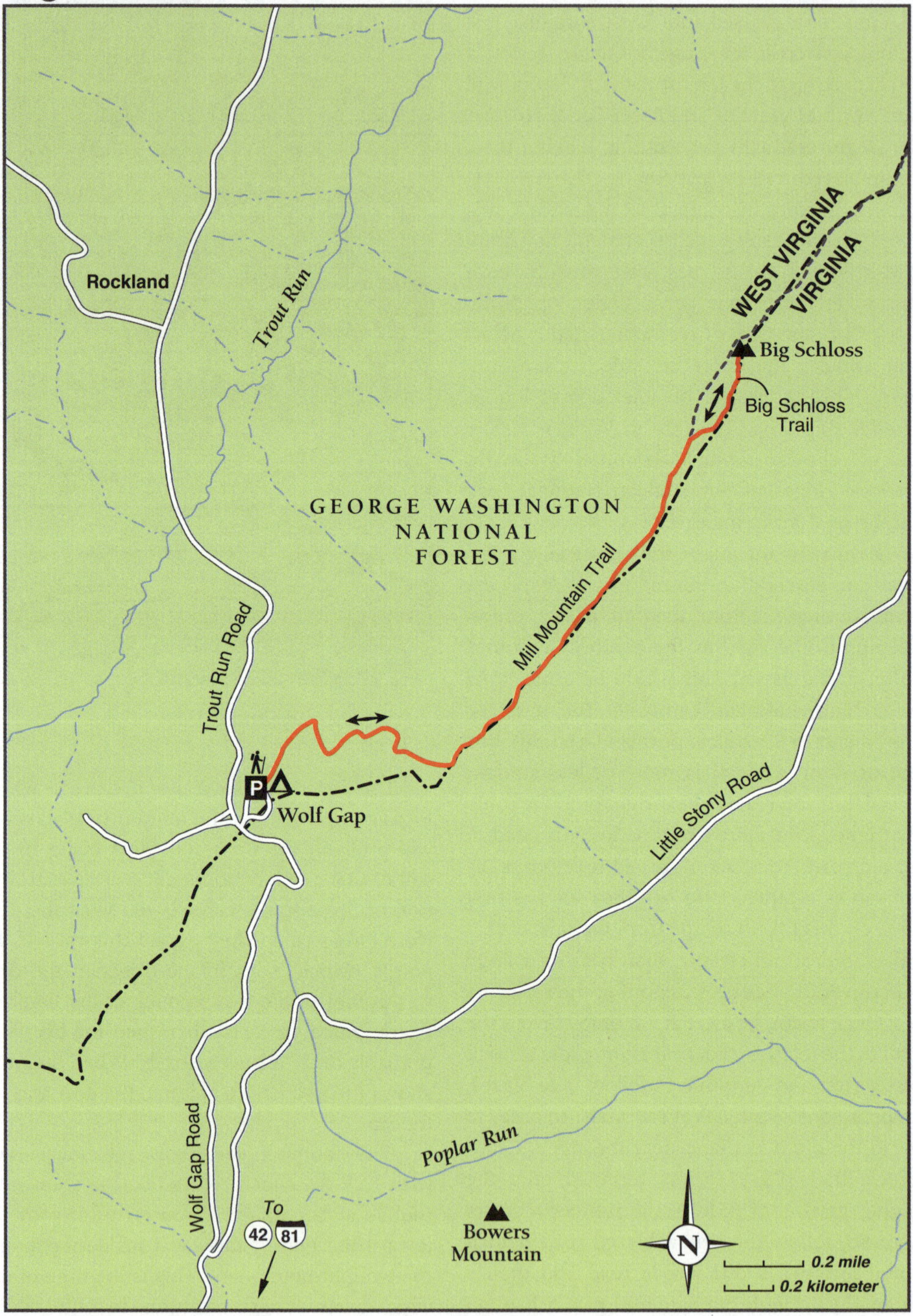

Rockland
Trout Run
WEST VIRGINIA
VIRGINIA
Big Schloss
Big Schloss Trail
GEORGE WASHINGTON NATIONAL FOREST
Mill Mountain Trail
Trout Run Road
P
Wolf Gap
Little Stony Road
Wolf Gap Road
Poplar Run
To
42
81
Bowers Mountain
N
0.2 mile
0.2 kilometer

18 Big Schloss

- **GPS:** N38.9251610 W78.6888668
- **TOTAL DISTANCE (round-trip):** 4.4 miles
- **HIKING TIME:** 2.5 hours
- **VERTICAL RISE:** 710 feet
- **MAPS:** USGS *Wolf Gap; National Geographic Trails Illustrated Map #792 Massanutten* and *Great North Mountain*
- **CONTACT:** Lee Ranger District
  95 Railroad Ave.
  Edinburg, VA 22824
  540-984-4101
  fs.usda.gov/gwj

The Hike at a Glance

0.25 Begin series of switchbacks
0.75 Attain ridgeline
1.9 Keep right onto Big Schloss Trail
2.2 Arrive at Big Schloss; retrace steps
4.4 Return to parking area

DIRECTIONS Take I-81 Exit 283 at Woodstock and follow VA 42 westward for about 7 miles. In Columbia Furnace turn onto and ascend VA 675 for 6.5 miles to Wolf Gap Recreation Area. Facilities include tent and trailer sites, picnic grounds, and pit toilets.

Big Schloss sits high atop the ridgeline that marks the border of Virginia with West Virginia. A short hike from Wolf Gap along the spine of Mill Mountain will bring you to this sandstone outcrop named by German immigrants. *Schloss* translates as a palace or castle, and once you stand on this natural structure you are sure to be as impressed as the early settlers were. The massive outcrop juts upward from the mixed hardwood forest, rising above the trees to permit a superb view of the surrounding countryside. Luckily, because most of the land surrounding Big Schloss is national forest, the scenery remains somewhat the same as it appeared back in the settlers' days. There are few places like this left in the eastern part of America—your eyes can gaze out upon ridgelines, forests, and valleys that show remarkably few signs of the 21st century.

Route Description

From the large parking area in the Wolf Gap Campground, walk to orange-blazed Mill Mountain Trail {FS 1004}, which is located close to campsite nine. Begin a series of switchbacks at 0.25 mile, as the ascent becomes a little steeper.

At 0.75 mile you will reach the ridge, where you should bear left onto a narrower pathway. In winter, your objective—the large rocks of Big Schloss—can be seen directly ahead through the trees. Soon a couple of rock outcrops to the right provide excellent views. Rolling out to the distance in the east are Little Sluice Mountain (see Hike 17), the Shenandoah Valley, Massanutten Mountain (see Hikes 19, 20, and 21), and the ridgelines of the mountains along Skyline Drive (see Hikes 22–29).

There are several obviously well-used campsites along this ridge. Because this is a national forest you could camp just about anywhere you wish. However, you should be conscious that this is a popular hike and that practicing no-trace camping will help preserve the beauty of the area. In addition, although campfires are always nice to sit around in the evening, they are very hard on the land. Fires not only leave charred spots but also destroy nutrients in the topsoil. Some places are so fragile that it could be years before any new growth will appear where a campfire has been. Be kind to the soil and carry a backpacking stove if you plan to do any camping. (The forest service has provided fire rings and grates at the Wolf Gap Recreation Area if you do wish to do your cooking over a fire.)

After walking level for a while, you will descend slightly at 1.3 miles, only to rise again along the rocky crest of the mountain. Pay attention at 1.9 miles, as the Mill Mountain Trail continues to the left, connecting with other trails of the George Washington and Jefferson National Forests; you want to bear right and ascend on white-blazed Big Schloss Trail {FS 1004A}.

Arrive at Big Schloss in 2.2 miles, take the wooden bridge across a cleft in the rock outcrop, and break out into the open. Walk all the way to the edge of Big Schloss for your outrageously wonderful reward. To the west is Trout Run Valley and Long Mountain in West Virginia, to the north is Anderson Ridge, and to the east is a repeat of the views you saw from the rock outcrops you passed earlier. To the south Tibet Knob rises like a cone from Great North Mountain's ridgeline. The first hatching box of the forest service project to reintroduce the peregrine falcon to the area was placed at Big Schloss. If you are extremely lucky, you may see one of these rare birds, also known as duck hawks, flying through the air with strong and rapid wing strokes. Return to your car by retracing your steps.

The relatively short hike to Big Schloss is well worth the splendid view.

photo: Jon Bilous/Shutterstock

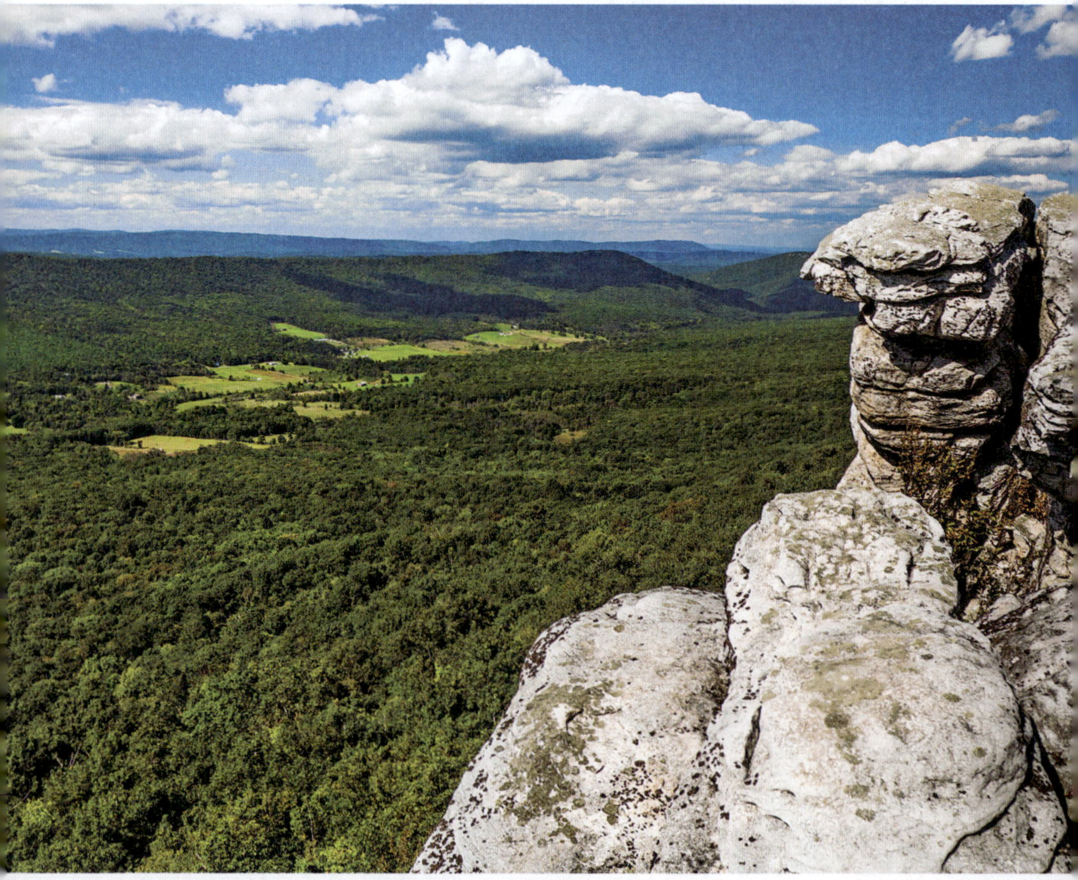

19 Signal Knob

- **GPS:** N38.9345473 W78.3200957
- **TOTAL DISTANCE (circuit):** 10.4 miles
- **HIKING TIME:** 7.0 hours
- **VERTICAL RISE:** 2,220 feet
- **MAPS:** USGS *Strasburg; National Geographic Trails Illustrated Map #792 Massanutten and Great North Mountain*
- **CONTACT:** Lee Ranger District
  95 Railroad Ave.
  Edinburg, VA 22824
  540-984-4101
  fs.usda.gov/gwj

The Hike at a Glance

- 1.5 Buzzard Rock
- 3.5 Meneka Peak Trail goes off to the left; stay right
- 4.4 Signal Knob; continue on orange-blazed Massanutten Trail
- 5.7 Four-way intersection; turn left, cross stream and Bear Wallow/Tuscarora Trail
- 9.2 The trail to the right leads to Elizabeth Furnace Recreation Area; stay left
- 9.9 Tuscarora Trail goes to right; stay left
- 10.4 Return to parking area

A walk to Signal Knob can bring you into a natural world of clear, flowing springs, succulent blueberries, deep woods, and quiet mountain streams. The walk can also help you appreciate the methods by which humans communicated in days before telephones, televisions, space-age satellites, and the internet created the worldwide, almost-instantaneous exchange of information.

Drums, in the form of hollow logs beaten with wooden sticks or stones, were probably the first means of long-distance communication. Once humans discovered how to make and control fire, smoke signals were employed. Later, as written languages became more precise and established, humans learned to use single symbols to convey concepts that would have taken many words to describe. Thus, flags came to be tools for signaling messages. Using flags, people could relay information from point to point, over and over again, to get the messages across great distances.

During the Civil War, the Confederacy used 2,106-foot Signal Knob, which overlooks a sweeping panorama of the Shenandoah Valley, to spot Union troops moving south from their encampments in Winchester and other places to the north. Information on these movements was signaled by flag to points farther south and then relayed numerous times, sometimes all the way to Richmond, the capital of the Confederacy.

DIRECTIONS You can reach the beginning of the Signal Knob hike by taking I-81 Exit 196 at Strasburg and following VA 55 eastward through Strasburg, continuing from town about 5 miles to a right onto VA 678. Driving 3.5 miles on VA 678 will bring you to the Signal Knob parking area, on the right. (See Hike 20 for directions to this hike from other points.)

Route Description

A white-blazed trail comes into the parking area from the left. As you will be returning via this route, ignore it now and take orange-blazed Massanutten Trail (some maps and other sources refer to it by its older name of Signal Knob Trail {FS 402}), leaving the parking lot to the right. Trail builders and maintainers have made your walking easier by doing a good job of removing boulders from the path, yet the treadway is on-and-off rough and rocky for the first 2.6 miles of the ascent. Despite the ruggedness, Signal Knob has become a popular mountain-bike destination, so be prepared to have to move aside at any moment.

Signal Knob

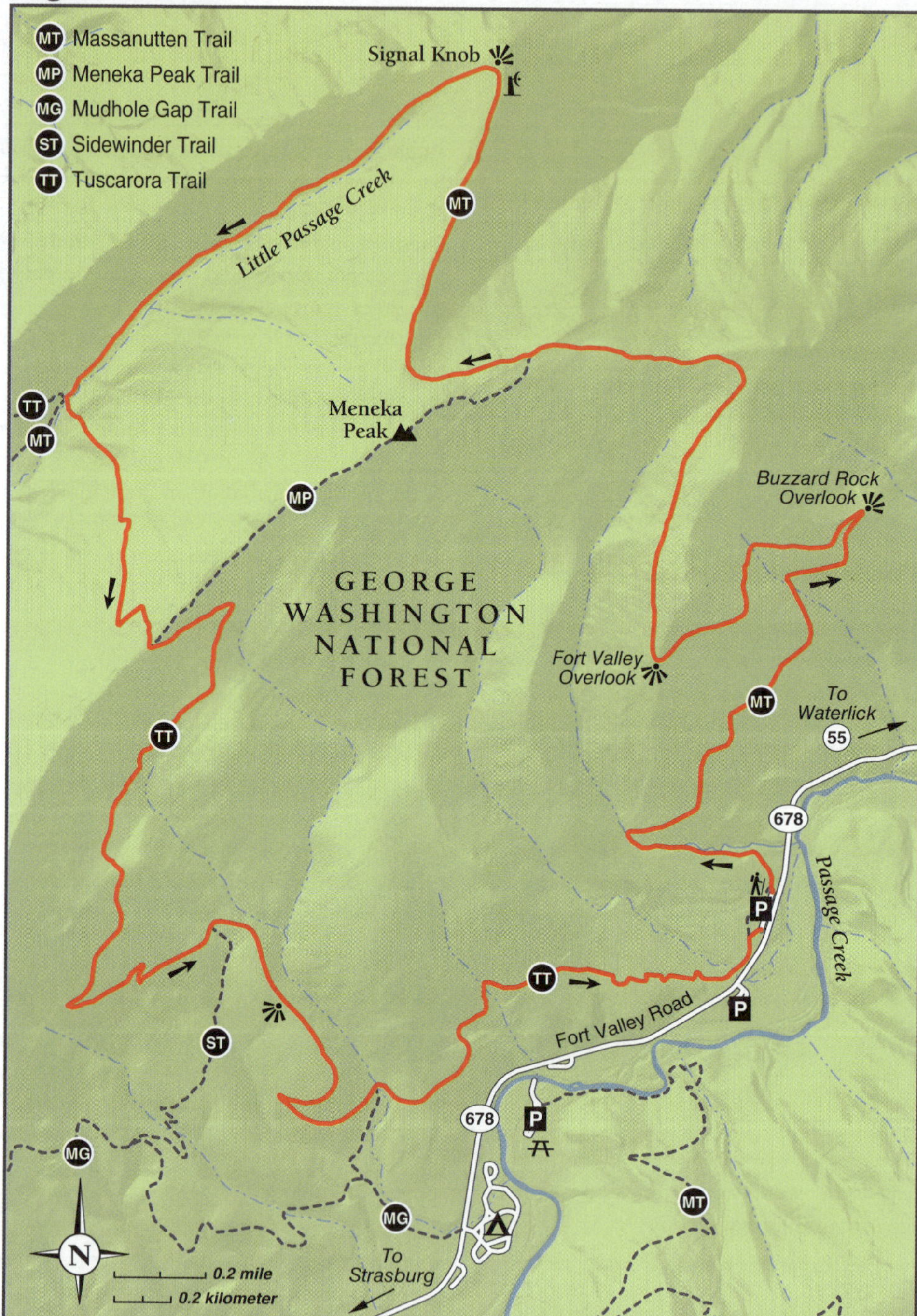
Massanutten Trail
Meneka Peak Trail
Mudhole Gap Trail
Sidewinder Trail
Tuscarora Trail
Signal Knob
Little Passage Creek
Meneka Peak
GEORGE WASHINGTON NATIONAL FOREST
Buzzard Rock Overlook
Fort Valley Overlook
To Waterlick
55
678
Passage Creek
Fort Valley Road
To Strasburg
0.2 mile
0.2 kilometer

Pass a forest service cabin (closed to the public) at 0.25 mile. In 0.4 mile, when you cross a small water run, look uphill a few feet for its source—a spring emanating from a stone-walled box. A rockslide, causing a break in the vegetation, gives a limited view to the southeast of shimmering Passage Creek in the valley directly below. Plan on abundant and irresistible blueberries at this spot in July and August to slow the forward progress of your hike.

Buzzard Rock, a prominent outcrop to the east, is visible at a natural overlook in 1.5 miles; the mountains of Shenandoah National Park are to the southeast. Small circular holes were made by sapsuckers in search of the insects that invaded the trees in order to feast on decaying wood. Swing around a spur ridge at 2.2 miles to another overlook, this one of bucolic Fort Valley, nestled between the eastern and western ridges of Massanutten Mountain. Kennedy Peak is the prominent point on the eastern ridge.

Shenandoah Valley Overlook Trail, no longer maintained, heads off to the right at 2.9 miles. You have just about reached the ridgeline and will be walking more or less level for a while. At 3.5 miles, white-blazed Meneka Peak Trail {FS 427} goes off to the left, crosses the peak, and rejoins this hike in about 1.5 miles at the 6.4-mile point; keep right. Greenbrier and sassafras are beginning to crowd out the rest of the undergrowth. Pass by the transmitter—the present-day means of communication that utilizes the mountain—and keep to the right to follow yellow blazes when a trail comes in from the left.

The far-reaching, commanding view of Shenandoah Valley from Signal Knob at 4.4 miles makes it easy to see why the Confederates used this vantage to observe Union troop activity. With a little searching, remains of the stone fortifications they built can be found on the knob. The Confederate army planned its strategy for the battle of Cedar Creek in 1864 from this point. Because of this advantage, the battle at first appeared to be going in their favor, but Union forces eventually rallied, forcing the Confederates under General Jubal A. Early's command to beat a hasty retreat southward. The Union wanted to ensure the valley would no longer be useful to the South, and the destruction by General P. H. Sheridan's troops was so complete that, in his words, "a crow would have to carry his rations if he flew over it." Turkey vultures are often seen hovering over Signal Knob, riding thermals rising from the valley.

Around the Signal Knob area is a trail that heads back to the transmitting towers. You need to look for the wide, descending, orange-blazed Massanutten Trail (some maps and other sources refer to it by its older name of Massanutten Mountain Trail {FS 408}), which will bring you to the headwaters of Little Passage Creek at 5.0 miles. In this valley is Sand Springs, the source of water for the troops on Signal Knob. Nearby is the grave of an unnamed soldier from Georgia.

Continue downstream to a four-way intersection at 5.7 miles. Orange-blazed Massanutten Mountain Trail continues straight, and the Tuscarora Trail (still identified on many maps and other resources by its older name of Big Blue Trail) is to the right. Take a left to cross Little Passage Creek and ascend the switchbacking, blue-blazed Bear Wallow Trail {FS 405.2}, which is also a part of the Tuscarora Trail at this point. (The Tuscarora Trail is a marked long-distance pathway of more than 250 miles. Its southern terminus is a junction with the Appalachian Trail a couple of miles north of Elk Wallow Gap in Shenandoah National Park. The trail crosses the Shenandoah Valley and continues through Virginia, West Virginia, Maryland, and Pennsylvania, where its northern terminus junctions with the AT, just north of Donnellytown, Pennsylvania.)

A trail to the right at 9.2 miles leads to the Elizabeth Furnace Recreation Area; keep left, cross a stream, and slab the hillside, following the blue and orange blazes. Larger trees, now making up a greater percentage of the forest, give the woods a deeper and darker feeling. Ascend a short distance to cross a spur ridge and descend through forest that may still be showing the scars of a 1984 fire and years of spongy moth invasions. A break in the vegetation lets you look out over the same farmland you observed from the Fort Valley Overlook; only now, with your lower elevation, you are able to make out more detail. Continue the descent, which is gentle at times but makes use of switchbacks at other spots. The Tuscarora Trail bears to the right at 9.9 miles; continue left to return to your car, at 10.4 miles. A right turn out of the parking area onto VA 678 for a drive of less than a mile will take you to two short (0.25-mile and 0.5-mile) interpretive trails in the Elizabeth Furnace Picnic Area. See the end of Hike 20 for additional walking opportunities in the nearby area.

Enjoy the view from Massanutten Mountain.

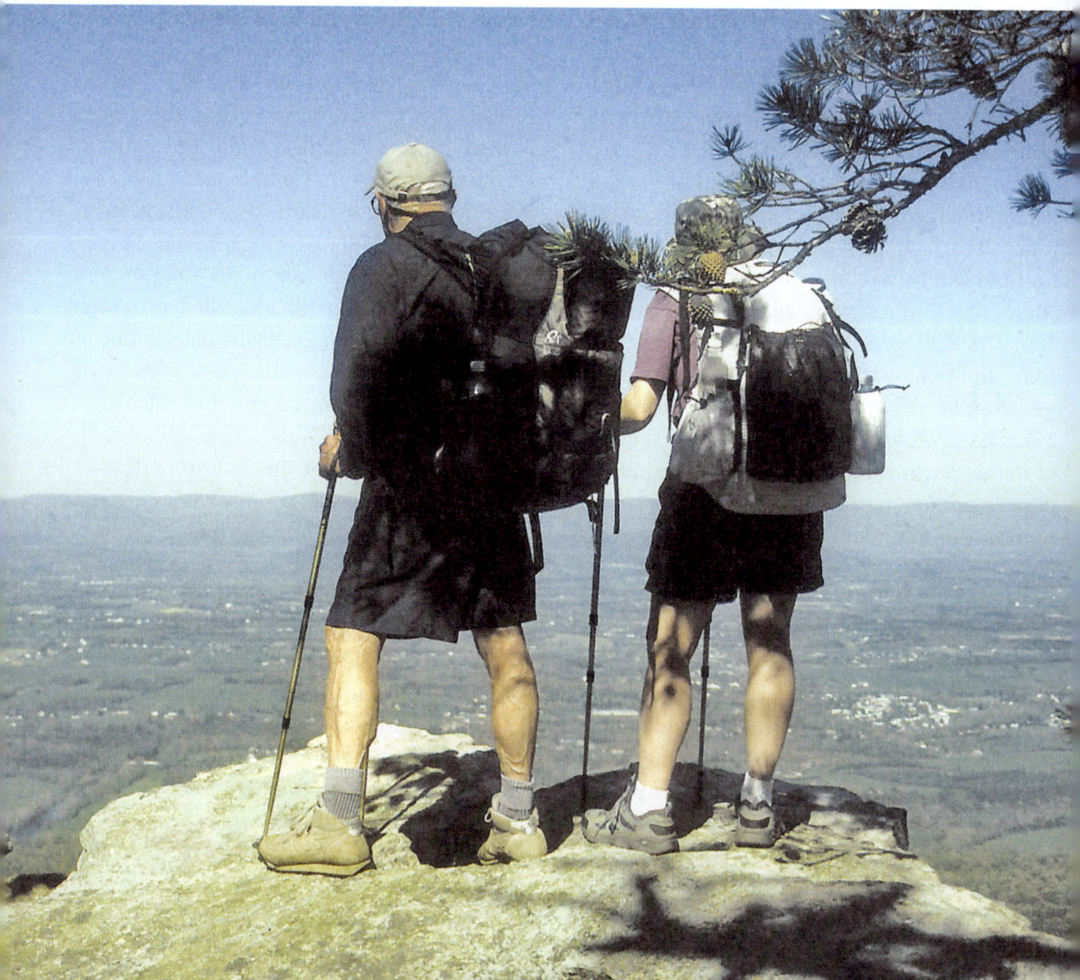

20 Woodstock Observation Tower

- **GPS:** N38.8719433 W78.4472781
- **TOTAL DISTANCE (round-trip):** 0.3 mile
- **HIKING TIME:** 15 minutes
- **VERTICAL RISE:** Less than 50 feet
- **MAPS:** USGS *Rileyville; National Geographic Trails Illustrated Map #792 Massanutten and Great North Mountain*
- **CONTACT:** Lee Ranger District
  95 Railroad Ave.
  Edinburg, VA 22824
  540-984-4101
  fs.usda.gov/gwj

The Hike at a Glance

0.15 Woodstock Observation Tower; retrace steps
0.3 Return to parking area

This little jaunt is so short it can barely be considered a hike. Nevertheless, if you are in the area, you shouldn't pass up the chance to walk to the Woodstock Observation Tower. It is so easy that even those who are out of shape can handle it—an excellent introduction for someone you are taking out on a hike for the first time. There are very, very few places in Virginia where you can reap such a marvelous and rewarding payback for the small amount of energy you will expend and the few minutes of time you will invest walking to this destination.

DIRECTIONS The drive to the trailhead is also simple and pleasurable. Take the I-81 Exit 283 at Woodstock, heading eastward to town, and turn left onto US 11. Despite the usual, modern-day strip of several service stations, motels, and restaurants next to the interstate, the town proper has retained much of the look of a previous era. The Shenandoah County Courthouse on Main Street, built in 1792, is the oldest courthouse still in use west of the Blue Ridge Mountains, and the inside of the building has been restored to its original design. Even having a meal in Woodstock can take on a historical aspect—one restaurant is in a former clothing factory from the 1920s and another in a 100-year-old home whose spring provided some of the water for the town.

Take VA 758 east out of town, entering the rich green, fertile, rolling pastoral landscape that has given the Shenandoah Valley much of its fame. Stay on VA 758 through several intersections, soon crossing the Shenandoah River. Observe and remember what the river looks like close up, for soon you will be treated to an aerial view that takes in many miles of its course. The road eventually turns to dirt and makes numerous switchbacks up the mountain, enabling you to use automobile power instead of leg muscles to gain the elevation necessary to reach the ridge on Powell Mountain. Leave your car at the signed parking area.

Route Description

Ascend a few stone steps on the right side of the road. Coming into intimate contact with a mountaintop environment of boulders, pines, and oaks, cross the white-blazed Wagon Road Trail {FS 552} in 200 feet. (Wagon Road Trail drops approximately 1 mile to the left to the Little Fort Recreation Area, a forest service campground and picnic area. A resort used to operate at Seven Fountains in Fort Valley (to the east). Most of its guests arrived in Woodstock by train from the metropolitan areas around Washington, D.C., and a stagecoach carried them from Woodstock, over the mountain, and to the resort. Wagon Road Trail actually follows the old stage route, and a meadow near

Woodstock Observation Tower

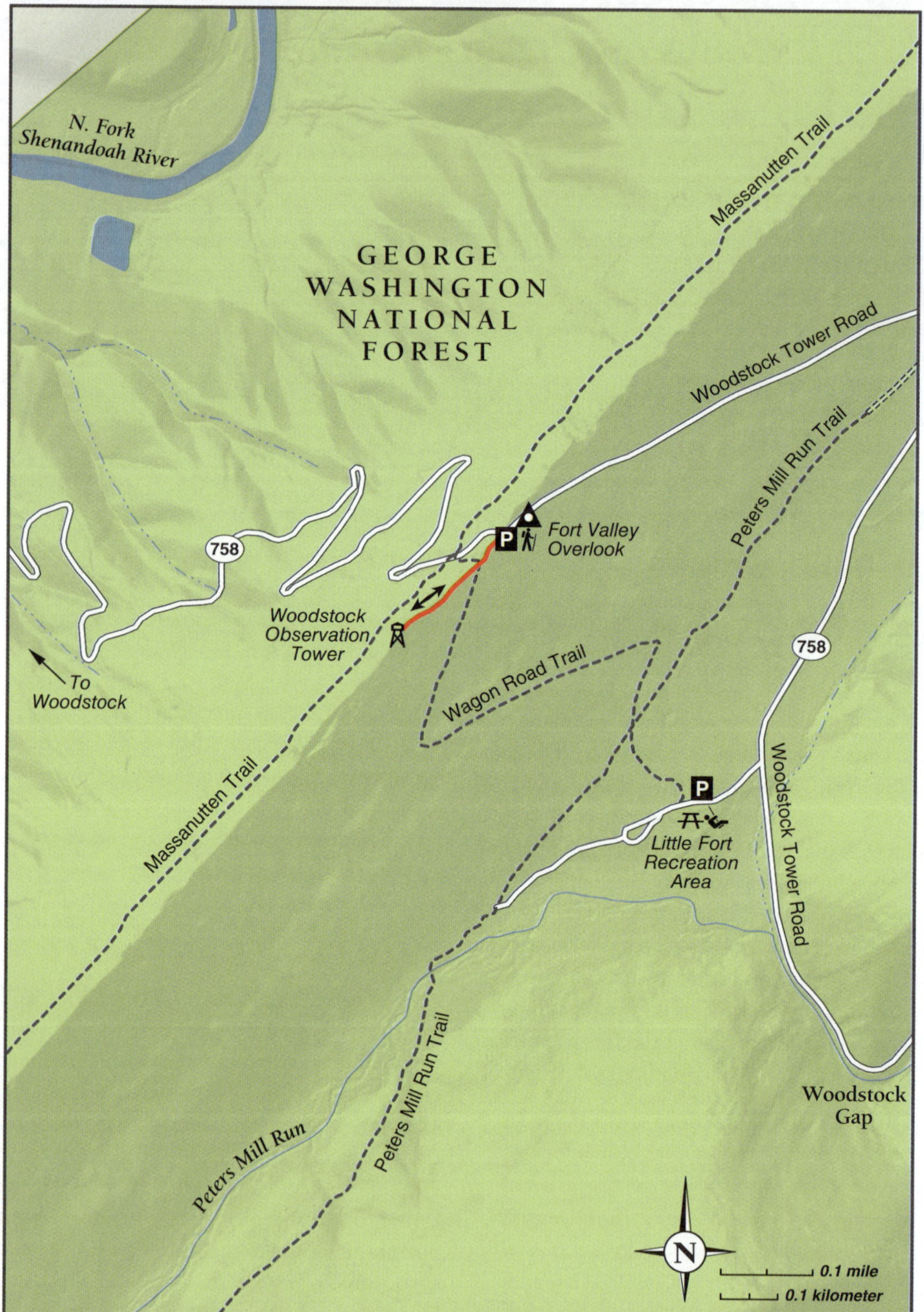

the Little Fort Recreation Area was used as a picnicking and rest stop.)

Continue on the ridgeline of the mountain to arrive at the Woodstock Observation Tower at 0.15 mile. Construction of the tower in 1935 was a cooperative effort by the Civilian Conservation Corps and the Woodstock Chamber of Commerce.

The 360-degree view from the tower is absolutely stunning. To the west, rising out of the wide, emerald expanse of Shenandoah Valley, are Little Sluice Mountain (see Hike 17), Mill Mountain (see Hike 18), and the higher Allegheny Mountains in West Virginia. At the base of Powell Mountain are the world-famous horseshoe bends of the Shenandoah River. The meandering course of the river between Edinburg and Strasburg is almost 50 miles, but a straight distance between the two towns is only about 15 miles! To the north and south are the ridgelines of Powell and Green Mountains, which, along with the eastern flank of Massanutten Mountain, completely surround Fort Valley, giving it the appearance of being a large volcanic crater. This "natural fort" was named by George Washington, who would have used the valley as a retreat had he been defeated at Yorktown. Farther east, beyond Massanutten Mountain and across Page Valley, are the Blue Ridge Mountains of Shenandoah National Park.

Let your eyes feast on this restful, visual treat. Maybe, just maybe, you shouldn't worry about the history of the area. Perhaps you shouldn't even try to pick out specific landmarks. Just relax and enjoy the splendor of this moment, a moment that you have been picked by the Fates to experience and possess.

The Massanutten Mountain area is rich with additional hiking opportunities. Continuing to drive east on VA 758 from the observation tower parking area brings you into the heart of Fort Valley and to the intersection with VA 678. Making a left turn onto VA 678 for several miles will bring you to the Elizabeth Furnace Recreation Area for two short interpretive trails and the Signal Knob hike (see Hike 19). A right onto VA 678 from its intersection with VA 758 and then continuing south via VA 675 and FSR 274 will take you past the Duncan Knob hike (see Hike 21), the Lion's Tale Trail—an interpretive trail for those with vision impairment—and the Massanutten Story Trail, a 0.5-mile paved pathway suitable for wheelchairs. Another paved trail and several other pedestrian routes emanate from the now-closed Massanutten Visitor Center in New Market Gap, where FSR 274 meets US 211.

Duncan Knob

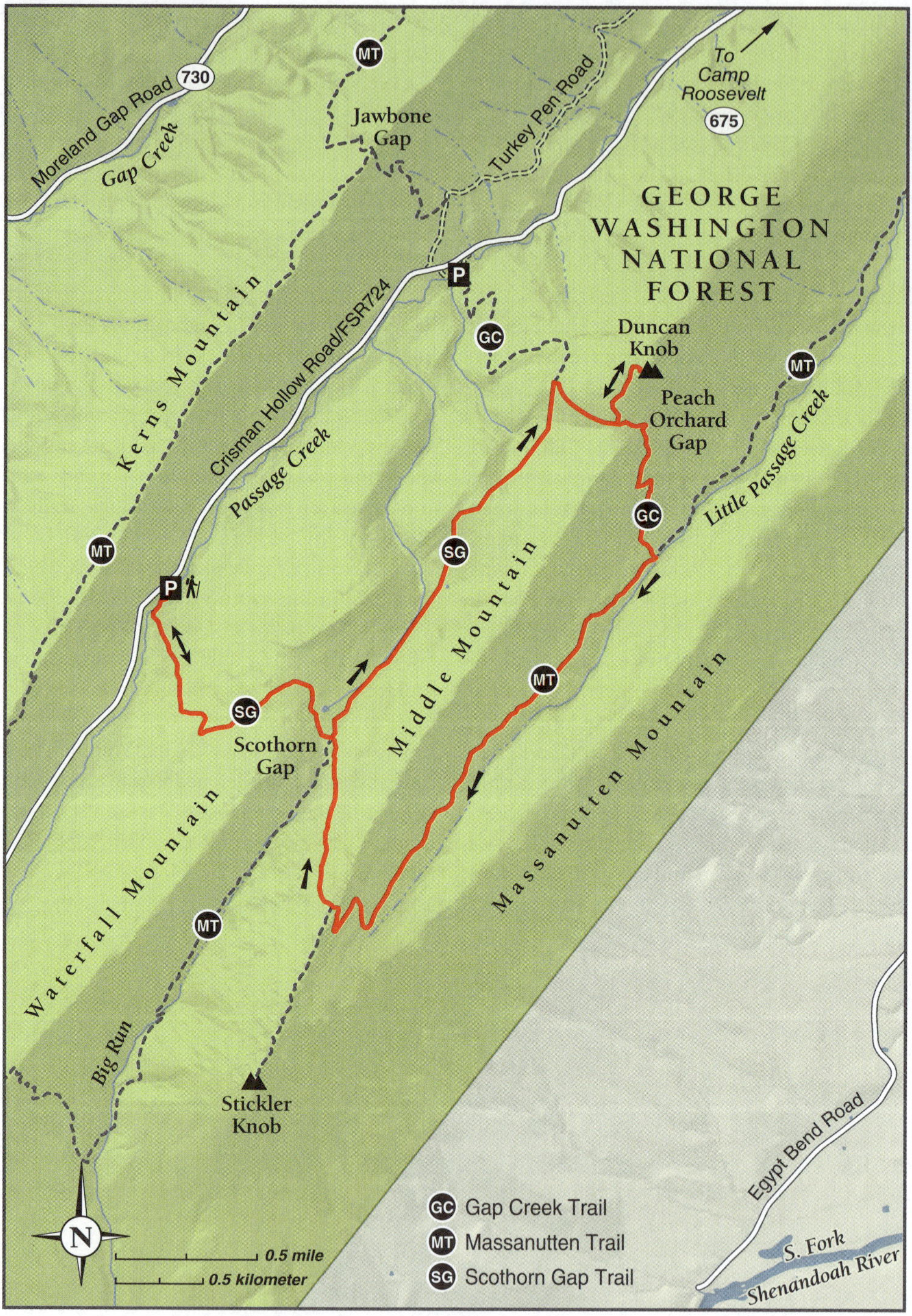

Moreland Gap Road
730
Gap Creek
MT
Jawbone Gap
Turkey Pen Road
To Camp Roosevelt
675
GEORGE WASHINGTON NATIONAL FOREST
P
GC
Duncan Knob
Peach Orchard Gap
MT
Kerns Mountain
Crisman Hollow Road/FSR724
Passage Creek
Little Passage Creek
GC
SG
MT
P
Middle Mountain
SG
Scothorn Gap
MT
Massanutten Mountain
Waterfall Mountain
MT
Big Run
Stickler Knob
Egypt Bend Road
S. Fork Shenandoah River
N
0.5 mile
0.5 kilometer
GC Gap Creek Trail
MT Massanutten Trail
SG Scothorn Gap Trail

21 Duncan Knob

- **GPS:** N38.6914856 W78.5799937
- **TOTAL DISTANCE (circuit):** 8.5 miles
- **HIKING TIME:** 6.0 hours
- **VERTICAL RISE:** 2,240 feet
- **MAPS:** USGS *Hamburg; National Geographic Trails Illustrated Map #792 Massanutten and Great North Mountain*
- **CONTACT:** Lee Ranger District
  95 Railroad Ave.
  Edinburg, VA 22824
  540-984-4101
  fs.usda.gov/gwj

The Hike at a Glance

1.3 Intersection with Massanutten Trail; bear left to stay on Scothorn Gap Trail

2.8 Right onto Gap Creek Trail

3.1 Peach Orchard Gap. At high point in gap, turn left to come to Duncan Knob. Then retrace steps to Gap Creek Trail, turn left, and descend to turn right onto Massanutten Trail

6.4 Attain Middle Mountain ridgeline

7.15 Intersection. Massanutten Trail makes a hard left. Turn left onto Scothorn Gap Trail

8.5 Return to parking area

At an elevation of 2,803 feet, Duncan Knob sits atop Catback Mountain, which is actually just one of the many ridges that make up 50-mile-long Massanutten Mountain. Standing alone and bisecting the Shenandoah Valley, Massanutten Mountain prevents the north and south branches of the Shenandoah River from meeting each other until the mountain comes to an end near Strasburg. The hike to Duncan Knob allows you to become familiar with the ridges and valleys of this great mountain and to gaze out upon a large expanse of land to see how the mountain has helped shape the surrounding topography.

This walk, which involves a short stretch of possibly unmarked trail and a bit of scrambling up a rocky slope for a few hundred feet, can be easily accomplished as a day hike. However, because the hike is all on public land where camping is permitted (sites abound throughout much of the hike), you might want to consider an overnight trip. Not only would this prolong your time on, and enjoyment of, the mountain, but it would also put you in position to be on top of Duncan Knob at the times of day when its view is best appreciated—early morning or early evening. It is at these times that rays of the sun strike the earth at just the right slant to produce a golden, glowing landscape—a great time to take photographs. Campsites are plentiful, especially in the first 3 miles or so. Just be sure to carry enough water, as sources may be scarce at the flattest or most choice sites.

DIRECTIONS Take I-81 Exit 264 at New Market and follow US 211 eastward for less than 10 miles to a left turn onto FSR 274 in New Market Gap. If you come to the now-closed Massanutten Visitor Center on the right side of US 211, you have gone just a few feet too far. Once on FSR 274, follow it past Massanutten Mountain Story Book and Waterfall Mountain trailheads to arrive at the Scothorn Gap Trail, {FS 555} on the right in 4.5 miles.

Route Description

Begin the hike by crossing Passage Creek and ascending the old red-blazed road (Scothorn Gap Trail {FS 555}). In 0.4 mile the road makes a little zigzag and ascends at a steeper grade; in one spot there are several switchbacks to modify the grade a bit before the road resumes the steep ascent. Mountain laurel becomes more dense, and maple and sassafras leaves add dashes of red to the forest in the fall. Level out on the ridgeline, passing through a wildlife clearing at 0.9 mile. Clearings such as this can be found in almost all of America's national forests. Usually they are not naturally occurring open spaces but are created by the forest service (many are remnants of old logging operations) to provide food or shelter sites for particular types of birds or animals. By designing the lay of the land and planting certain trees, shrubs, grasses, and flowers, the forest service can attract a variety of wildlife, such as deer, turkeys, grouse, squirrels, and quail to an area. Camp in the woods next to a clearing, be quiet and still, and odds are—especially at dusk—you will be able to watch several birds or animals as they go about their daily activities. Take the proper precautions, though, as these clearings are popular hunting spots during the season.

Skirt the corner of another clearing at 1.3 miles and bear to the right, looking for the red blazes as your route reenters the woods to junction with the orange-blazed Massanutten Trail {FS 408} coming in from the right. You will return on this trail. Turn left now and descend along the old woods road. At 1.8 miles, an unmarked trail to the right leads to a small pond that can provide wildlife with water during dry seasons. At 2.1 miles, skirt the right side of a clearing and continue to descend, sometimes quickly. The forest you are walking through must be home to a great assortment of wildlife, judging by the wide variety of scat seen on rocks. At 2.6 miles, the route crosses a small draw and ascends slightly, becoming more of a trail than an old roadway.

Scothorn Gap Trail ends as you come to blue-blazed Gap Creek Trail {FS 409} at 2.8 miles. Part of this trail drops to the left for about a mile to FSR 274, but you want to follow it uphill to the right. Come onto the ridgeline in Peach Orchard Gap at 3.1 miles. At the high point in the gap is what may be an unmarked but discernible trail off to the left. Follow this trail (if you lose it, just keep going uphill) through the woods for a little more than 1,000 feet to come to the rock scree facing of Duncan Knob. Scramble up the rocks (going a bit to the left is the easiest) to the knob. Take a well-deserved break on top; the Olympian view more than makes up for the few calories you've burned to reach here.

Directly southwest is Middle Mountain—you have just walked along its western flank and will soon explore its eastern side. To the west are rocky outcrops on Kerns Mountain, and beyond is I-81 winding through the Shenandoah Valley. Southeast and almost directly below are the oxbow bends of the South Branch of the Shenandoah River. On the eastern horizon, across Page Valley, are the Blue Ridge Mountains of Shenandoah National Park.

Return to the Gap Creek Trail and turn left (eastward) to descend a rocky pathway through abundant sassafras. Gap Creek Trail ends as it meets up with the orange-blazed Massanutten Trail {FS 408} in Duncan Hollow. To the left it is about 3 miles to Camp Roosevelt (site of the first Civilian Conservation Corps camp in America; building foundations still exist) and VA 675. You need to make a right and gradually ascend. Despite the presence of an old roadway, Duncan Hollow is a wonderful valley, showing few signs of human activity and isolated from traffic noise and other sounds of modern society. The hollow also supports a luxuriant growth of mountain laurel, especially beautiful from May to June when the clusters of rich pink-to-white flowers contrast with deep-green leaves.

Be on the lookout for small, cone-shaped holes made by ant lions in the sandy soil of the roadbed. These enterprising larvae make use of the "angle of repose" by crafting the sides of their dens at about a 30-degree angle, the steepest slant at which dry sand can sustain a slope. Unsuspecting insects stepping onto this sand steepen the slope by just a degree or two and are sent tumbling into the clutches of the lion hiding in the sand below.

Ascend more quickly at 4.7 miles for a short distance before the road mellows again and you pass through a forest of large oaks and maples. Several trees may bear the scars of violent lightning strikes. At 6.1 miles, the road deteriorates into a rough and rocky pathway that swings to the right (soon passing the

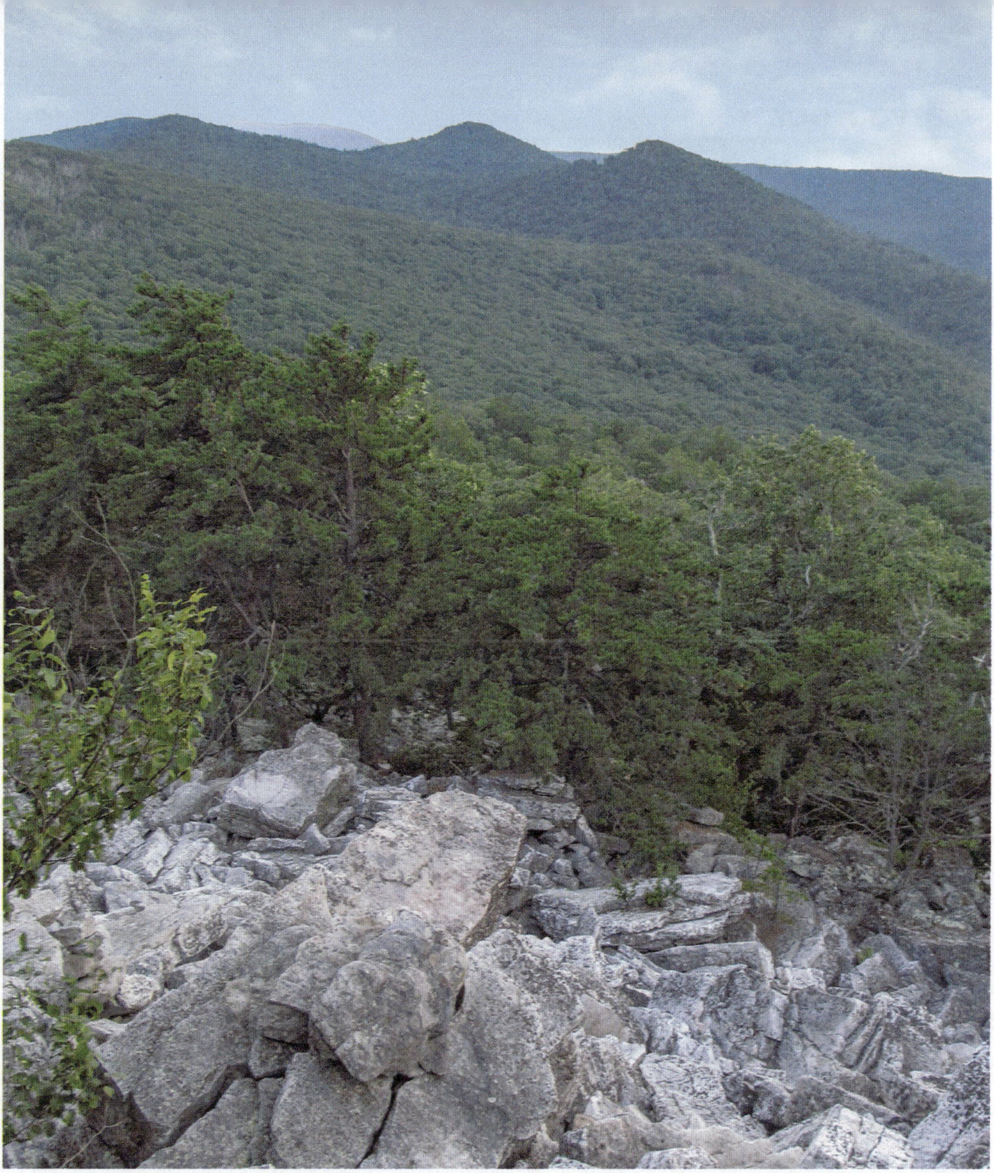

Looking out from the rock field on Duncan Knob

photo: Johnny Molloy

possibly unmarked trail to Stickler Knob) and ascends steeply to attain the boulder-strewn and mountain laurel–covered ridge of Middle Mountain at 6.4 miles. If you are hiking in the fall, stop to examine the small capsules on the mountain laurel. Break open one of these capsules, which were the plant's flowers earlier in the year, and you will discover what looks to be brown dust. Each dust speck is actually a seed of the mountain laurel and is so small that more than 1,000 of these seeds could easily fit into something about the size of a pea.

Come to an intersection at 7.15 miles. The Massanutten Trail makes a hard left; you want to make the left turn back onto the red-blazed Scothorn Gap Trail and retrace your steps on the same old road on which you began this hike. Arrive back at Passage Creek and your automobile at 8.5 miles. See the end of Hike 20 for additional walking opportunities in the area.

Marys Rock

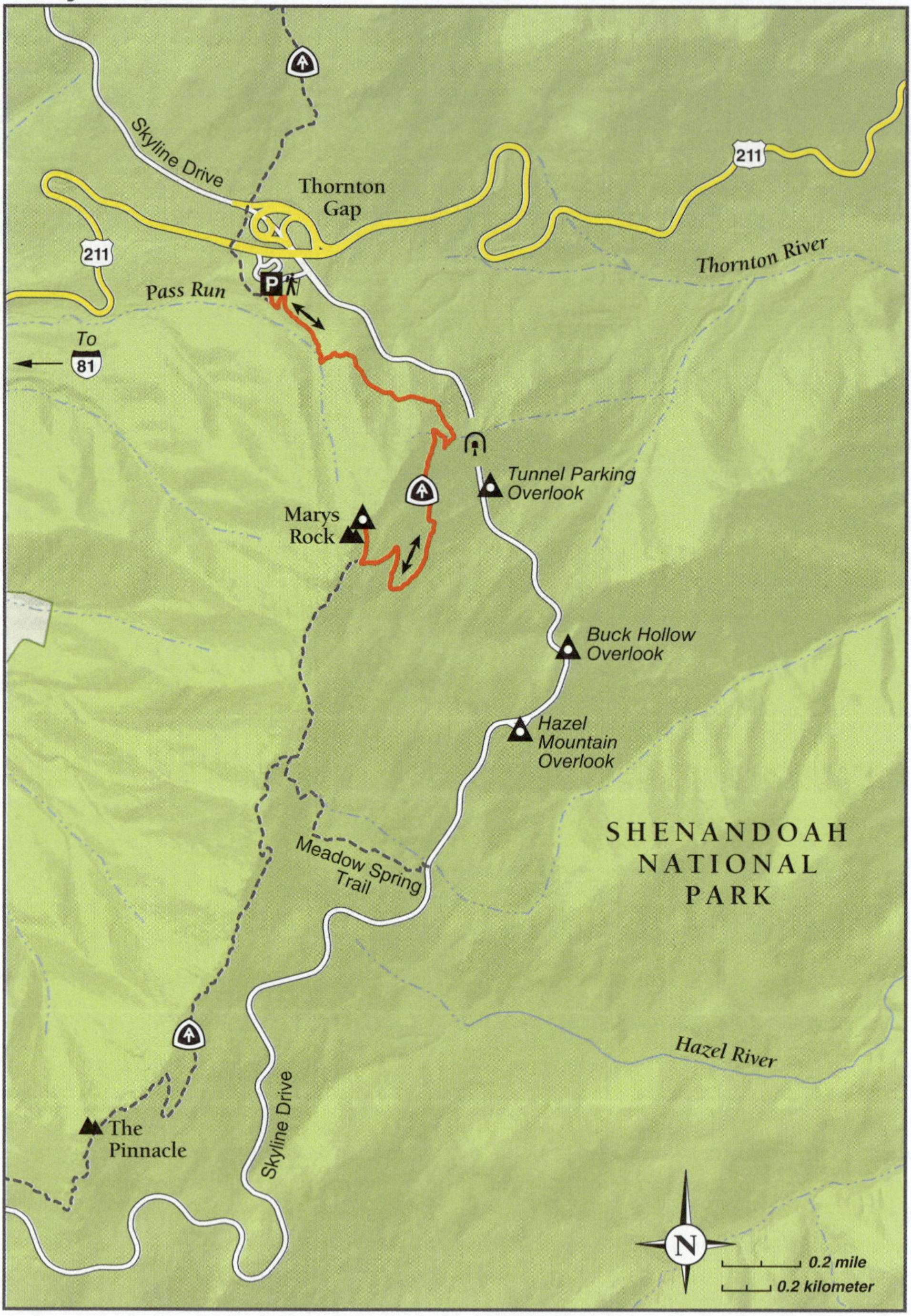

Skyline Drive
Thornton Gap
211
211
Thornton River
Pass Run
P
To
81
Tunnel Parking Overlook
Marys Rock
Buck Hollow Overlook
Hazel Mountain Overlook
SHENANDOAH NATIONAL PARK
Meadow Spring Trail
Hazel River
The Pinnacle
Skyline Drive
N
0.2 mile
0.2 kilometer

22 Marys Rock

- **GPS:** N38.6598821 W78.3215220
- **TOTAL DISTANCE (round-trip):** 3.6 miles
- **HIKING TIME:** 2.5 hours
- **VERTICAL RISE:** 1,240 feet
- **MAPS:** USGS *Thornton Gap; National Geographic Trails Illustrated Map #228 Shenandoah National Park*
- **CONTACT:** Shenandoah National Park
  3655 US 211 E.
  Luray, VA 22835-9036
  540-999-3500
  nps.gov/shen

The Hike at a Glance

- 0.0 Turn left onto the AT just a few feet after starting the hike
- 1.7 AT goes off to the left; keep right
- 1.8 Arrive at Marys Rock; retrace steps
- 3.6 Return to parking area

Encompassing the present-day crest of the Blue Ridge Mountains and its hundreds of attendant spur ridges, which spread in all directions like twisted and gnarled fingers, Shenandoah National Park stretches from Front Royal to Waynesboro, a distance of almost 75 miles and an area of nearly 200,000 acres. Congress authorized the establishment of the park in 1926 but provided no funds for land acquisition. We can thank the Commonwealth of Virginia for making it a reality. The Virginia Assembly appropriated $1 million, and about $1.2 million in donations from various sources (much of it from individual citizens) made it possible to purchase nearly 4,000 tracts of private land, which were deeded to the federal government in 1935. Some of this land was not sold willingly, and there is still a deep-seated resentment of the government by some of the families who were relocated from their ancestral homes. We should not minimize the loss experienced by these families, yet the establishment of the park has provided many overall benefits to the land.

As the 20th century began, second- and third-growth forests, logged since the early 1700s, covered much of what is now the park. Today, most signs of lumbering, as well as those of grazing and farming, have been largely erased through the growth of the forests. First came shrubs, pines, and black locusts; now 95% of the park is nearing a climax forest of oak, hickory, yellow poplar, and other hardwoods. This regeneration is so complete that 40% of the park was designated a wilderness area in 1976. Through the years, countless millions of Americans and foreign visitors have been able to enjoy these parklands, which, if they had remained in the hands of a few, would have either continued to deteriorate or, based upon what has happened in other mountain areas of Virginia, been turned into housing developments or high-priced resorts. Today, through law, the park cannot spend any funds to acquire new lands.

President Franklin Roosevelt officially dedicated the park in 1936, as men of the Civilian Conservation Corps (CCC) busily built trails, shelters, fire roads, and various visitors' facilities. The 105-mile Skyline Drive was essentially completed in 1939. Today the park has campgrounds, modern lodging facilities and a set of rustic cabins, two visitor centers, and picnic areas.

There are many legends and stories about the origin of the name *Shenandoah*, but perhaps the most romantic and beautiful is that it is a derivative of a Native American word meaning "daughter of the stars." When applied to Shenandoah National Park, those words seem more than appropriate, for the park is truly a stellar treasure in the vast system of public lands that citizens of the United States own in common. More than a dozen waterfalls crash down steep slopes; more than 200 species of birds, including 35 kinds of warblers, have been recorded in the park; and more than 1,200 species of vascular plants can be found within its borders. Turkeys, bobcats, raccoons, and skunks inhabit the region in significant numbers, and you have a chance of seeing black bears on backcountry hikes. There are so many deer that it has almost become common knowledge in Virginia that if you want to see a deer, you simply go to Shenandoah. The best feature of the park for walkers and hikers is that its network of more than 500 miles of trails makes its vast acreage easily navigable. Because the pathways are so well marked, and many of them are graded for gradual ascents and descents, the park is a good breaking-in place for novice hikers.

While hiking, please be sure to obey the regulations instituted by the park service in order to reduce the impact of well over 1 million visitors a year. Wood fires are permitted only in fireplaces in developed campgrounds, picnic areas, and certain trail shelters. No fires are allowed in the backcountry, so bring your backpacking stove if you want any hot meals on your hikes. You must obtain a backcountry camping permit (available at entrance stations, visitor centers, and some self-registering trailheads) before taking off on any overnight trips. The Old Rag Shelter and the four Byrds Nest shelters are for picnics only and may not be used for overnight accommodations except in the case of extreme weather conditions. Huts along the Appalachian Trail (AT) are intended to be used only by long-distance hikers. All dogs must be kept on a leash and are prohibited on certain trails. There are, of course, numerous other regulations, and you will be given a list of the most pertinent ones when you receive your camping permit. In addition, be sure to employ leave-no-trace hiking and camping methods.

DIRECTIONS The majority of the park's trails originate on or near the Skyline Drive, which is accessible from US 340 in Front Royal and US 250 and I-64 east of Waynesboro. US 211 crosses the drive at milepost 31.5 and US 33 crosses it at milepost 65.7. The trailhead for Marys Rock is in Thornton Gap, at the intersection of US 211 and Skyline Drive.

Route Description

The trek to Marys Rock is a good introduction to the park's trails. Using a section of the AT, the hike gains its elevation on a well-graded, switchbacked pathway leading to one of the most easily reached 360-degree views in the park. Along the way you will pass through tunnels of mountain laurel and, except during the coldest months of the year, a grand array of wildflowers.

Enter the woods on a wide trail from the turnaround circle at the end of the parking lot and intersect the AT in a few feet. The AT descends right for 0.1 mile to US 211, but you want to follow it to the left, ascending through a profuse growth of mountain laurel, whose blossoms will burst forth in late spring. A little farther up the trail, stinging nettle can be almost as abundant as the laurel. Brushing up against the nettle will give the tiny, stiff hairs an opportunity to scratch your skin and deposit an irritant that may itch for the rest of the day. One experience of this kind will, no doubt, keep you on the watch for the nettle.

At 0.6 mile, a break in the vegetation provides a view of Thornton Gap and some of the mountains of the park to the north. At 0.9 mile, after switchbacking a couple of times, pass by several overhanging rocks that could become small emergency shelters in case of a rain shower. Cushiony moss growing on boulders along the trail helps soften the look and feel of the rock field you walk through.

Although most of the trail you have been walking on was built by the CCC in the 1930s, the section at 1.2 miles in particular bears the unmistakable signs of the Corps' high-quality handiwork. The pathway rises at a more-or-less gradual rate and is almost wide enough for two people to walk abreast in some places. The rock walls that were built during the Great Depression to shore up this sidehill trail are still performing their duty. Trail crews of today do an admirable job of maintaining, rehabilitating, and reconstructing pathways, but trails of the CCC will still be with us for a long time.

After making a couple more switchbacks, come to an intersection at 1.7 miles. (If you can arrange a car shuttle, you could turn this walk into a one-way hike. After visiting Marys Rock, return to this point and follow the AT south to a left turn onto Meadow Spring Trail, which will drop you to Skyline Drive at mile point 33.5. Total distance of the full hike would be about 3.5 miles.) Turn right and at 1.8 miles arrive at Marys Rock, made up of granodiorite that geologists believe to be at least 1 billion years old.

Marys Rock is a favorite birders' perch to watch the fall hawk migration. The annual procession may begin as early as August, when one or two hawks a day have been spotted heading south. The watching becomes most spectacular in mid-September through early October as, in some years, several thousand broad-winged hawks a day have been seen. Various other hawks, such as the red-tailed and the red-shouldered, keep bird-watchers coming back to Marys Rock into November and even December.

The 360-degree view is obtained by scrambling 80 feet up to the top of the huge rock outcrop—not advisable in wet or windy weather. (Rare plants that are sensitive to trampling grow along the ridge to the south, so please do not venture into that area.) To the north is the road intersection from which you began the hike. Pass Mountain makes up the ridgeline closest to you, and behind it are the Three Sisters and Neighbor, Knob, and Hogback Mountains. Scanning to the east, you may be able to make out the gorge of Little Devils Stairs between Little Hogback and Mount Marshall. The Piedmont is clearly visible beyond Oventop and Jenkins Mountain. Southward are the Pinnacle and Stony Man (see Hike 23), while to the west is Massanutten Mountain (see Hikes 19–21), rising up to bisect the Shenandoah Valley.

I must admit that, after having visited here countless times, my favorite activity at Marys Rock now has little to do with bird-watching or identifying distant mountains. Rather, it involves picking the perfect-weather day; beginning the hike early in the morning; and carrying a big lunch, gobs of munchies, a quart or two of lemonade, and a good book up to the summit. I pick a nice, flat spot on the rock and spend the rest of the day soaking up warm sunshine, eating, reading, and glancing up every so often to gaze upon the serene beauty in which I've enveloped myself.

Simply retrace your steps to return to the parking area when you're ready.

Once you visit Marys Rock, you'll find that you want to go there often.

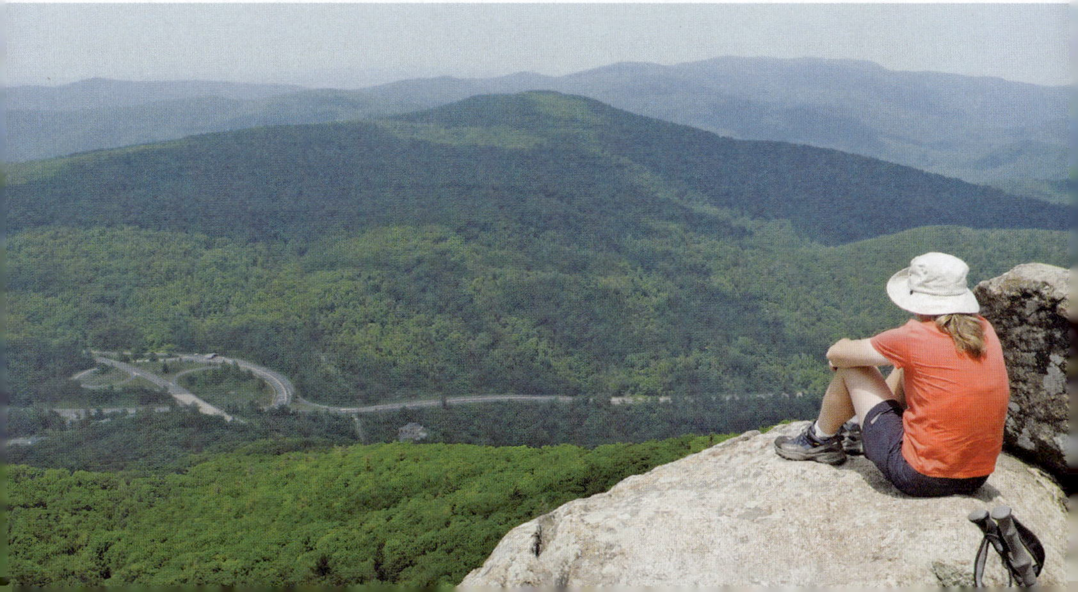

Stony Man

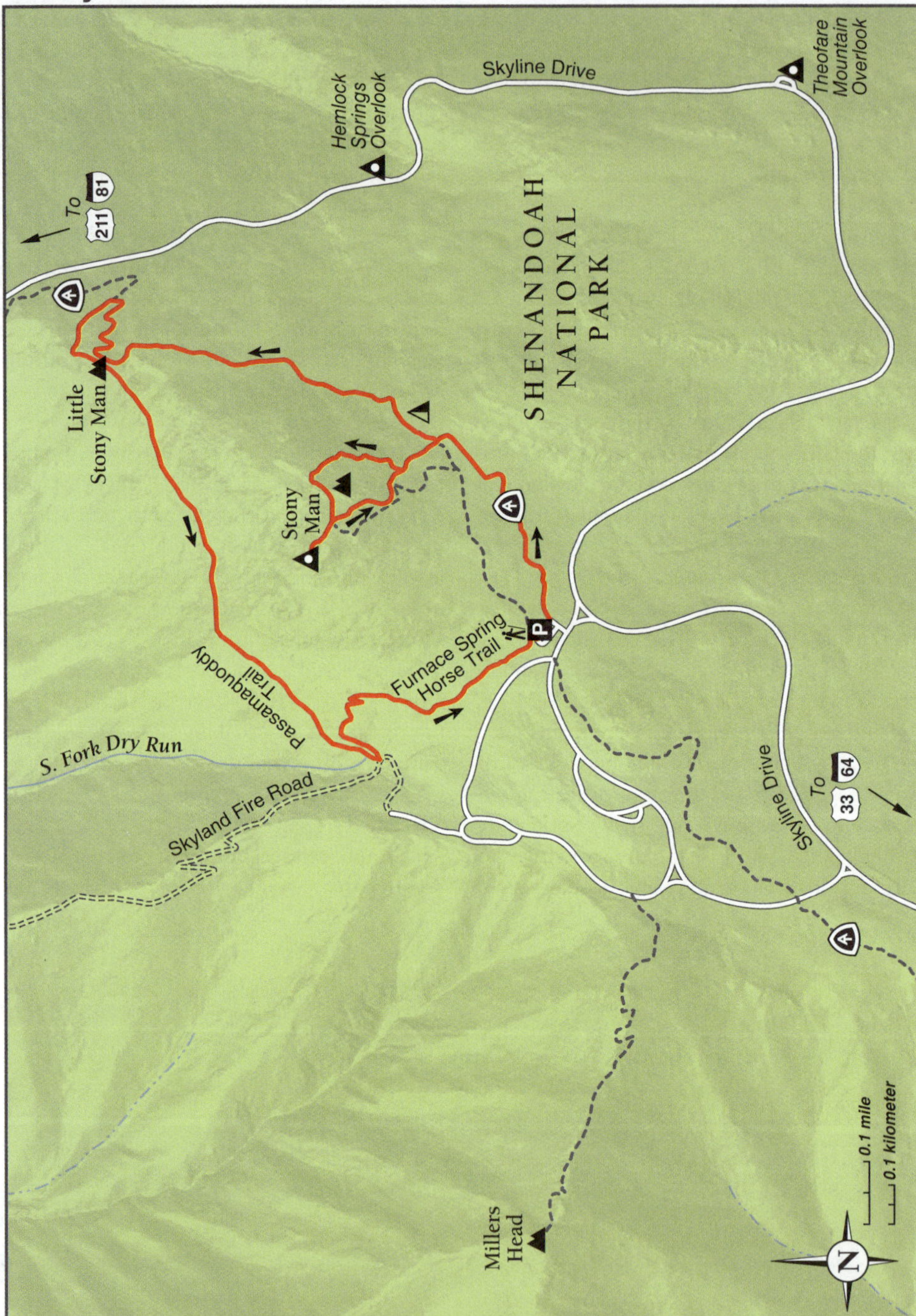

Skyline Drive
Hemlock Springs Overlook
Theofare Mountain Overlook
To 211 81
SHENANDOAH NATIONAL PARK
Little Stony Man
Stony Man
Passamaquoddy Trail
Furnace Spring Horse Trail
S. Fork Dry Run
Skyland Fire Road
Skyline Drive
To 33 64
Millers Head
0.1 mile
0.1 kilometer
N

23 Stony Man

- **GPS:** N38.5931509 W78.3757694
- **TOTAL DISTANCE (circuit):** 3.5 miles
- **HIKING TIME:** 2.0 hours
- **VERTICAL RISE:** 760 feet
- **MAPS:** USGS *Big Meadows* and *Old Rag Mountain; Shenandoah National Park Whiteoak Canyon* and *Skyland* maps; *National Geographic Trails Illustrated Map #228 Shenandoah National Park*
- **CONTACT:** Shenandoah National Park
  3655 US 211 E.
  Luray, VA 22835-9036
  540-999-3500
  nps.gov/shen

The Hike at a Glance

- **0.4** Stay straight at four-way intersection; soon keeping right at loop trail intersection
- **0.7** Right at second four-way intersection and arrive at face of Stony Man; retrace steps to the four-way intersection and continue straight ahead
- **1.0** Keep more or less straight upon having returned to loop trail intersection; keep left onto the AT at the next intersection
- **1.7** Cliffs of Little Stony Man
- **1.9** Left onto Passamaquoddy Trail
- **2.9** Left onto Furnace Spring Horse Trail
- **3.5** Make a left just a few feet before returning the parking area

George Freeman Pollock opened his mountain resort, Skyland, to the public in 1888. A carriage road from Luray wound up the western slope of the Blue Ridge, carrying his guests to the lodge sitting below Stony Man. (The road is still in fairly good shape and can be walked from the resort down to the park boundary on the edge of Page Valley.) The resort was an almost immediate success, as flatlanders, politicians, and business leaders found it to be a congenial place to enjoy the beauty of the mountains and escape the heat of summers in the cities, valleys, and Piedmont. Yet, unlike many private landowners who, even today, oppose the establishment of federal- or state-protected lands, Pollock was a loyal supporter of Shenandoah National Park and worked diligently to make it become a reality. Today's visitors to Skyland have their choice of nearly 200 rooms (some in cabins) in which to stay, can enjoy their meals in the dining room, and can take guided horseback trips originating from the resort's stables.

Park service history records show that Pollock first came to the mountains on a scientific expedition to study mammal life on Stony Man for the Smithsonian Institution. Pollock's father had been part owner of a mining operation that had begun around the turn of the 19th century, when chunks of copper were found scattered about the summit of Stony Man. The ore, however, proved to be hard to work and operations ceased by the mid-1800s. Evidence of the mining can still be found, but only by those willing to search for it, as the land has had well over a century to hide the scars.

The first part of this hike to 4,010-foot Stony Man, the second-highest point in the park, is an extremely popular one, as you have to gain only about 300 feet in order to reach an Olympian 180-degree view. Most people, though, just follow what is known as the Stony Man Trail (it has signs keyed to a brochure) to the summit and retrace their steps back to the parking area. However, in this hike you will continue northward from Stony Man on the Appalachian Trail (which reaches its highest point in the park on the side of the mountain), leaving the bulk of the crowd behind, to come to another viewpoint on Little Stony Man, before following a historic route through a jade forest of evergreens and mountain laurels to return to the point of origin.

DIRECTIONS To reach the trailhead, drive into the north entrance of Skyland (Skyline Drive mile 41.7) and make a right into the first parking lot. White blazes mark the pathway you want to take as the Appalachian Trail, in addition to a trailhead sign that identifies it as the Stony Man Trail. Pick up a trail pamphlet from the dispenser and begin the gradual ascent into an oak forest. (If there are no brochures in the container, you can obtain one from the Byrd Visitor Center at Skyline Drive mile 51.0.)

Route Description

When the first version of this guidebook was written, there were still numerous silvery-gray logs scattered about the ground. Alas, there are currently very, very few of these reminders that are all that are left of the once-mighty chestnut trees that used to be so numerous that they made up more than 25% of the trees in Shenandoah's forest. The chestnut blight, a fungus disease accidentally introduced into North America from Asia near the beginning of the 20th century, removed the chestnuts from the landscape of the continent by the end of the 1930s. The chestnut had played an important role in the daily life of Blue Ridge Mountain residents. Being plentiful, the nuts were easily gathered in the fall, providing the mountain people with a supplement to their diet and a quick source of cash when sold by the bushel. The tree's timber was used to build log homes and durable fences to keep livestock from roaming too far. Its bark, rich in tannin, was stripped and sold to tanneries for the processing of hides. The inner bark also contains the tannin, which makes the wood resistant to decay. The roots and stumps of these fallen trees still produce sprouts that grow for a while before they become fungus-infected and die. The hope is that someday the sprouts will be able to resist the disease, or that scientists will develop a strain that will not succumb to the blight.

Just as the chestnuts have disappeared, there are now not as many fir and spruce trees

View from Little Stony Man Cliffs

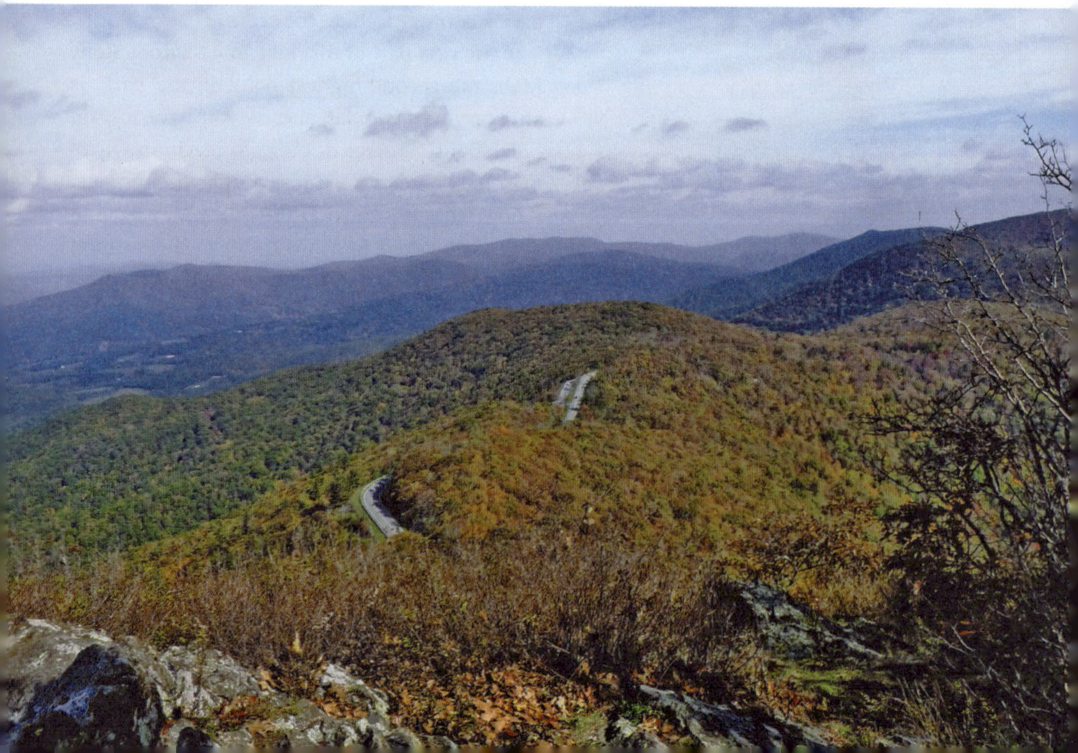

as there once were on Stony Man, but there are enough that this is your chance to learn how to tell them apart. The easiest way is to shake hands with their branches: the balsam fir will feel soft and welcoming to the touch, and while the red spruce's sharp, stiff needles won't puncture your skin, you certainly will not want to give it a firm handshake. Another way to distinguish the two is that the spruce's needles extend out from all sides of the branch, while the fir's needles have two white stripes on the bottom and grow with only two rows, one on each side of the branch.

Come to a four-way intersection at 0.4 mile. To the left it is 0.4 mile to the Skyland road; to the right, it's 0.6 mile to Little Stony Man Cliffs. You want to continue straight ahead on the trail, following blue blazes and keeping to the right at the next intersection to begin the loop trail toward the summit. This is a harsher environment, as evidenced by the stunted trees and, possibly, those struck by lightning. At 0.5 mile there is a wintertime view to the northeast of Nicholson Hollow. According to Pollock, years before the establishment of the national park, Aaron Nicholson and his relatives declared the hollow to be a "free state" and not subject to the laws and taxes of Virginia.

Arrive at another four-way intersection at 0.7 mile, where you want to make a right to come to the "face" of Stony Man for a grand view. Below is Page Valley, with Massanutten Mountain on its far side, and the town of Luray, with its nearby caverns that are the largest in the Shenandoah Valley. The buildings of Skyland are nearby, while the prominent peak to the south is Hawksbill (see Hike 26). The rocky summit you see to the north is Marys Rock (see Hike 22), and the cliffs closer by are Little Stony Man, where you will be standing a short time from now.

Retrace your steps back to the four-way intersection. Left is the way you came up and right is the horse trail; you want to keep straight, walking by gnarled tree trunks. Soon, bypass the horse trail that is paralleling on the right. At 1.0 mile you'll have returned to the loop-trail intersection, where you don't want to make the hard left but instead keep more or less straight to come to another four-way intersection. Straight ahead is the Stony Man Trail going back to the parking lot; to the right is the horse trail, which leads 0.4 mile to the road. You want to take the AT to the left, descending north through a heavy oak forest. The oak trees became dominant once the chestnuts had been killed by the blight.

Arrive at the cliffs of Little Stony Man at 1.7 miles, where you can look back up to the rock "face" of Stony Man. Switchback down, away from the cliffs. At 1.9 miles the AT goes right for 0.4 mile to the Little Stony Man Parking Area (Skyline Drive mile 39.1); you will go left to begin following blue-blazed Passamaquoddy Trail. The present-day path follows the general route of the original trail Pollock laid out in the 1930s. He evidently named the trail after himself, stating that the word means "abounding in pollock" in the language of Maine's Passamaquoddy. You'll soon pass by the lower cliffs of Little Stony Man and begin walking into a grand and deep forest of large oaks and evergreens. When the mountain laurel begins to become abundant, you may find it hard to believe there were once mining operations going on in the area.

Pay attention when you come to the intersection at 2.9 miles. Do not continue with the blue blazes, which follow the road 0.4 mile to the Skyland dining room. Instead, bear left onto the yellow-blazed Furnace Spring Horse Trail, still passing through a wonderful evergreen forest. This is one of my favorite spots because it is so quickly accessible from either the dining room or the Stony Man Trail parking lot, yet it seems as if almost no one ever walks this portion of the trail. Even horse traffic appears to be somewhat light on the ascending pathway. Make a left at the next intersection to return to your car, finishing this 3.5-mile walk.

Old Rag

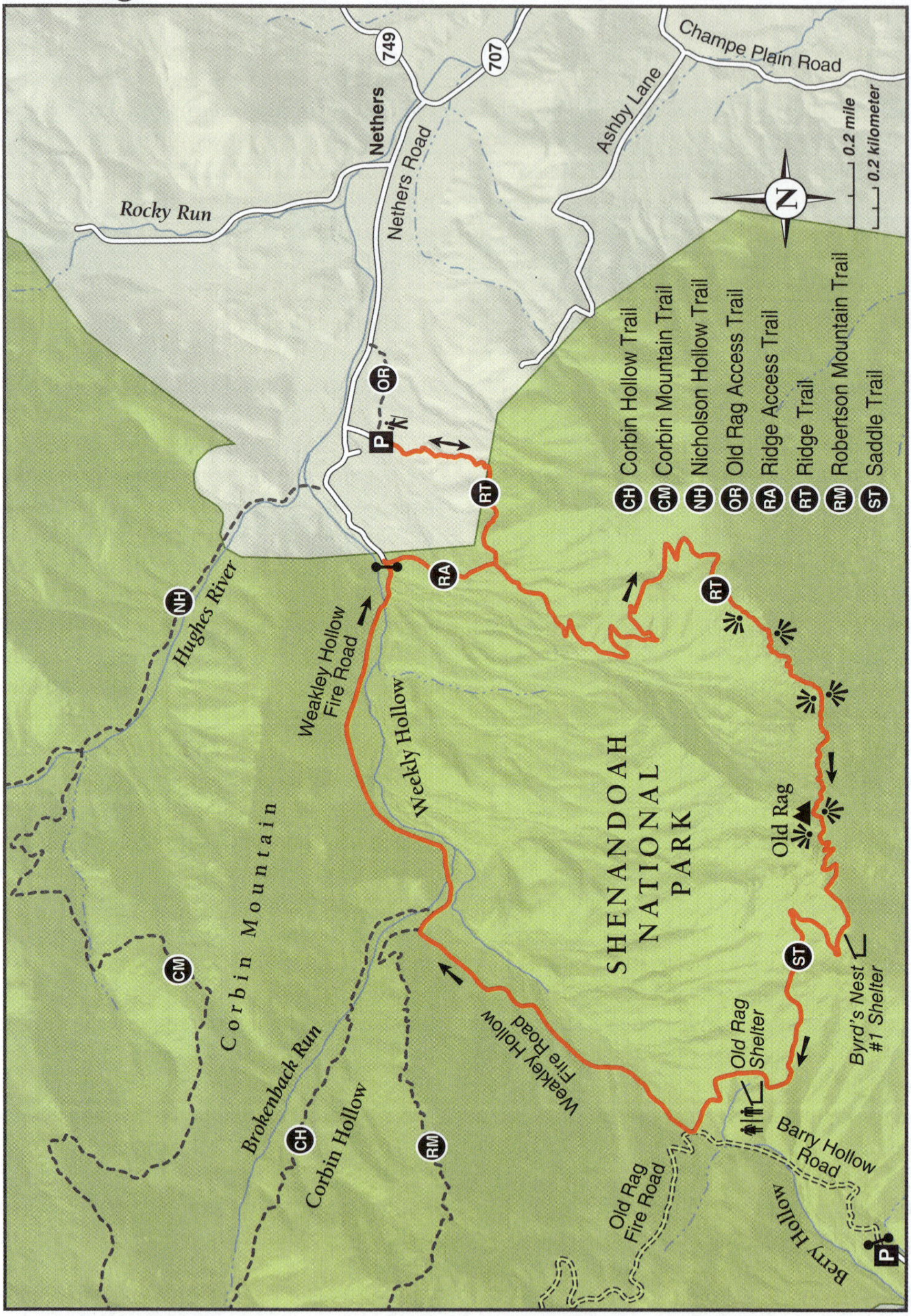

Champe Plain Road
749
707
Nethers
Nethers Road
Ashby Lane
Rocky Run
0.2 mile
0.2 kilometer
N
OR
P
RT
RA
NH
Hughes River
Weakley Hollow Fire Road
Weakly Hollow
SHENANDOAH NATIONAL PARK
Old Rag
Corbin Mountain
CM
Brokenback Run
CH
Corbin Hollow
RM
Weakley Hollow Fire Road
ST
Old Rag Shelter
Byrd's Nest #1 Shelter
Barry Hollow Road
Old Rag Fire Road
Berry Hollow
CH Corbin Hollow Trail
CM Corbin Mountain Trail
NH Nicholson Hollow Trail
OR Old Rag Access Trail
RA Ridge Access Trail
RT Ridge Trail
RM Robertson Mountain Trail
ST Saddle Trail

24 Old Rag

- **GPS:** N38.5708287 W78.2869461
- **TOTAL DISTANCE (circuit):** 9.2 miles
- **HIKING TIME:** 6.25 hours
- **VERTICAL RISE:** 2,380 feet
- **MAPS:** USGS *Old Rag Mountain; Shenandoah National Park Old Rag Trail* map; *National Geographic Trails Illustrated Map #228 Shenandoah National Park*
- **CONTACT:** Shenandoah National Park
  3655 US 211 E.
  Luray, VA 22835-9036
  540-999-3500
  nps.gov/shen

The Hike at a Glance

- 0.8 Ridge Access Trail comes in from the right; stay left
- 3.0 Crawl through 40-foot boulder tunnel; then ascend staircase into a narrow cleft
- 3.6 Old Rag summit
- 4.2 Byrd's Nest 1; begin following Saddle Trail
- 5.2 Old Rag Shelter
- 5.6 Begin following Weakly Hollow Road
- 6.0 Bypass Robertson Mountain Trail
- 6.8 Bypass Corbin Hollow Trail
- 8.0 Right onto Ridge Access Trail
- 8.4 Left onto Ridge Trail
- 9.2 Return to your automobile

The hike up the Ridge Trail to the summit of Old Rag is one of the most exhausting miles-long climbs in all of Virginia. Many people who have done the trip also say that it is by far one of the most fun excursions they have ever made. In order to reach the mountaintop, you're going to scramble over giant boulders, slide down bare rocks, crawl through narrow tunnels, and climb a unique staircase. If you are mentally prepared for these stone formations, you will feel like a kid again, bouncing around on a giant playground. If you view them as obstacles, you'll probably have a miserable time. As a bit of compensation, the route down the mountain is relatively easy, dropping first on a well-graded trail and then descending along gently sloping fire roads.

Be forewarned. This is an extremely popular hike. So popular, in fact, that the park service has had to build several parking lots to keep people from parking on private property or leaving automobiles beside the road while the owners went on a hike. Like the Cedar Run and Whiteoak Canyon hike (see Hike 25), I contemplated not including Old Rag in this book because of its heavy use, but I decided that the mountain is such a wonderful experience that excluding it would be a disservice to you. To avoid the largest crowds, I suggest you undertake the hike during the middle of the week and don't even consider it anytime during the autumn "leaf season." Also, to impact this heavily used area as little as possible, please make this just a day trip and don't camp anywhere along the route. (Park regulations prohibit camping above 2,800 feet in elevation.) Although you should do so on any hike you take, the park service asks that you "please stay on the official trail in order to avoid damaging the sensitive plant communities that grow on Old Rag's thin rocky soils."

DIRECTIONS Old Rag is an outlying mountain, not a part of the main crest of the Blue Ridge. To reach the trailhead, take VA 231 for 12.5 miles north of Madison (coming from the north this would be about 8 miles south of Sperryville); then turn onto VA 602, heading west toward Nethers. (There's a small spot next to the road, where you can pull off to eyeball the craggy ridgeline of Old Rag as it rises high above fields of planted crops.) You want to keep left 0.5 mile beyond the turn (do not cross the bridge) as VA 602 ends and becomes VA 601.

A short distance later, VA 601 ends and you want to stay straight, with the road designation becoming VA 707. Once more, this time in Nethers, you'll want to keep to the left, now taking VA 600 instead of continuing on VA 707, which goes off to the right. At 0.4 mile from this intersection you'll reach the first parking area, which is the overflow lot. (If you end up having to park here, you will take a pathway from it to the main parking area, adding about three-quarters of a mile to the overall length of the hike.) About 0.3 mile beyond the overflow lot is the main parking lot on the left where you will leave your car. (Just a bit beyond this lot is a horse trailer/RV parking lot.)

Note: There may be a fee to hike in this area, in addition to the usual park entrance fee.

Route Description

The park service contact station and bulletin board are at the end of the parking area just before you walk onto the trail and begin the ascent. The Ridge Access Trail comes in from the right (you will be returning via this route) at 0.8 mile; stay left on the Ridge Trail. Continuing with the ascent, you can see, through the leaves and at rock outcrops, the various hollows—Corbin, Weakley, and Nicholson—north of Old Rag. In the spring, the hillside at 2.1 miles is covered by a great field of trillium, just before you step over a water run lined with skunk cabbage.

Your gentle stroll is now over, as the trail becomes steeper and the rock scramble begins. The rocks at 2.7 miles allow you to survey the lands in and around Nicholson Hollow, where the Hughes River begins its journey from the Blue Ridge to meet the Hazel River in the Piedmont, about 10 miles east of the park boundary. Look above you to see a part of the rugged ridgeline and some of the rock outcrops you'll soon be traversing. A few steps farther on will give you a different perspective on the flatter lands to the southeast. As you continue to ascend, think of the huge boulders that you're going to have to use your hands, arms, legs, knees, and feet to climb over, under, and around as nature's giant "jungle gym." Doing so will keep you from becoming frustrated by how slowly you're now progressing up the mountain. At 3.0 miles, crawl through a 40-foot boulder tunnel and then take a staircase into a narrow cleft. The forces of wind, rain, ice, snow, and sunshine have weathered ages-old hardened lava into these 11 nicely spaced steps.

Advance, with periods of boulder-climbing, until you reach the sign marking the 3,268-foot summit of Old Rag at 3.6 miles. Park personnel have told me that they know of only four places in the national park where it's possible to obtain a 360-degree view—and you're now standing at one of them. Just about due west is Hawksbill (see Hike 26) and to the right of it and below Bettys Rock you will see the whitewater of the falls tumbling down Whiteoak Canyon (see Hike 25). Stony Man (see Hike 23) is a little farther to the right, while almost due north you can make out the granite bluffs of Marys Rock (see Hike 22). Below you is Weakley Hollow, which you will be following to return to your car. To the east and south is the great expanse of the Piedmont. As your gaze circles back around to the mountains, spot outlying Big Tom and Doubletop Mountains before your eyes come to rest on the green fields of Big Meadows on the main crest of the Blue Ridge.

After enjoying your lunch (please practice Leave No Trace ethics), take in the various viewpoints (avoiding the west summit, which is closed due to rare plant concerns) and study the rock under your feet. The Old Rag granite contains peanut-sized bits of feldspar and blue quartz. The quartz erodes more quickly, leaving little bits of the feldspar jutting up from the surface of the rock. Please don't be tempted to take any samples as souvenirs; in any case, rock in the park is just as protected by law as are the plants, animals, and artifacts.

After you have explored the mountaintop to your heart's content, return to the trail, following the blazes through mountain laurel on the southwest side of Old Rag, where you look down onto Byrds Nest 1. When you arrive at that structure at 4.2 miles, climb the rock behind it for some additional views. From the structure, you'll follow the Saddle Trail, passing a place where you can observe Whiteoak Canyon in greater detail than you did from the summit. You will also see the effect of thousands of people a year using the Old Rag Shelter (no overnight camping permitted) at 5.2 miles. The entire little knob that the shelter sits on is nearly devoid of any undergrowth. Rainwater is unable to soak into the hard-packed, bare ground, meaning the soil will continue to erode away in some areas near the shelter. It is because of this heavy use throughout the Old Rag area that I request that you refrain from camping anywhere along this entire hike route. Perhaps, in order to protect resources, the time has come for the park service to dismantle the Old Rag and Byrds Nest 1 shelters and totally ban camping within several miles of Old Rag.

Continue to follow blazes, now walking along the Old Rag Fire Road, which is lined by showy orchids in the spring. Also beside the road is running cedar, which resembles tiny hemlock or pine trees. This small club moss can trace its roots back more than 300 million years to when its ancestors grew to be more than 100 feet tall. Come to a four-way intersection at 5.6 miles. The Berry Hollow Fire Road descends to the left to go to a parking area on the park boundary. You want to keep straight for just a few feet so that you can make a right turn to descend along the Weakley Hollow Road. The Robertson Mountain Trail comes in from the left at 6.7 miles, as does the Corbin Hollow Trail at 6.8 miles. Continue downstream, passing hundreds of wildflowers, and cross Brokenback Run and side streams on footbridges. Just as you come to a gate at 8.0 miles, turn right and ascend along the Ridge Access Trail to the intersection with the Ridge Trail at 8.4 miles. Turn left onto it and retrace your steps back to your car at 9.2 miles. It's time to leaf through this guidebook again and begin planning your next walkabout.

The highest rock on the summit of Old Rag

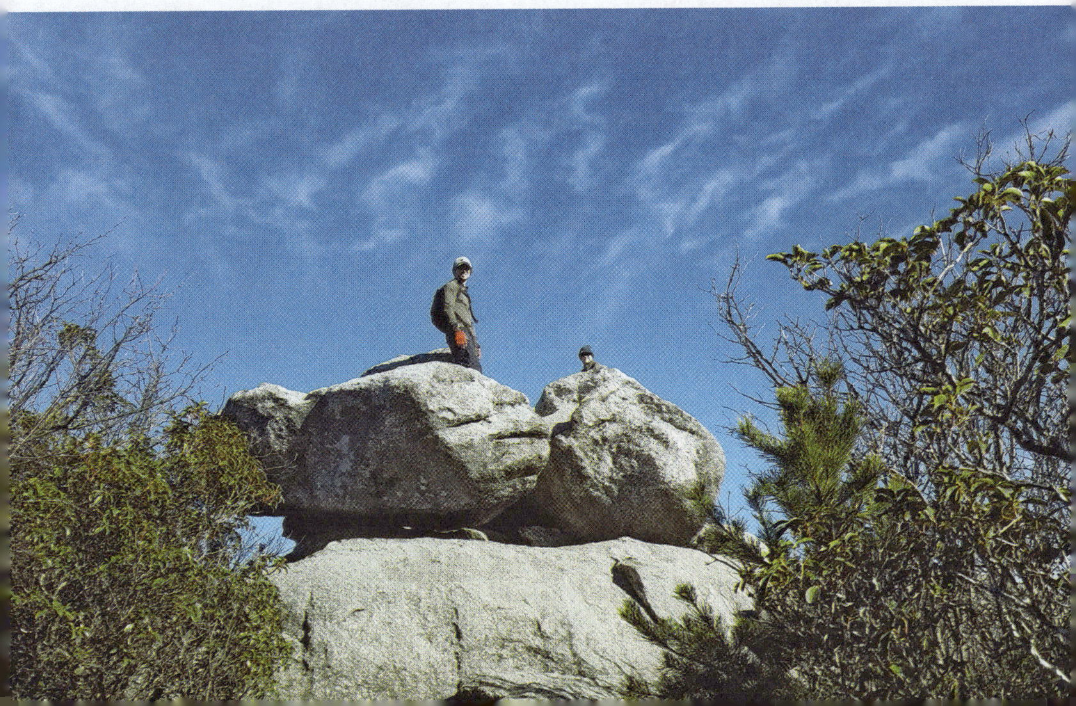

Cedar Run and Whiteoak Canyon

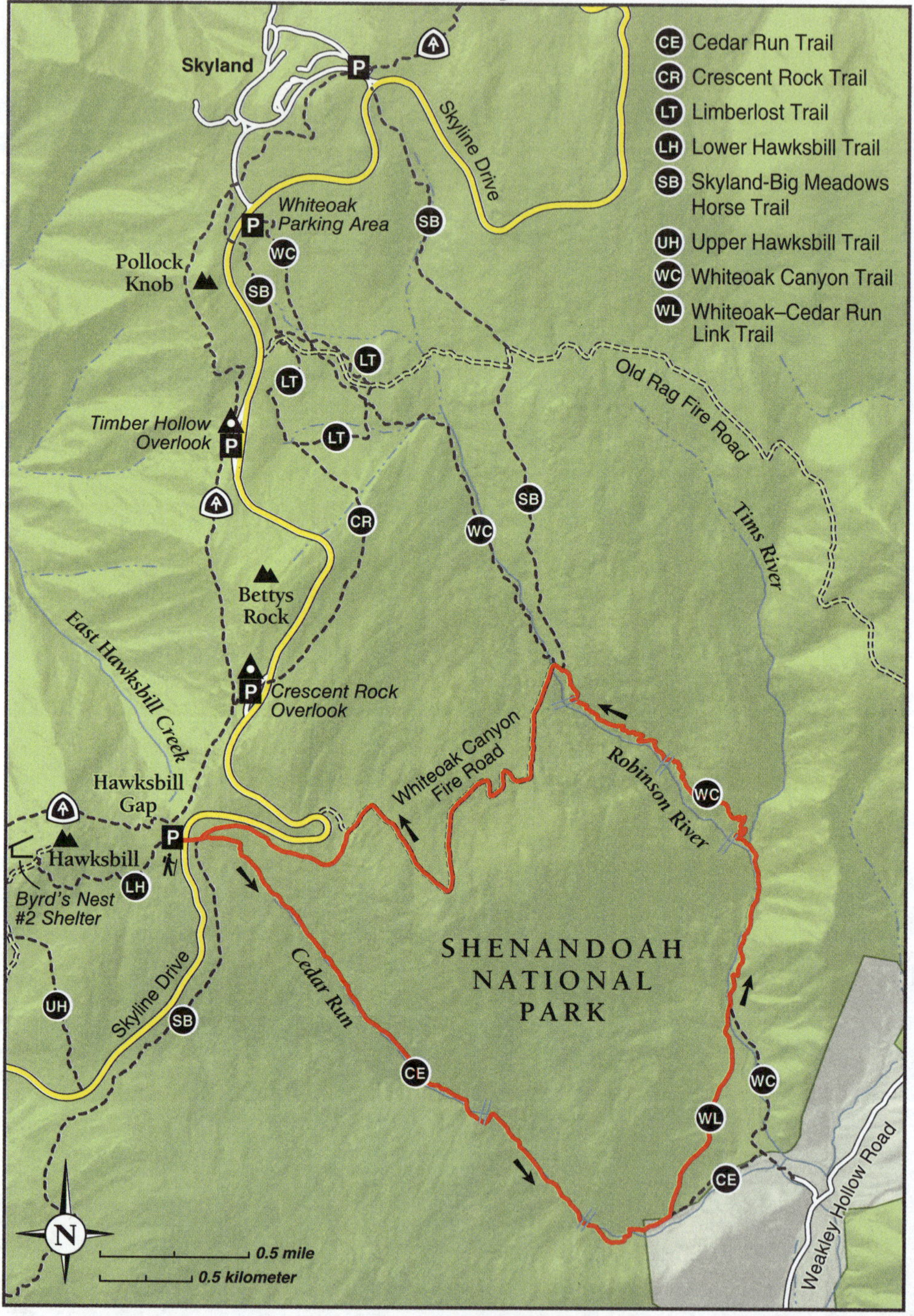

25 Cedar Run and Whiteoak Canyon

- **GPS:** N38.5561247 W78.3868561
- **TOTAL DISTANCE (circuit):** 8.0 or 9.3 miles
- **HIKING TIME:** 6.0 or 7.0 hours
- **VERTICAL RISE:** 2,320 or 2,560 feet
- **MAPS:** USGS *Big Meadows* and *Old Rag Mountain; Shenandoah National Park Old Rag Trail* map; *National Geographic Trails Illustrated Map #228 Shenandoah National Park*
- **CONTACT:** Shenandoah National Park
  3655 US 211 E.
  Luray, VA 22835-9036
  540-999-3500
  nps.gov/shen

The Hike at a Glance

- 1.5 Ford Cedar Run
- 2.5 Ford Cedar Run
- 2.6 Left onto Whiteoak–Cedar Run Link Trail
- 3.4 Come to Whiteoak Run; soon cross it and turn left onto Whiteoak Canyon Trail
- 4.1 Cross Whiteoak Run's largest tributary
- 5.4 Short side trail left to largest falls; return to main trail and continue to ascend. At next intersection is the departure of the longer hike (see below). To continue on shorter hike at this intersection, go upstream a few feet, cross Whiteoak Run on footbridge, go downstream, and turn right to ascend on Whiteoak Canyon Road
- 7.3 Take pathway to left
- 8.0 Right onto Cedar Run Trail; stay right at next intersection to return to parking area

The Hike at a Glance *(longer hike option)*

From intersection described in 5.4 above, continue upstream to top of Upper Falls and cross Whiteoak Run

- 7.1 Left onto Limberlost Trail
- 7.5 Left onto Crescent Rock Trail
- 8.6 Arrive at Crescent Rock Overlook; take connector trail to AT and turn left onto it
- 9.3 End of hike

The trails along Cedar Run and in Whiteoak Canyon are so popular that I debated for a long time about whether or not they should be included in this guidebook. The pathways are worn and eroded from thousands of feet tramping on them year after year, and the crowds during weekends in the summer and fall are so large that it may feel like you're going to a circus instead of taking a walk in the woods. Yet the waterfalls and scenery on this hike are so impressive that it would be gross negligence not to include it in a hiking guide to Virginia.

During the course of the trek, Cedar Run drops about 2,000 feet, creating numerous cascades and pools, while Whiteoak Canyon's six waterfalls are rated among the 13 highest in Shenandoah National Park. I have you descending along Cedar Run and, because I believe you can better observe waterfalls when walking up to them instead of looking back at them, ascending Whiteoak Run. When you reach Upper Falls in Whiteoak Canyon you will have the option of choosing one of two different routes. The first option is shorter and follows a dirt road for a distance, making the final ascent a bit easier. The longer option is a bit steeper but extends your time in the woods. No matter which option you choose, the ruggedness of terrain, rough conditions of the trails, slippery footing, and the fact that almost every bit of the vertical rise is accomplished in the 2-mile climb along Whiteoak Run make this a strenuous excursion.

DIRECTIONS Leave your car at the Lower Hawksbill Parking Area (Skyline Drive mile 45.6).

Route Description

Cross the road to begin descending on blue-blazed Cedar Run Trail. In less than 100 yards the Skyland–Big Meadows Horse Trail comes in from the right and, in a few feet, goes off to the left. You'll want to keep following the blue blazes. Pass by a spring at 0.3 mile; be careful about any off-trail wanderings because the stinging nettle is usually waist high by the middle of June. The trail continues to get rougher and rockier. At 0.5 mile, you'll begin walking next to Cedar Run as it descends the mountain in a series of small falls, passing one that drops about 25 feet at 0.7 mile.

At 1.0 mile, you will come to another series of cascades, some with the water spreading out across the full length of the streambed, others channeling the creek through narrow slots in the bedrock. You've walked 1.4 miles when you reach the spot where two streams meet the creek, so you deserve a break. Besides, Cedar Run has leveled out a bit here, and there is a small pebble beach and a deep pool made just for swimming. (Do be careful swimming in any stream. The water may be very cold, the rocks slippery, pools deeper than they appear, and the currents swift.) The large flat rock next to the pool provides a good place to soak up some sun after a quick dip in the cool, clear water.

There is another great swimming hole where you ford Cedar Run at 1.5 miles. You can go downstream a bit to overlook the largest falls of the run. Return to the trail to ascend 200 feet above the stream before descending steeply, almost straight down, on rough rock steps. By the time you've hiked 1.7 miles, the falls have become so numerous that it is nearly impossible to distinguish one from another; just enjoy all of this water dropping down the narrow gorge as the trail climbs high above the stream once more. Be alert at 2.5 miles, where the trail drops back down to the stream. The route makes a sudden switchback to the left to ford Cedar Run for the final time—avoid the mistake of continuing straight on a pathway that enters private property.

At an intersection at 2.6 miles, bear left onto Whiteoak–Cedar Run Link Trail. (The Cedar Run Trail to the right goes to the Berry Hollow Parking Area on VA 600. It also joins up with the Whiteoak Canyon Trail, but at a point a little lower than you need to go.) Now that you have swung away from the sound of rushing water, things seem quieter and more relaxed. The trail has only minor ups and downs, woodpeckers chip away at the trunks of hardwood trees, and the songs of other birds can now be heard coming from spots both near and far in the forest.

Come to Whiteoak Run at 3.4 miles, crossing it in just a few minutes to turn left and follow Whiteoak Canyon Trail upstream. (The trail also goes downstream about 0.8 mile to VA 600.) Remember that camping is not permitted anywhere in Whiteoak Canyon. You have now entered a land ruled by water. Contemplate the steep canyon walls high above you. Thousands of years of water rushing over prehistoric lava beds have carved out this deep and narrow gorge. The stream down here carries the cumulative flow of numerous springs that break forth from their underground flows near the crest of the Blue Ridge Mountains. Even in times of drought, water makes an impact here. The gorge is well protected from direct sunlight, meaning the floor of the canyon is less susceptible to evaporation, enabling plants to survive during times when their counterparts in other portions of the park are struggling to live.

The route back up to Skyline Drive will be almost as steep, rough, and rocky as the one you descended upon. At 4.1 miles, cross over the largest tributary of Whiteoak Run (look upstream to see that it has its own set of small falls) and come to the first of many falls (this one has about a 60-foot drop) you will be treated to while on the Whiteoak Canyon Trail. After viewing the falls, negotiate a series of switchbacks and a section that involves some steep climbing. A rock facing permits a view through the canyon and across to some of the mountains along the eastern edge of the park. A few cedar trees are found along this section of the trail, and the ones that grow in the open are gnarled and twisted, reminiscent of trees exposed to the harsh conditions of the high Rocky Mountains.

Pass another falls at 4.7 miles; so much water is draining into this gorge that the liquid seems to just ooze out of the canyon walls. In five minutes you will be standing at the top of one falls and then, almost immediately, at the base of another. It may sound like the stream is getting larger and noisier as you walk by the large boulder at 5.1 miles. Once you get past it and the sound drops back to its normal level, you'll realize that the face of this giant rock echoes the sounds of the rushing water. Ascend some concrete and stone steps where, once again, the rock walls have water running down them. Come to an intersection at 5.4 miles; take the short side trail to the left to view the largest of the falls, which drop nearly 90 feet into the canyon. If by some miracle you have not met anyone on the hike so far, you are almost guaranteed to do so here. Upper Falls is one of the most popular spots in the park, and the majority of people who visit Whiteoak Canyon from Skyline Drive go no farther downstream. Return to the main trail and continue your ascent to a bit of level land at the top of the falls. This place was a popular attraction years before Shenandoah National Park was established. A wagon road extending from Skyland brought in visitors by the hundreds. George Freeman Pollock, who founded Skyland in the 1890s, became known for the fabulous and elaborate picnics he supplied for his guests when they came here to enjoy the falls and take a dip in the stream.

There is an intersection here, and this is the place at which you will have to decide whether to take the longer or the shorter hike. The longer trek is detailed in the final two paragraphs below; to continue with the shorter hike, go upstream a few feet to cross Whiteoak Run on a footbridge. Once on the other side, go downstream to turn right and ascend on the yellow-blazed Whiteoak Canyon Road.

At a right-hand switchback at 7.3 miles, the road goes 0.1 mile to Skyline Drive near mile 45. You want to continue following the yellow blazes by taking the pathway that heads off to the left. At 8.0 miles you'll arrive back at the Cedar Run Trail. Make a right onto it and stay right at the next intersection to end the hike in less than five more minutes in Hawksbill Gap.

If you are doing the longer hike, you will continue upstream from the intersection at the top of Upper Falls to cross Whiteoak Run in a few minutes and ascend along the left side of the creek. At 7.1 miles you want to leave Whiteoak Canyon Trail and turn left onto Limberlost Trail. Slow down and take in the drama of this place.

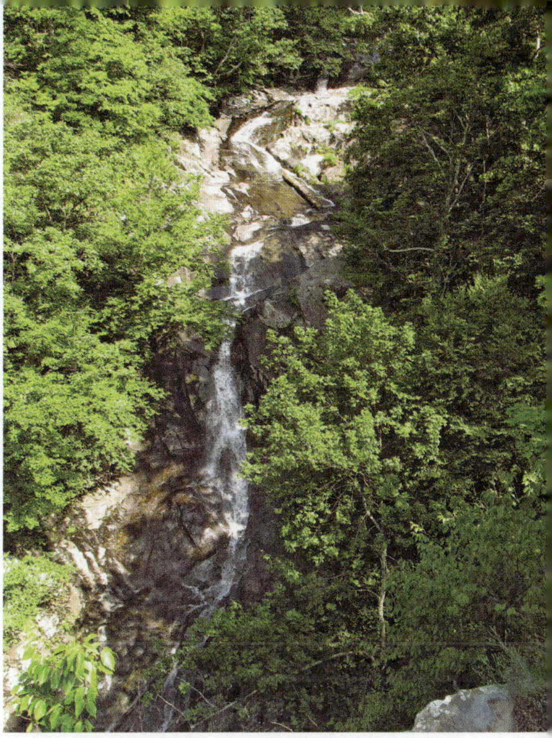

View of Upper Falls photo: Johnny Molloy

Before they started dying due to the infestations of the hemlock woolly adelgid, giant hemlocks in this forest were believed to be 270–370 years old. The often-heard cry of a barred owl simply adds to the romance of the woods. Pollock gave the area its name because it reminded him of Gene Stratton Porter's *Girl of the Limberlost.* Pollock was not only the founder of Skyland but also an ardent supporter of the establishment of Shenandoah National Park. His wife, Addy, purchased the hemlocks to save them from timbering. Sadly, almost all the trees are dead; the park service is treating some in the hope that at least a few may survive. An excellent account of the Pollocks' story is told in Reed L. Engle's book *In the Light of the Mountain Moon: An Illustrated History of Skyland.*

At the next intersection at 7.5 miles, the Limberlost Trail goes off to the right and you want to keep to the left, ascending on the Crescent Rock Trail. Arrive at Crescent Rock Overlook (Skyline Drive mile 44.4) at 8.6 miles and take the connector pathway to intersect the Appalachian Trail (AT). Turn left on the AT, passing underneath Crescent Rock and on to the next intersection, where you'll make another left to end the hike in Hawksbill Gap at 9.3 miles.

Hawksbill

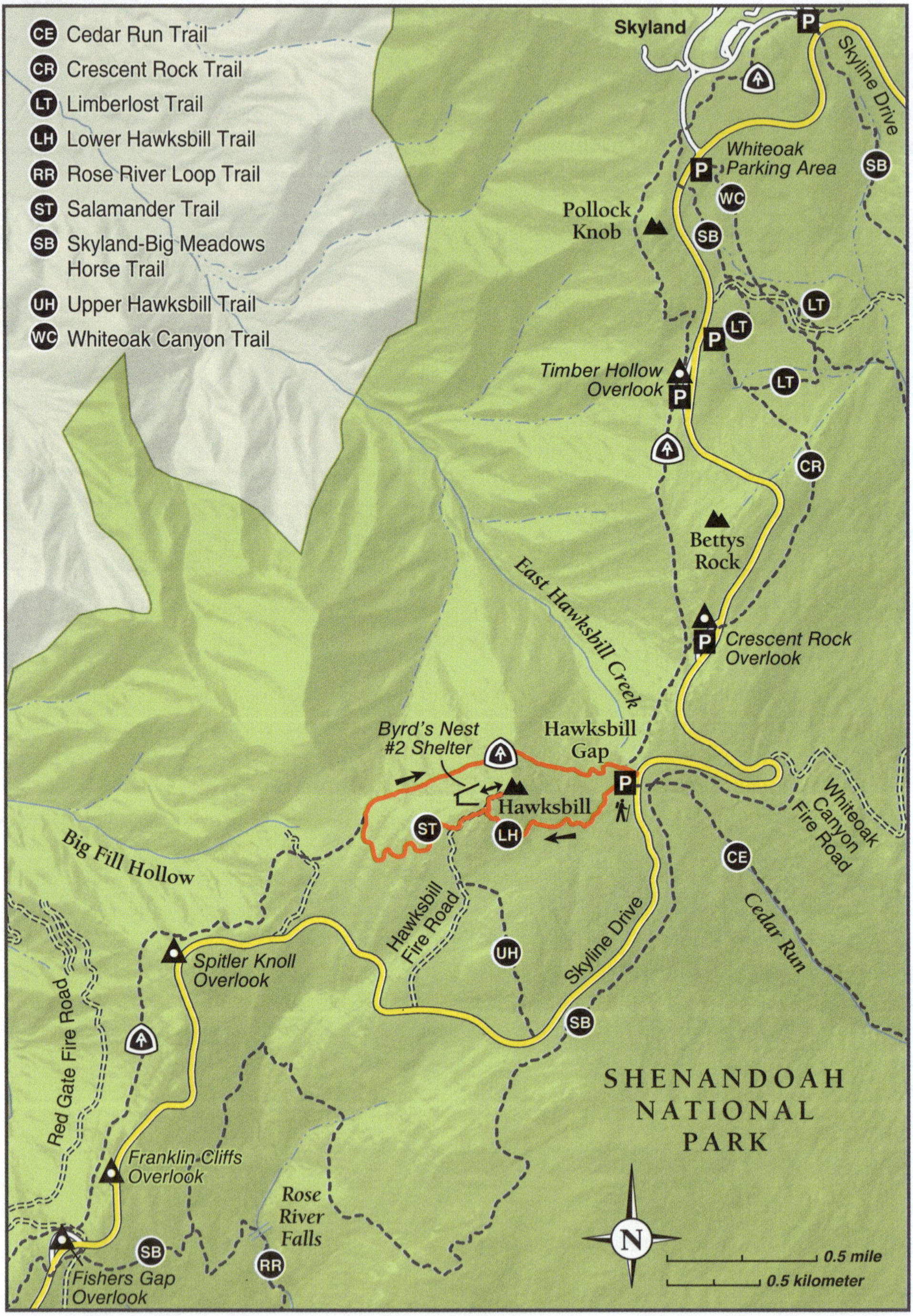

CE Cedar Run Trail
CR Crescent Rock Trail
LT Limberlost Trail
LH Lower Hawksbill Trail
RR Rose River Loop Trail
ST Salamander Trail
SB Skyland-Big Meadows Horse Trail
UH Upper Hawksbill Trail
WC Whiteoak Canyon Trail
Skyland
Skyline Drive
Whiteoak Parking Area
Pollock Knob
Timber Hollow Overlook
Bettys Rock
Crescent Rock Overlook
East Hawksbill Creek
Byrd's Nest #2 Shelter
Hawksbill Gap
Hawksbill
Whiteoak Canyon Fire Road
Big Fill Hollow
Hawksbill Fire Road
Cedar Run
Spitler Knoll Overlook
Skyline Drive
Red Gate Fire Road
SHENANDOAH NATIONAL PARK
Franklin Cliffs Overlook
Rose River Falls
Fishers Gap Overlook
N
0.5 mile
0.5 kilometer

26 Hawksbill

- **GPS:** N38.5561247 W78.3868561
- **TOTAL DISTANCE (circuit):** 2.8 miles
- **HIKING TIME:** 1.75 hours
- **VERTICAL RISE:** 740 feet
- **MAPS:** USGS *Big Meadows; National Geographic Trails Illustrated Map #228 Shenandoah National Park*
- **CONTACT:** Shenandoah National Park
  3655 US 211 E.
  Luray, VA 22835-9036
  540-999-3500
  nps.gov/shen

The Hike at a Glance

0.7 Right onto trail that leads to shelter and Hawksbill summit; after enjoying the summit, retrace steps to intersection and make a right onto Salamander Trail

1.7 Right onto AT

2.7 Leave AT and bear right

2.8 Return to parking area

There is an attraction about the "most" of something that fascinates humans and tends to draw us toward these famous entities. Tourists visit One World Trade Center in New York because, in part, it is the "tallest" building in the country. We idolize athletes who are the "best" in their chosen sport. Bloomington, Minnesota, has a mall that has drawn thousands of shoppers yearly ever since it became known as the "largest" in America. Spelunkers are always looking for the "deepest" cavern, and, conversely, hikers often have the desire to top the "highest" summit. Hawksbill is not the tallest mountain in the Old Dominion (Mount Rogers in southern Virginia has that honor), but it does have the distinction of being the loftiest peak within the boundaries of Shenandoah National Park.

Unlike the long and involved climbs that you must undertake in order to attain many other paramount pinnacles, the nice thing about Hawksbill is that it may be reached in a moderately easy ascent of less than 700 feet in elevation from where you leave your car. Like Marys Rock (see Hike 22), Hawksbill is a grand spot from which to watch the annual fall hawk migration. The circuit hike is, in fact, a good birder's walk year-round. Evening grosbeaks—not often seen during the warmer months in the mid-Atlantic states—and pine siskins have been spotted fluttering around the evergreens in winter, while ruffed grouse go about their mating rituals in the spring. Warblers and juncos usually become quite common as the temperatures warm up. In the past, the park service has used Hawksbill to participate in a program of reintroducing peregrine falcons to the Blue Ridge Mountains. Up until the mid-1950s, these raptors could be seen rocketing about the North American skies at speeds of more than 100 miles per hour. Yet, like the osprey and the bald eagle, they fell victims to the cumulative effects of DDT. The insecticide caused some hatchlings to be born deformed, but more commonly it weakened the shells of the birds' eggs to the point that the eggs simply could not hold together long enough for the chicks to be born. Now that DDT has been banned in the United States, breeding the birds in captivity and then releasing them into the wild has proven somewhat successful in preserving the species.

DIRECTIONS The hike begins from the Hawksbill Gap Parking Area (Skyline Drive mile point 45.6), about 15 miles south of US 211 in Thornton Gap or approximately 20 miles north of US 33 in Swift Run Gap.

Route Description

Take the trail from the parking lot, following it to the left, as you will be returning on the pathway coming in from the right.

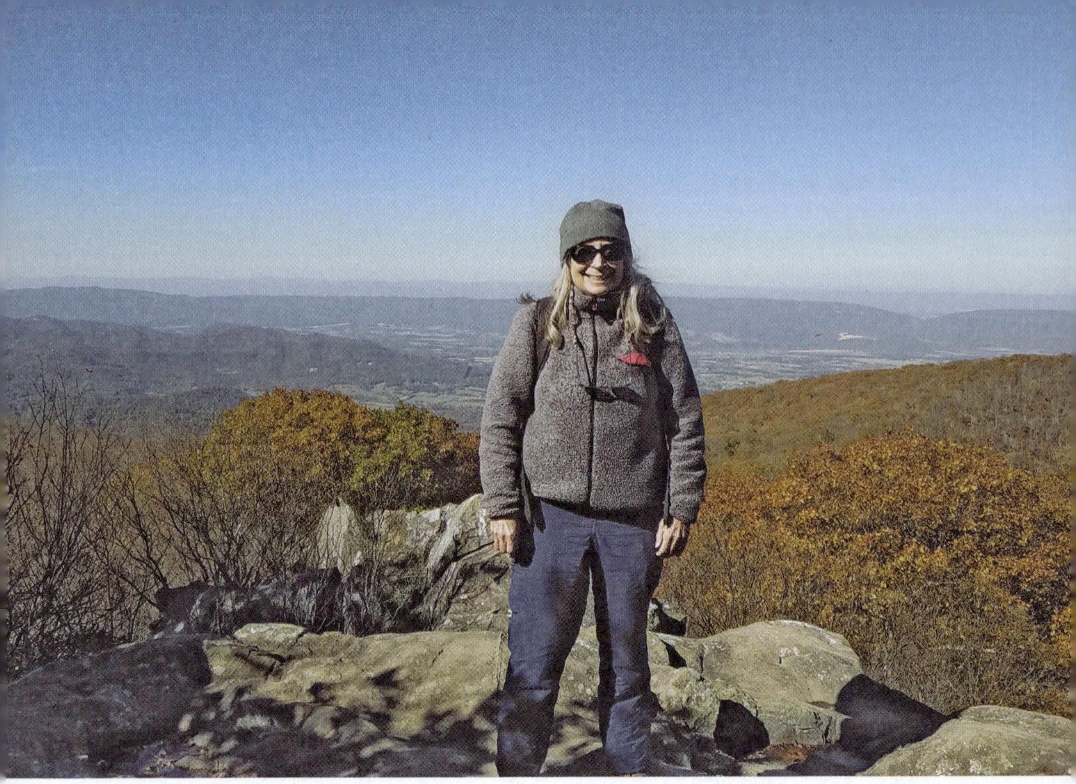

On the summit of Hawksbill

Your route ascends through balsam fir and red spruce, holdovers from another time. The Ice Age's cooler temperatures permitted these trees, more typical of New England and Canada, to begin to compete with, and even gain a foothold against, the traditional southern hardwoods such as oaks and poplars. Once the northern glaciers receded and warmer temperatures returned, most of the northern plants died out, unable to tolerate a southern climate. However, the cooler temperatures on the higher peaks and ridges of the Blue Ridge, such as Hawksbill, have allowed some of these trees to remain and prosper, separated from their relatives several hundred miles to the north. Look at the range map of a tree identification guide and you will see that a tree mixed in with the evergreens here, the mountain ash, extends itself as far south as northern Georgia only by clinging to the high elevations of the Appalachian Mountain chain.

A side trail to the left at 0.2 mile runs less than 100 feet to a spring that can usually be counted on to flow throughout the year. The trail makes several switchbacks before leveling out somewhat at 0.5 mile; striped maple is abundant in the understory. Its bright-yellow flowers, hanging as long-stemmed clusters, make their appearance at just about the time of year when warm temperatures become a daily occurrence. At 0.6 mile enter the no-camping zone, and at 0.7 mile make a right turn at a trail intersection to come to Byrds Nest Shelter 2 and the Hawksbill's summit at 0.8 mile.

Continue to the stone-walled outlook for the almost, but not quite, 360-degree panorama for which you've gained this elevation. Almost directly beneath you are Timber and Buracker hollows, funneling and dropping East Hawksbill Creek out to the town of Luray, some 3,000 feet below where you are standing. (East Hawksbill Creek, accessible by bushwhacking from Hawksbill Gap, is highly recommended as a native-trout fishing stream by Harry Slone in his *Trout Streams of Virginia*.) The view westward is of Page Valley, which, except for those who are sticklers for technicalities, is really just the easternmost portion of the Shenandoah

Valley. The two sections of the valley come back together near Harrisonburg, where Massanutten Mountain (see Hikes 19–21), the massive ridge due west, comes to an end. Northward you can see Skyline Drive making a wide swing eastward around a prominent rock outcrop, Stony Man (see Hike 23). To the east is Old Rag (see Hike 24), bristling with its noticeable rocky ridgeline and jagged summit. To the south is Spitler Hill, and closer (to the southwest) is rounded Naked Top.

After your picnic-lunch break at 4,049 feet above sea level, return to the shelter, walking past it to turn right onto the blue-blazed Salamander Trail and soon walking out of the no-camping zone.

Intersect the Appalachian Trail (AT) at 1.7 miles. To the left it goes 2.2 miles to Fishers Gap and Skyline Drive mile point 49.3. You need to make a right, descending and then ascending on the fern-lined AT and listening for the cry of a pileated woodpecker. If you don't know how one sounds, just think of Woody Woodpecker; he and his laugh were patterned after the pileated woodpecker (although some ornithologists claim it is more akin to the acorn woodpecker's call). If, as many ornithologists believe, the ivory-billed woodpecker may be extinct, then the nearly 20-inch pileated will inherit the status of being North America's largest woodpecker. At 2.2 miles, you will swing around a large rock promontory to cross a series of rockslides, or talus slopes, whose openings in the forest canopy can provide limited views of Stony Man to the north. For the second time on this hike, mountain ash trees are part of the forest. Not really an ash but, rather, a member of the rose family, it has red berries that usually hang on the tree well into winter, providing food for grosbeaks and other birds. People of the southern Appalachians used to make a tonic from the juice of the berry to treat a variety of ailments.

You will soon begin a quick switchbacking descent along a spur ridge to arrive at an intersection at 2.7 miles. The AT keeps to the left and reaches Stony Man in 2.7 miles. You want to make a right turn and go 500 feet to return to the parking area in Hawksbill Gap at 2.8 miles.

The ascent to Hawksbill is relatively easy, despite it being the highest point in Shenandoah National Park.

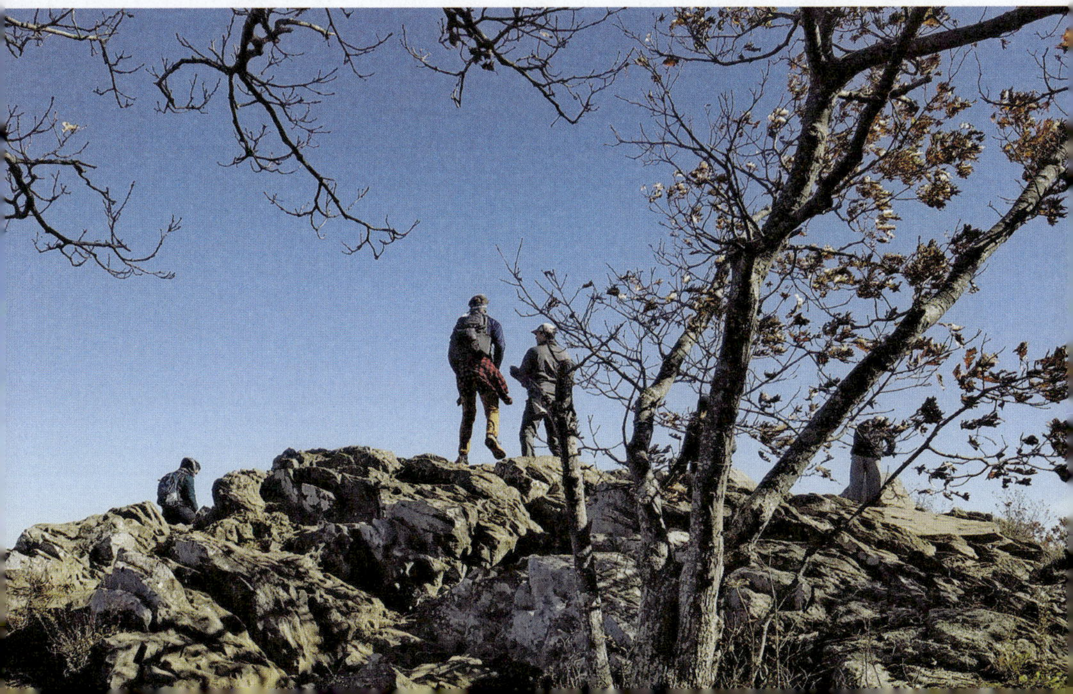

Rapidan Camp

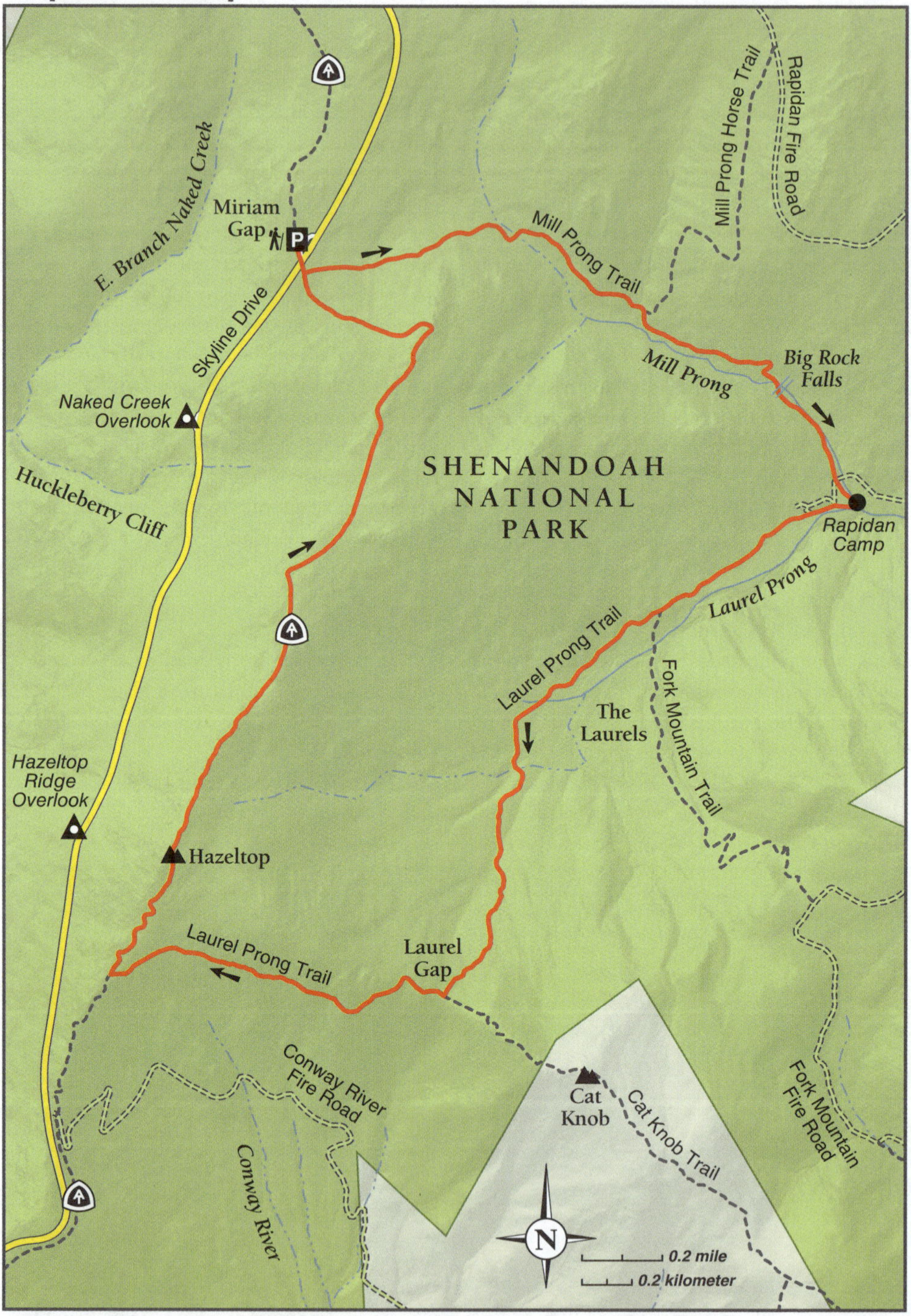

27 Rapidan Camp

- **GPS:** N38.5002967 W78.4457049
- **TOTAL DISTANCE (circuit):** 7.4 miles
- **HIKING TIME:** 5.0 hours
- **VERTICAL RISE:** 1,480 feet
- **MAPS:** USGS *Fletcher* and *Big Meadows; National Geographic Trails Illustrated Map #228 Shenandoah National Park*
- **CONTACT:** Shenandoah National Park
  3655 US 211 E.
  Luray, VA 22835-9036
  540-999-3500
  nps.gov/shen

The Hike at a Glance

0.0 Cross Skyline Drive and in a few feet bear left on Mill Prong Trail
1.1 Cross stream and keep to right at intersection
1.9 Arrive at Rapidan Camp and follow interpretive trail
2.2 Walk away from camp on Laurel Prong Trail (gravel road)
2.5 Keep right on Laurel Prong Trail
3.8 Keep right on Laurel Prong Trail
4.9 Bear right onto AT
5.4 Hazeltop Mountain summit
7.3 Left at intersection
7.4 Return to parking area

Shortly after he was elected president in 1928, Herbert Hoover sent his personal staff on a search for the perfect site for a weekend retreat. He stipulated that it had to be within a day's drive from Washington, D.C., and, in order to be an escape from the heat of summer and as free of mosquitoes as possible, above 2,500 feet in elevation. Being an ardent angler, Hoover's most stringent requirement was that the site had to contain favorable trout-fishing streams. The location of Rapidan Camp on the eastern edge of the Blue Ridge Mountains next to the Rapidan River met all these requirements. Hoover, declining to use federal funds or offers of assistance from the Commonwealth of Virginia, purchased the land and building materials himself.

The Marine Corps, as part of a training exercise, constructed roads and 13 buildings, completing the major portion of Rapidan Camp in 1929. Hoover and his wife, Lou, came to the camp often during his term to escape the rigors of being America's First Family, but the president also used the retreat to meet with high-level government officials and foreign dignitaries. Probably the most memorable of such meetings was with the prime minister of Great Britain, Ramsey MacDonald, in which world armaments and limits on naval power were discussed. Upon losing a bid for reelection in 1932, the Hoovers donated the camp and 164 acres to the Commonwealth of Virginia for inclusion in the proposed Shenandoah National Park, which was established in 1935. He had hoped that future presidents would continue to use his camp, but Franklin Delano Roosevelt, due to having polio, could not negotiate the topography and established a new retreat in Maryland, Camp David.

Interpretive tours of Rapidan Camp are available during the season. Check at visitor centers for the latest information. The grounds of the camp are open to the public year-round and can be reached by way of this circuit hike. The trip takes in the two streams that come together at the camp to form the Rapidan River, the short interpretive trail winding through the camp that gives bits of information about the area, and a lush stand of mountain laurel.

DIRECTIONS If you have two cars and wish to shorten the hike by 2.0 miles, you can leave one car at Booten's Gap (Skyline Drive mile 55.1). To begin the hike, leave your car in the Milam Gap Parking Area (Skyline Drive mile 52.8).

Route Description

Cross the drive and enter the woods on the Appalachian Trail (AT). In a few hundred feet you will want to take the blue-blazed Mill Prong Trail, which heads off to the left and passes through an overgrown orchard. Amazingly, despite this spot's proximity to the road and all of the developments around Big Meadows Lodge, I have twice seen black bears lumbering around these old fruit trees. Bears are omnivores, and vegetative matter is the largest part of their diet, so these bears may have been enjoying fruit from trees that were planted in the 1920s or earlier. Actually, it seems like bears will consume just about anything, including twigs, leaves, roots, nuts, insects, carrion, and berries. They tear the bark off a tree in order to consume the cambium, or the living inner bark of the tree. Everyone knows that bears love honey and the honeycomb, but they will also eat the bees and their larvae. Most of the animal protein in their diet comes from grubs, ants, termites, beetles, and other insects, with fish and small mammals, such as mice and voles, comprising the bulk of the small amount of meat they do consume.

Cross Mill Prong at 0.7 mile. At 1.1 miles, cross a side stream and come to a T-intersection. The trail to the left goes about 0.8 mile to the Rapidan Fire Road and then 2.2 miles to Big Meadows. You, however, want to bear right, following the trail, which at this point is open to horses and is identified as such by being blazed yellow. You will soon be walking along Mill Prong, where in times of plentiful rainfall there are small cascading waterfalls and pools that may entice you to soak your feet for a while. Stinging nettle and jewelweed, as they often do, grow side by side. In the fall you can find out why jewelweed is also known as touch-me-not. When its seedpods are good and ripe, just touching them will cause them to explode open, casting the seeds in all directions.

At 1.5 miles, you will begin a switchback and quick descent, entering a no-camping zone. A couple of minutes later you'll cross Mill Prong a few feet below 10-foot Big Rock Falls. Continue descending in this pretty little green stream valley of moss, boulders, hardwoods, and hemlocks. The Rapidan Fire Road comes in from the left at 1.9 miles, where you'll bear right to arrive in Rapidan Camp. Three of the original 13 buildings are still standing. The one in the middle is the President's Cabin, and the Prime Minister's Cabin (where MacDonald stayed during his visits) is on the right. President Hoover's guard, secretary, and manager, Larry Richey, and the president's physician, Dr. Joel T. Boone Jr., stayed in the Creel Cabin, the smaller building to the left. Take the signed interpretive trail through the grounds, and perhaps you can recapture the days when government policy was decided while casting fishing lines into the water and international politics were discussed while sitting on an old log. Just behind the cabins, Mill Prong and Laurel Prong meet to form the Rapidan River. The Rapidan flows eastward to join up with the Rappahannock River a few miles northwest of Fredericksburg. In turn, the Rappahannock continues the march, becoming miles wide before it finally deposits the water you see flowing past you at Rapidan Camp into the Chesapeake Bay.

Finishing the interpretive trail, walk away from the camp on a gravel road, the yellow-blazed Laurel Prong Trail. At 2.2 miles the road forks—take the one to the left and not the one going directly uphill. At 2.5 miles the road becomes Fork Mountain Trail and heads off to the left. You will need to follow the now blue-blazed Laurel Prong Trail to the right as you leave the no-camping zone. After crossing Laurel Prong, come to a zone of transition at 3.5 miles, where mountain laurel appears in abundance for the first time on this hike. The ascent also becomes a bit steeper.

At the top of the ridgeline, at 3.8 miles, arrive at a T-intersection. To the left, Cat Knob Trail goes about half a mile to meet the Jones Mountain Trail. Bear right, continuing on Laurel Prong Trail to a break in the vegetation that permits a view of Booten's Gap and the Shenandoah Valley beyond. There is some interesting-looking rock tripe on the rock formations you pass at 4.2 miles. While tripe is not the best-tasting of foods, stories abound of people lost or trapped in alpine areas who have survived for days by eating nothing but lichen such as this. (Please don't taste the rock tripe here. Remember, it is against the law to pick any vegetation in the park.)

You will come to another T-intersection at 4.9 miles. If you have been able to arrange for an automobile at Booten's Gap (Skyline Drive mile 55.1), you can turn left to follow the AT to end the walk in half a mile. To continue on the circuit hike, bear right and follow the AT up the southern flank of Hazeltop Mountain to the 3,812-foot summit at 5.4 miles. This is a totally different environment from that at Rapidan Camp. The soil is drier, the forest is almost exclusively hardwoods, the rocks of the ridgeline are uplifted and tilted, and there are gooseberries and fields of cow parsnip. Pass through a grove of hawthorns on sloping land at 6.2 miles. Because of the complexity and difficulty of distinguishing one type of hawthorn from another, there is no agreement as to how many different kinds there are throughout the world. Some botanists say 120, while others declare there are more than 1,200. Be that as it may, the heavy foliage and sharp-tipped thorns of the trees provide a well-protected nesting site for many different species of birds. Arrive back at the Mill Prong–AT intersection at 7.3 miles, where you'll turn left to return to Milam Gap and the Skyline Drive to finish the hike at 7.4 miles.

The Byrd Visitor Center is less than 2 miles to the north on Skyline Drive and is certainly worth a visit now that you're in the area. You can obtain information on various aspects of the park, pick up a backcountry camping permit, study the exhibits showing the human and natural history of the area, and watch movies or attend ranger-led programs about the park. Books, maps, and more are sold here; if you want more information on Rapidan Camp, you can pick up a copy of Darwin Lambert's *Herbert Hoover's Hideaway*.

Adjacent to the visitor center is the Big Meadows complex, containing a lodge, picnic area, campground, and wayside camp store and restaurant. In-season, interpretive programs are given in the amphitheater, and if you're lucky, you might happen to catch a lap dulcimer concert or a bit of mountain music in the lodge's taproom.

You might spot a black bear at Rapidan Camp.

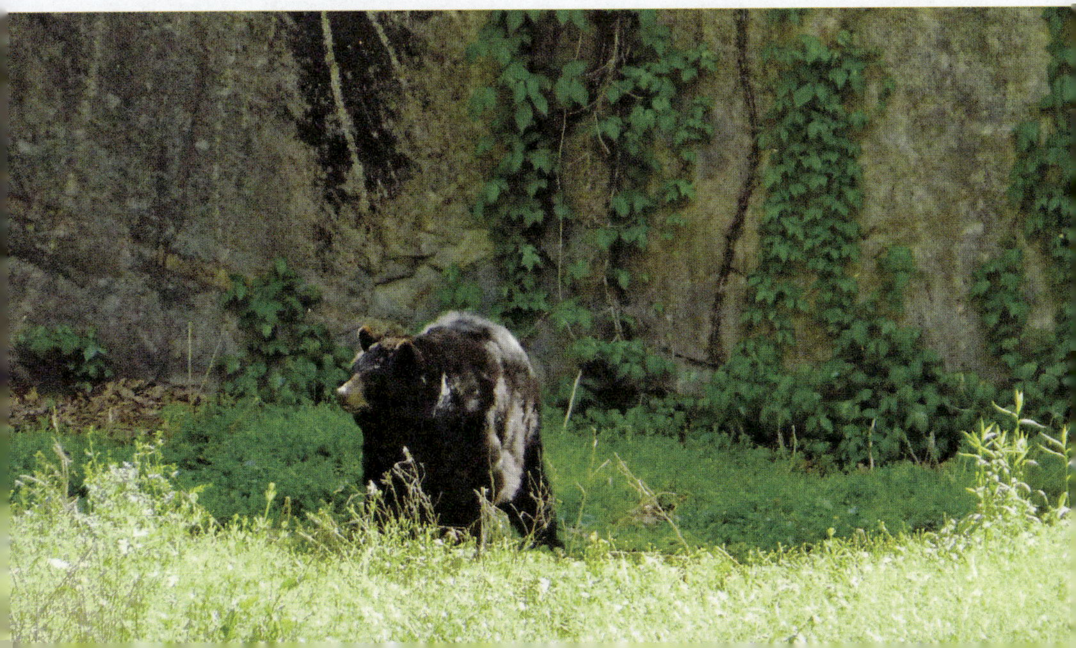

Rocky Mountain, Brown Mountain, and Rockytop

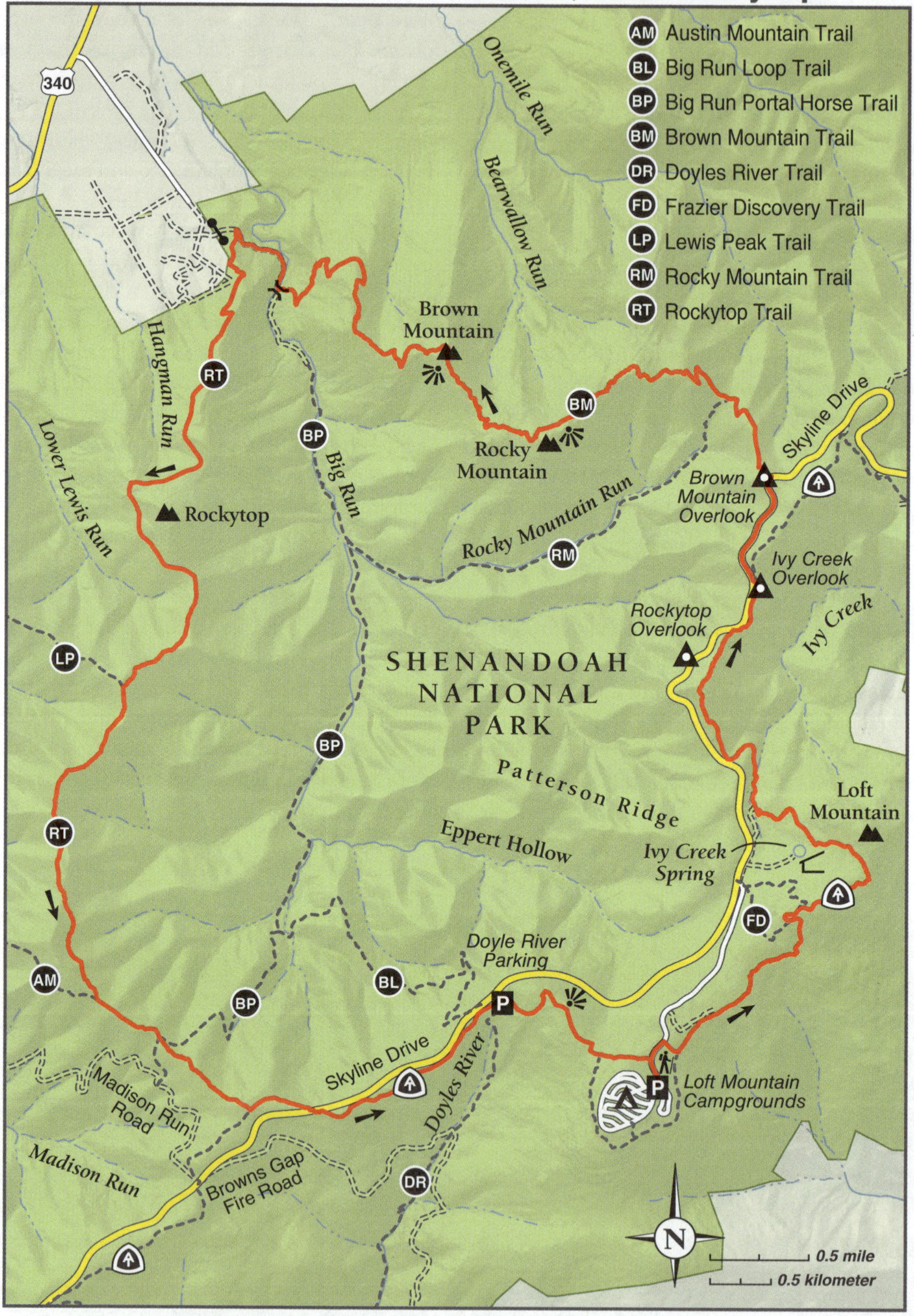

28 Rocky Mountain, Brown Mountain, and Rockytop

- **GPS:** N38.2475100 W78.6677926
- **TOTAL DISTANCE (circuit):** 20.0 miles
- **HIKING TIME:** 12 hours; recommended as a 2-day backpacking trip
- **VERTICAL RISE:** About 4,000 feet
- **MAPS:** USGS *McGaheysville* and *Browns Cove; National Geographic Trails Illustrated Map #228 Shenandoah National Park*
- **CONTACT:** Shenandoah National Park
  3655 US 211 E.
  Luray, VA 22835-9036
  540-999-3500
  nps.gov/shen

The Hike at a Glance

0.4 Left onto the AT

1.5 Frazier Discovery Trail is on the left; stay right on AT

1.6 Frazier Discovery Trail is on the left; stay right on AT

2.5 Trail to left goes to Ivy Creek Spring; stay right on AT

3.2 Cross Ivy Creek

4.6 Come to Ivy Creek Overlook and begin to follow Skyline Drive northward

5.2 Come to Brown Mountain Overlook and begin to follow Brown Mountain Trail

5.9 Rocky Mountain Trail comes in from left; stay right

6.8 Rocky Mountain summit

8.2 Brown Mountain summit

10.3 Intersect the Big Run Portal Trail, turn left, but make a right turn in a few feet, so as to not stay on the Big Run Portal Trail

10.9 Do not take trail to right that goes to park boundary; stay left

14.2 Lewis Peak Trail goes off to right; stay left

16.1 Austin Mountain Trail goes off to right; stay left

16.5 Four-way intersection; continue straight

17.2 Left onto AT

18.7 Step over Doyles River Trail and continue on AT

19.6 Left to ascend on unnamed connector trail

20.0 End of hike

Big Run watershed is the largest in Shenandoah National Park—1 inch of rainfall translates into 200 million gallons of water falling into the drainage system! A rugged topography—made up of Rocky Mountain, Brown Mountain, Rockytop, and the main crest of the Blue Ridge—encircles Big Run and invites exploration, but there are so many miles to cover that it is best to plan an overnight hike to have enough time to enjoy yourself. As you go to sleep, snug and comfortable in your tent, you will have the satisfaction of enjoying peace and quiet because the great majority of backcountry hikers in the park overlook this area as a camping destination. Carry plenty of water and be sure that you have obtained information about and know the current park regulations concerning backcountry campsites.

DIRECTIONS Having obtained a backcountry camping permit at an entrance station or visitor center, you can reach the beginning of the hike by turning off Skyline Drive at the Loft Mountain Wayside (mile 79.5) and taking the service road to the campground. Leave your car in the auxiliary parking area just above the camp store. This way you will be able to have a junk-food feast at the camp store just before, and after, the hike. If you are doing the hike at a time of year when the campground is closed and you are unable to gain access to the parking lot, probably the best place to leave your automobile, and begin and end the hike, is the Doyles River Parking Area (Skyline Drive mile 81.1), which is at the 18.7-mile point of this hike.

Route Description

From the parking lot, walk to the camp store, take the pathway behind it for a good view of the Piedmont, and follow it out to the Appalachian Trail (AT). At 0.4 mile, turn left onto the AT, where open areas continue to give views to the east. Butter-and-eggs, a European flower that has spread from cultivated gardens, blooms throughout the summer months. During the fall, when the thistle is in flower, the unmistakable seedpods of milkweed cover a large percentage of these open fields. Enter a wooded area where some grand, old, gnarled trees deserve your respect for being able to survive year in and year out in this harsh upland environment.

At 1.5 miles the Frazier Discovery Trail comes in from the left. You will keep right, soon coming to an outcrop on the left to present you with a view of the Big Run drainage, the area into which you are heading. At 1.6 miles the Frazier Discovery Trail takes leave of the AT to go left 0.6 mile to the Wayside coffee shop. Once again, keep right, this time beginning a long, switchbacked descent. After an open area where you can enjoy blackberries in season, you will enter the woods and descend more rapidly to intersect a trail at 2.5 miles. This one goes left about 200 yards to Ivy Creek Spring and 0.6 mile to the Wayside. Stay to the right on the AT.

By the time you cross Ivy Creek at 3.2 miles, it will have become large enough to have a small cascade and pools. Take a break and look into the water to find a few small trout and maybe even a crayfish or two crawling from one submerged crevice to another. Tiny, harmless ring-necked snakes sometimes take advantage of the flat rocks to warm themselves in the bit of sunshine that manages to make it through the forest canopy. After you have

Looking out from the Rockytop Trail

photo: Johnny Molloy

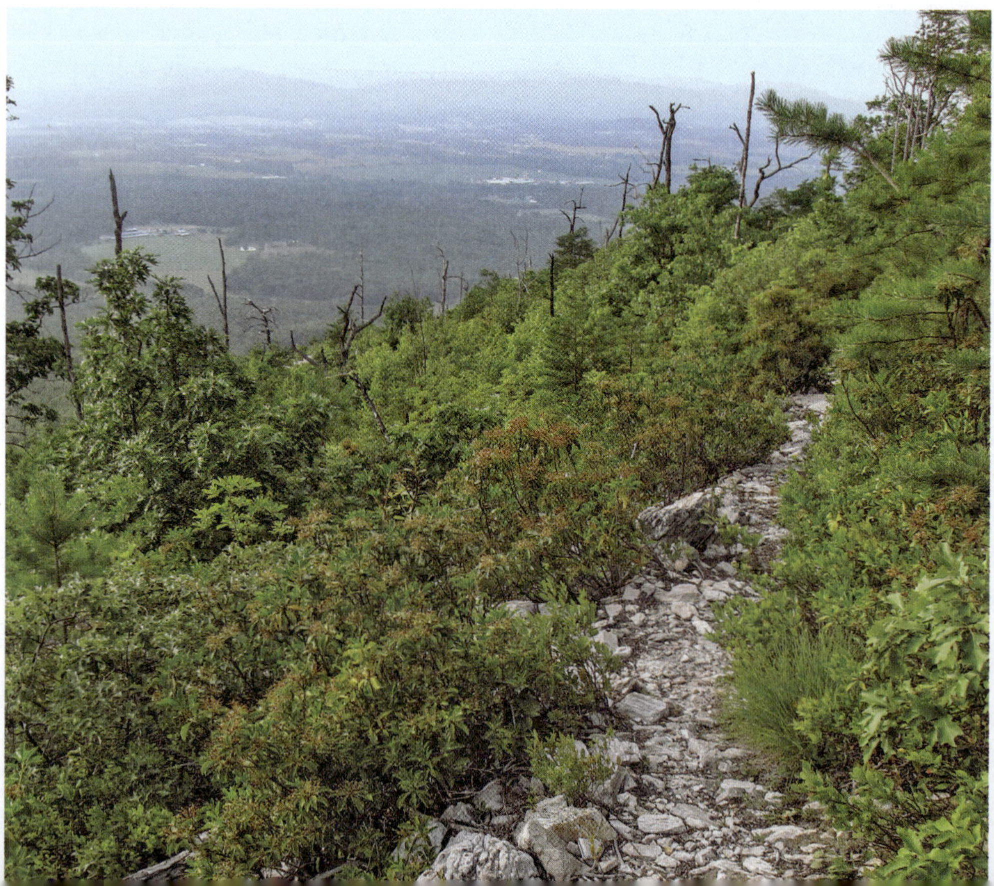

gobbled down a few handfuls of gorp and several swigs of water, you'll begin to ascend through a typical Virginia woods of mountain laurel, pines, and blueberries.

At 3.7 miles you will have a view that takes in Rockytop, whose heights you will be standing on later in the hike, and Trayfoot Mountain. Descend to come to the Ivy Creek Overlook at 4.6 miles (Skyline Drive mile 77.5), where you leave the AT to walk northward on the grassy shoulder of the drive. As you walk along the roadway you can survey what is going to be your domain for the rest of the day and part of tomorrow—Rocky and Brown Mountains, Rockytop, and the numerous tributarial hollows of Big Run. At 5.2 miles come to the Brown Mountain Overlook and begin to follow blue-blazed Brown Mountain Trail along a narrow ridgeline that often carries the tunes of various songbirds.

Come to an intersection at 5.9 miles where the Rocky Mountain Run Trail descends left 2.7 miles to Big Run Portal Trail. You want to ascend to the right, slabbing a hillside covered with heavy undergrowth and dead trees, a sign of past spongy moth (*Lymantria dispar dispar*) infestation. The spongy moth was brought to Massachusetts in 1869 from France for experimental crossbreeding with silkworms. Unfortunately, some escaped and the moth has now spread throughout much of North America, with some being found even as far away as California and Washington. It is when they are in the larval, or caterpillar, stage that they feed on the leaves of trees and other foliage, sometimes completely defoliating vast acreages. A healthy tree can usually withstand one or two consecutive years of defoliation, but any more than this and the tree will probably die. Natural forces, such as the nucleopolyhedrosis virus and the spongy moth fungus, can help bring the moths under control. One thing is certain, though: Just as surely as the chestnut blight cleared the way for oaks to become one of the dominant trees in the southern highlands, the spongy moth is changing the look of our forests once again. It will be interesting to see what the vegetative cover of the Blue Ridge Mountains will be in decades to come.

After going up and down and back and forth along the undulating ridgeline, you'll reach the 2,800-foot summit of Rocky Mountain at 6.8 miles for one heck of a view. The whole Big Run watershed is laid out below you, and across the valley is Rockytop with Trayfoot Mountain behind it. You can make out your route back along the entire ridgeline you have just walked from Skyline Drive. Look at the rock beneath your feet and you can see the fossilized bore holes of the scolithus, a worm believed to have lived 500 million years ago. Look for these signs of ancient life just about any time this hike passes by rock outcrops or talus slopes.

Attain the summit of Brown Mountain at 8.2 miles for a view much like you had from Rocky Mountain, except that the valley floor appears much closer. The descent is now via switchbacks, and breaks in the vegetation will give you an interesting perspective on the very southern peak of Massanutten Mountain to the northwest.

Intersect Big Run Portal Trail at 10.3 miles and turn left so that you can make a right turn in just a few more feet, so as to not stay on Big Run Portal Trail. There are some great swimming holes when you cross Big Run. As I was beginning a hike once in mid-May, a ranger jokingly dared me by saying, "You'll be a real man if you take a dip in one of those mountain creeks!" By the end of July the water should have warmed up enough that just about anyone can enjoy submersing themselves for a while. Just remember, in addition to cold water, any mountain stream is likely to have deep holes, slippery rocks, and swift currents. (After your swim, it is worthwhile to take a short walk downstream a few hundred yards to Big Run Portal, where the stream impressively rushes through a narrow ravine in the bedrock.)

From the bridge, ascend along the rocky trail, veering away from the stream. Pay attention at 10.9 miles, where the trail continues ahead 0.2 mile to the park boundary; you want to make a left and begin the long and sometimes switchbacked ascent of blue-blazed Rockytop Trail. Looking out through the vegetation you should be able to make out Brown and Rocky Mountains and mark your progress as you rise from the valley floor. At 12.6 miles, cross one rock field, and soon after, another. Above you is the highest peak on the ridge—the one that most people refer to as Rockytop, although USGS maps give another knob farther up the trail that distinction. The view you have is to the west, most notably Lewis Peak. It is estimated that there are anywhere from 300 to 600 black bears at any given time in the park, and judging from the amount of scat I've seen when crossing these talus slopes, the Big Run watershed must provide food for quite a few of them. The scat is usually cylindrical, somewhat like that of a dog's, and often contains remnants of what the bears have eaten—seeds, leaves of grass, rodent bones and fur, and nutshells. During the time of year when the bears are gorging themselves on the abundant variety of berries in the park, the scat is no longer solid but resembles a large, black or dark blue, liquid cow pie.

The Lewis Peak Trail takes off to the right at 14.2 miles, so you want to keep to the left. Walking sticks (the insects, not the hiking aid) are so perfectly camouflaged that you have to keep a sharp eye out to spot one, even though thousands feed on the park's foliage. You'll now be making minor ups and downs on the ridgeline, walking in and out of patches of turkeybeard, pokeweed, and wild rose, until you stay to the left when you come to the Austin Mountain Trail going off to the right at 16.1 miles. The Rockytop Trail ends at a four-way intersection at 16.5 miles. The Madison Run Spur Trail makes a hard right to descend to Madison Run Road in about 0.3 mile. Big Run Loop Trail descends left to Big Run. You want to go straight toward Skyline Drive and the AT, which you will intersect at 17.2 miles. Turn left and follow its white blazes, descending to cross Skyline Drive (mile 82.2) and then walking on the rocky backbone of a ridge, passing some interesting rock formations. Shallow remains of trenches built during the Civil War are overgrown with trees and underbrush on the right side of the pathway.

Hike by the Doyles River Overlook (Skyline Drive mile 81.9) and descend to the intersection with the Doyles River Trail at 18.7 miles. A parking area and the Skyline Drive are 120 feet to the left; you want to continue straight and ascend on the AT, but be on the lookout for poison ivy overtaking the pathway. A rock outcrop will present you with a view of just about every place you've been on this hike—Loft, Brown, and Rocky Mountains and Rockytop. Here, on Big Flat Mountain, the apple trees you walk under are evidence of an old orchard. Deer are attracted to this area, and you will no doubt see a few close to where you leave the AT at 19.6 miles to make a left onto an unnamed connector trail. With the large number of deer seen in the Blue Ridge Mountains, it is hard to believe that the population near the turn of the 20th century was almost wiped out. Some historical accounts say that domestic dogs ran down and destroyed (as they still do today in many rural and suburban areas) almost as many as were killed for human consumption. Loss of habitat from farming and timbering only compounded the decline in numbers. To rectify this assault on the natural order of things, white-tailed deer were reintroduced into the park in 1934, and it is estimated that 6,000 now live within its borders. When you come to the campground's amphitheater you'll want to make a right to ascend to the road and your car, ending the hike at exactly 20.0 miles.

The camp store, with its cold liquid refreshments and shelves of high-calorie snacks, is only a few hundred steps beyond the parking lot.

29 Riprap Hollow

- **GPS:** N38.1530850 W78.7724587
- **TOTAL DISTANCE (circuit):** 9.6 miles
- **HIKING TIME:** 6.0 hours
- **VERTICAL RISE:** 2,260 feet
- **MAPS:** USGS *Crimora; National Geographic Trails Illustrated Map #228 Shenandoah National Park*
- **CONTACT:** Shenandoah National Park
  3655 US 211 E.
  Luray, VA 22835-9036
  540-999-3500
  nps.gov/shen

The Hike at a Glance

0.1 Right onto AT
2.7 Riprap Parking Area is to the right; stay left on AT
3.2 Left onto Riprap Trail
4.4 Chimney Rocks
6.9 Left to cross stream and ascend on Wildcat Ridge Trail
9.5 Step across AT and continue straight
9.6 End of hike

Hot summer days are not meant for working in office buildings or for toiling in the bright sunshine. They are better spent peering off into the distance while standing on lofty ridges with soft breezes blowing through your hair, having picnics with family and friends in quiet shady groves, or walking into narrow ravines to take dips in cool mountain streams. A hike into Riprap Hollow can provide you with places to experience all of this and more. It provides the perfect excuse for you and a few compatriots to chuck work for the day; fill up the day packs with sandwiches, gorp, and other goodies; and go wandering about in the southern section of Shenandoah National Park.

DIRECTIONS You could just as readily start this circuit hike from the Riprap Parking Area (Skyline Drive mile point 90.0), but I have you beginning and ending the hike from the Wildcat Ridge Parking Area (Skyline Drive mile point 92.1; about 15 miles north of US 250 and I-64 in Rockfish Gap). I've done this so that after you have made the 1,300-plus-foot, 2.7-mile climb out of Riprap Hollow, you won't face 2.8 more miles of ups and downs in order to reach your automobile. If you have two cars, you could completely eliminate those miles (making it about a 7-mile hike) by first leaving one car at Wildcat Ridge and then beginning from Riprap parking. After obtaining your backcountry permit and obtaining current camping regulations, you could make this into a backpacking trip easily walked in two days.

Route Description

Take the trail from the Wildcat Ridge Parking Area. In 0.1 mile, come to a four-way intersection where the Wildcat Ridge Trail is straight ahead (you will be returning on it) and the Appalachian Trail (AT) runs left and right. You want to turn right onto the AT, walking through an understory of mountain laurel, sassafras, and azalea. Azalea, like mountain laurel and rhododendron, is a member of the heath family and grows well throughout the mountains of Virginia. The national park seems to have more than its fair share of azaleas, and if you are lucky enough to be walking in the woods during that short period of the year (usually late May and early June) when it and the mountain laurel are both in full bloom, your eyes will have a visual color feast. The laurel's clumps of white to rich-pink flowers mix nicely with the azalea's deeper pink blossoms.

The Riprap Hollow area was the scene of three wildland fires during the 1990s; the

Riprap Hollow

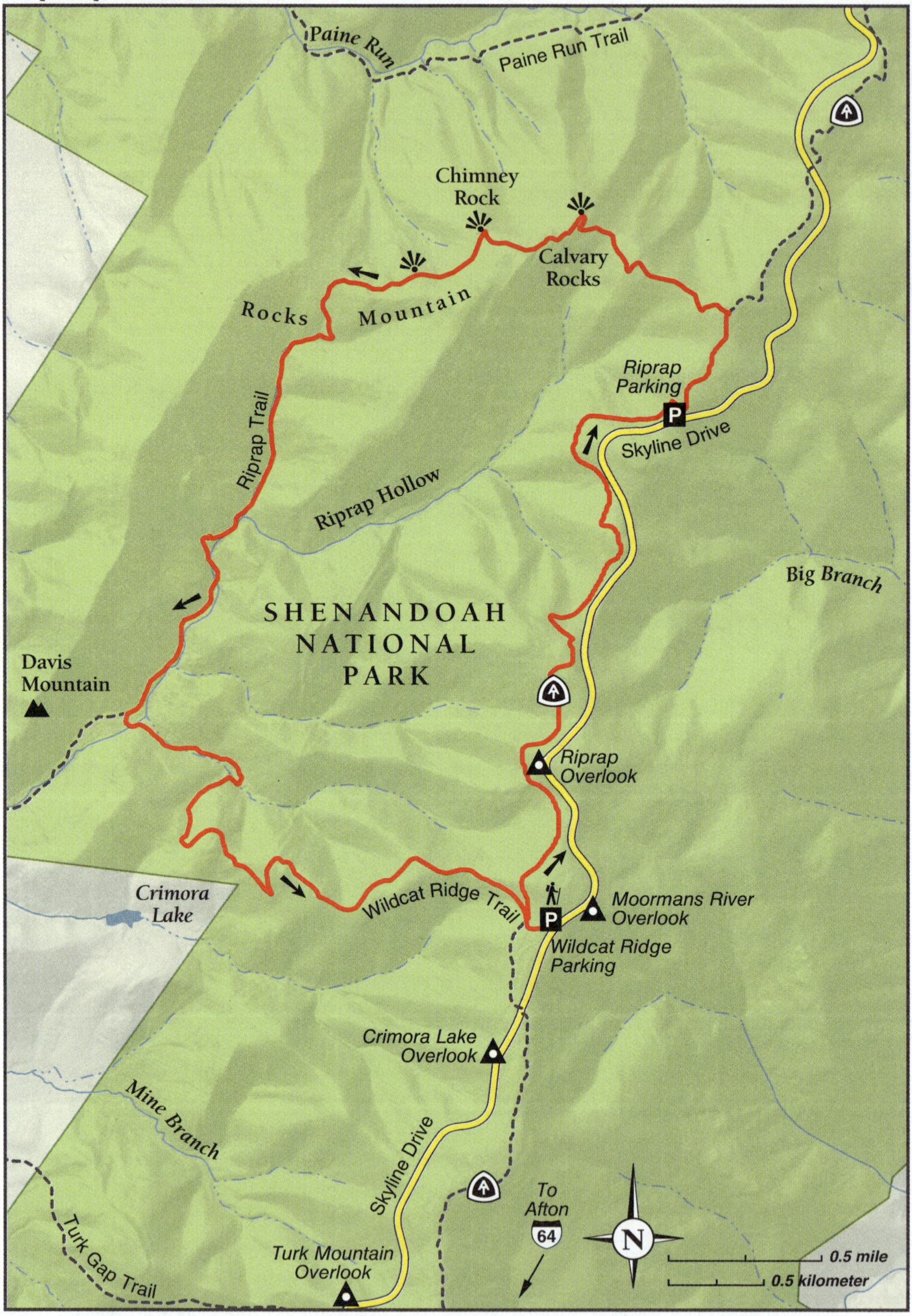

portion of the AT you are now walking upon was burned in 1999, when ashes from a controlled burn by national park personnel were rekindled by strong winds. Within a week, the fire grew to 3,200 acres, and it took 500 firefighters, aided by engines, helicopters, and air tankers, to control the flames. Luckily, it was mostly just undergrowth that burned along the AT (the effects of the fire might not even be noticeable by the time you walk here), but the interior area of Riprap Hollow sustained major losses. The large number of spongy moth–damaged trees was a major factor in the fire's rapid spread, and you may see a number of dead trees when looking onto the lower elevations from some of the hike's viewpoints.

At 0.7 mile, low growth permits a view of the Shenandoah Valley and of the place you are eventually going to enter, Riprap Hollow. Pass by an occasional rhododendron shrub as you gradually rise to cross a flat ridge and begin descending on switchbacks at 1.2 miles. Repeat this up-and-down process a couple of times until, at 2.4 miles, you can spot the ridgeline you will use to descend into the hollow. At 2.7 miles the Riprap Parking Area is a few feet to the right; you want to stay left, continuing on the AT, to come to another intersection at 3.2 miles. Leave the AT and make a left onto blue-blazed Riprap Trail as it descends with limited views of the valley created by Paine Run. The rocks to the right at 4.0 miles provide a wonderful grandstand view. North is Horsehead Mountain and beyond it is Trayfoot Mountain, but the most spectacular view is of the Shenandoah Valley as it stretches north and south and west. From here it is obvious why the wide, rolling expanse of the valley, bordered on the east by the Blue Ridge Mountains and on the west by the Allegheny Mountains (somewhat hidden here by Massanutten Mountain), was the natural conduit for early settlers as they made their way to southern Virginia and points westward from Pennsylvania, Maryland, and northeastern Virginia.

By the time you reach Chimney Rock at 4.4 miles, you have lost more elevation and the valley will appear much closer. Gaze back up to your right and you can see the Skyline Drive near the crest of the mountains—that's how far down you have come since you turned off the AT. The hillside trail you continue to descend is well graded and wide; keep looking through the vegetation and you'll be able to monitor the progress of your descent in relation to the surrounding mountains. The next rock outcrop at 4.8 miles gives a completely unobstructed view of the Paine Run watershed. The very southern peak of Massanutten Mountain is visible to the northwest as it juts above the ridge of Trayfoot Mountain. You are so close to the floor of the Shenandoah Valley that it seems as if you could be walking on it in just a few minutes. In addition to the wind rustling the leaves, your ears should now be able to make out the sound of the stream dropping into Cold Spring Hollow.

Drop quickly into the hollow, where the trail becomes rough and rocky in this exceptionally beautiful gorge. Don't take the old, washed-out path going left and downhill after you've passed the small falls at 6.1 miles. Rather, you should ascend up to the right and then drop back down to cross the stream. You have entered Riprap Hollow when, after 6.3 miles of walking, you reach what many consider to be one of the prettiest spots in the park. The water of the stream has worn a large, deep hole into the bedrock, creating an absolutely lovely swimming pool where you can relax, propped up against smooth rocks, while the waters of a small falls massage tired muscles. A more perfect place to while away a few hours would be hard to find. The silvery water drops around soft-looking, moss-covered boulders; sunlight is filtered through hundreds of tree branches; and the pool mirrors the evergreen leaves of mountain laurel and rhododendron thickets. Although catawba rhododendron can often be found in abundance almost anywhere else in the mountains of Virginia, this is one of the very few places in Shenandoah National Park that it thrives in great numbers. Something else to contemplate while you are relaxing here—about 1 mile beyond the park boundary,

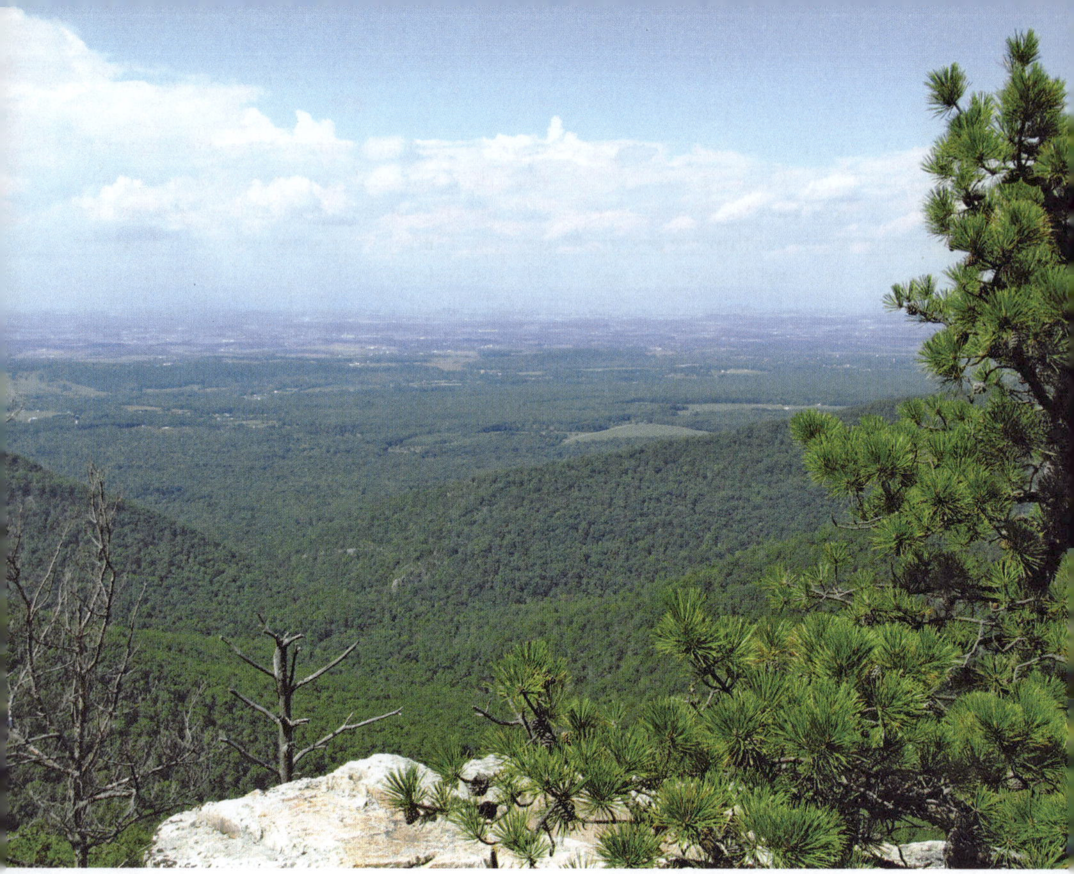

View of the Shenandoah Valley

photo: Johnny Molloy

this stream disappears from the surface of the earth, joining Shenandoah Valley's subterranean water system.

Unfortunately, no matter how lovely this spot is, you are eventually going to have to leave. At 6.5 miles, cross over to the west side of the stream, beginning to follow the old fire road. Be sure to pay attention at 6.9 miles because the fire road continues straight, but you want to make a left to cross the stream and begin to rise out of Riprap Hollow on the Wildcat Ridge Trail. You will first ascend on an old road, crisscrossing a side stream before the road ends and you ascend steeply to obtain the ridgeline in 7.8 miles. If you have ever had the pleasure of walking through a field of beargrass in the northern Rockies, you'll be excited to see turkeybeard scattered about. While it doesn't grow quite as tall as its western relative in the lily family, the turkeybeard's cluster of tiny white flowers at the top of its stem can be almost as large and impressive.

The use of this sidehill trail makes for a more gradual ascent to where you come into a gap to cross over to the other side of the ridge for a view of the cliffs and talus slopes near the summit of Turk Mountain to the south. Take in your last good view of the Shenandoah Valley from the trail. From here you will crisscross the ridgeline a few times, coming to the intersection with the AT at 9.5 miles. Cross the AT and continue straight to the Wildcat Parking Area at 9.6 miles.

Aren't you glad you didn't go to work today?

30 Blue Ridge Tunnel

- **GPS:**
  N38.0435157 W78.8575178 **(western trailhead)**
  N38.0333273 W78.8424495 **(eastern trailhead)**
- **TOTAL DISTANCE (one-way):** 2.3 miles; **(round-trip)** 4.6 miles
- **HIKING TIME: (one way)** 1.25 hours; **(round-trip)** 2.25 hours
- **VERTICAL RISE: (one way)** 300 feet; **(round-trip)** 480 feet
- **MAP:** *Blue Ridge Tunnel Trail map*
- **CONTACT:** Claudius Crozet Blue Ridge Tunnel Foundation/Nelson County Economic Development and Tourism
  8579 Thomas Nelson Hwy.
  Lovingston, VA 22949
  434-263-7015
  blueridgetunnel.org

The Hike at a Glance

0.6 Enter the tunnel
1.45 Exit the tunnel
1.7 Leave the old railroad grade
2.3 Arrive at western trailhead

The Blue Ridge Tunnel is at the meeting place of the northern end of the Blue Ridge Parkway, the southern end of Skyline Drive, the Appalachian Trail, the US Bicycle Route 76 (a part of the TransAmerica Trail), Interstate 64, and US 250. However, all of these things will be about 700 feet above you when you're walking the Blue Ridge Tunnel Trail as it cuts through the mountain at Rockfish Gap.

In the early 1800s, settlers west of the Blue Ridge Mountains were still quite isolated from those in the east. The James River and Kanawha Canal had been started with grand dreams to connect the eastern seaboard with the Ohio River. Yet, by 1851, it had only reached as far west as Buchanan, Virginia. By that time, railroads had become a more popular and less expensive way of moving people and goods.

Laborers, primarily Irish immigrants and Black slaves rented out by nearby landowners, began working on the Blue Ridge Tunnel in 1850. It was thought that construction would be completed within three years, but there were unexpected conditions. Extremely hard rock, known as greenstone (volcanic in origin), frequent water drainage problems, and rockslides, along with diseases, worker strife, and funding problems, delayed completion. It was the longest railroad tunnel in the United States when it finally opened in 1858. It remained in use until a newer, adjacent tunnel was completed in 1944.

In 2001, Nelson County began exploring a way to turn the tunnel into a trail and, in 2007, was able to obtain the tunnel from the CSX Corporation for only $1. Through a series of grants, donations, and other sources that totaled almost $6 million, the county and a coalition with governmental agencies in Albemarle and Augusta counties, along with other entities, were able to accomplish their goal, opening the trail to the public in November 2020. It was an immediate success and is now one of the most popular hikes in Virginia. (Within six months of opening, the trail's eastern trailhead parking lot had to be expanded from only about a dozen spaces to more than 50!)

Be sure to bring a flashlight with good batteries, as the tunnel is not lighted and it gets quite dark in there. Also, be prepared for cooler temperatures (it's a great place to be on a hot summer day), and remember that the trail is open to bicyclists too.

DIRECTIONS Take I-64 Exit 107 near Crozet, head westward on US 250, and go 6.7 miles (keep straight at this point for 2.0 more miles if you are going to leave a shuttled car at the western trailhead). Turn left onto VA 6, continue another 0.5 mile, make a right onto Afton Depot Lane, and follow it to the parking area.

Blue Ridge Tunnel

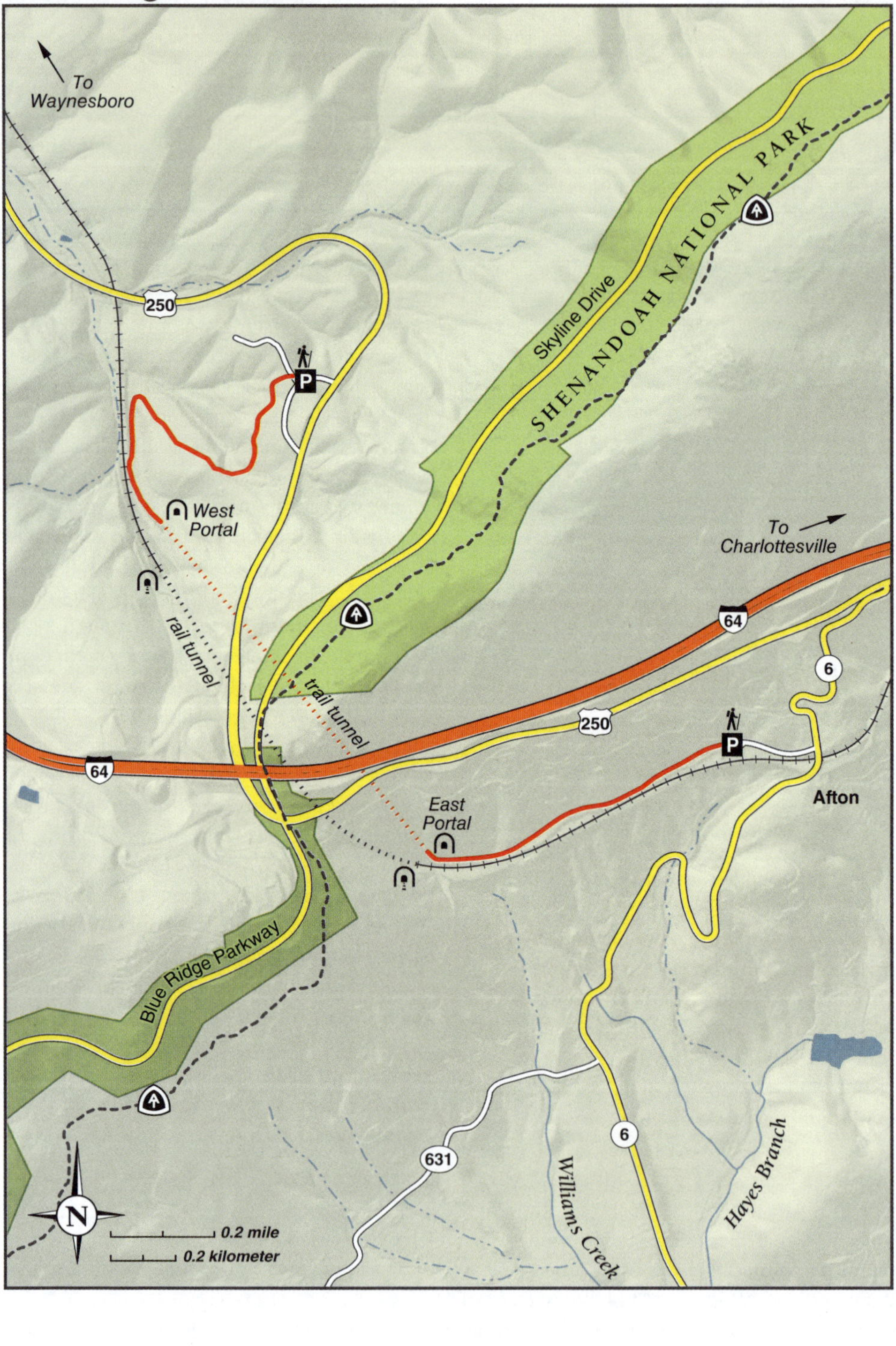

Route Description

The trail ascends at a gradual rate from the parking area, paralleling railroad tracks to the left that are currently used by freight trains and Amtrak's passenger train, the *Cardinal.* Interpretive signs provide an amazing amount of detailed historical information about the tunnel and its construction, including the project's overseer, Claudius Crozet.

Colorful assortments of wildflowers grow along the embankment in spring and summer, including mountain phlox, mint, thistle, and chicory. The latter's blossoms, which may grow well into autumn and appear at intervals along the upper portion of the stem, open early in the morning to entice passing bees and other insects. Yet, each flower lasts but a day. By early afternoon the petals have begun to wither and will have completely fallen off by the time darkness approaches. New blossoms will appear at a different spot along the stem the next morning. The plant was imported by early settlers to the New World from the Old World, where it had been cultivated for centuries. Chicory's leaves, which resemble those of one of the plant's relative's, endive, have been added to salads. Its roots are dried and roasted to be used as a substitute for, or an additive to, coffee.

The sound of dripping water and small drafts of cooler air greet you as you enter the tunnel's eastern portal at 0.6 mile where—even though the tunnel is 4,273 feet long—you can see the tiny bit of light at the tunnel's far end. Get the flashlight out and enjoy this now natural world that was created by humans more than a century and a half ago. Salamanders, crayfish, snakes, bats, and more make their homes here, while water drips almost continually from the ceiling and walls (be sure to search out the "gushing rock"; you will hear it long before you reach it).

Distances can be deceiving. The portal at the far end can appear to be close by, but if you turn around you will see that you are still closer to the eastern portal. It's at about the halfway point that you are directly below I-64, the Appalachian Trail, and Skyline Drive. This is also a good point to let out a yell or a loud whistle to enjoy hearing it echo throughout the tunnel. Don't be afraid or ashamed of being a kid again. Besides, it's a good bet you won't be the only person having fun with these sound waves.

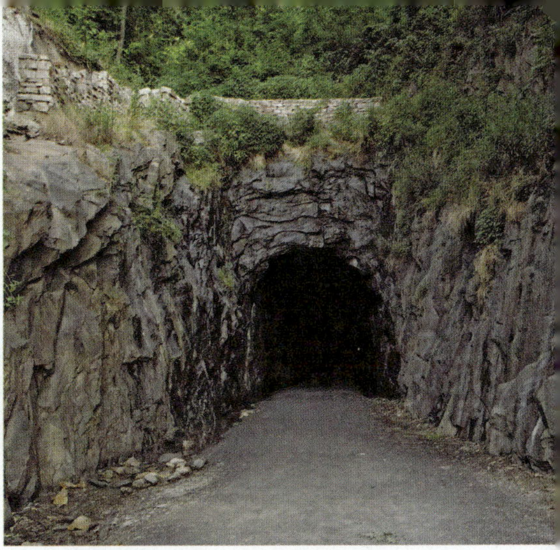

The eastern portal

Look at the walls of the tunnel and you can't help but be amazed that the tunnel was ever built. It was constructed in the days before dynamite, so workers had to carve out the rock using just hand tools, such as pickaxes and drills, along with some black powder. Those working from the western end had a bit of an easier job, as the rock there was slightly softer. However, that meant it was less stable and that's why the tunnel is lined with bricks for the last 0.25 mile. It was dangerous employment no matter which part of the tunnel was being worked on, and more than a dozen men died during construction.

Emerge from the tunnel at 1.45 miles and descend to 1.7 miles where the trail takes its leave of the old railroad bed and makes a series of steep ups and downs. One ascent is at a 19% grade, but it does not last long. Now that you are away from the narrow cut of the railroad bed, you can gaze into the hardwood forest as you go over one small ridgeline after another.

The one-way journey comes to an end at 2.3 miles at the western trailhead parking lot. Those who did not shuttle a car now have the pleasure of turning around and doing the hike in reverse.

Whetstone Ridge

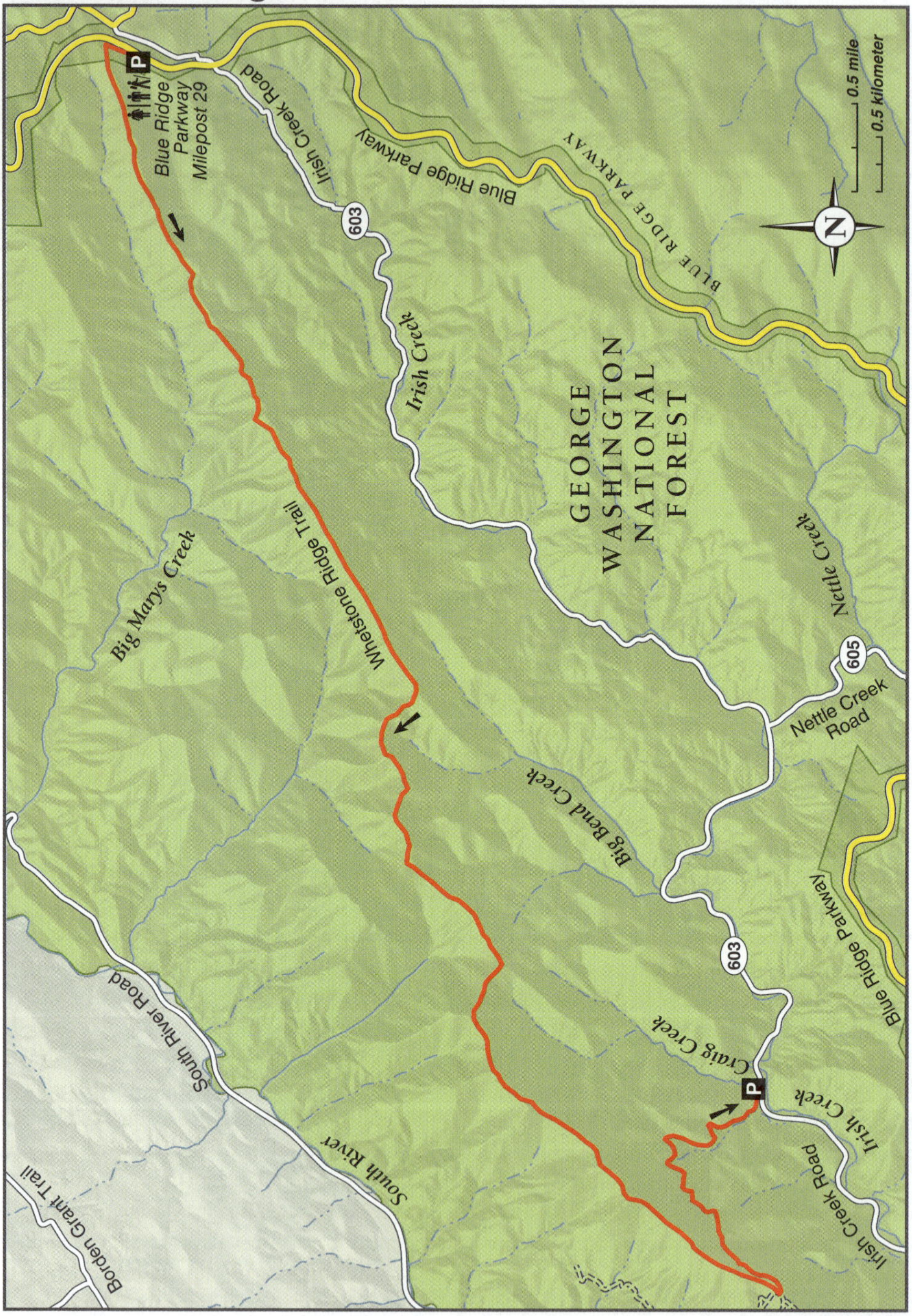

31 Whetstone Ridge

- **GPS:** N37.8691117 W79.1485523
- **TOTAL DISTANCE (one-way):** 11.8 miles
- **HIKING TIME:** 7.75 hours
- **VERTICAL RISE:** 4,500 feet
- **MAPS:** USGS *Montebello* and *Cornwall; National Geographic Trails Illustrated #789 Lexington/Blue Ridge Mountains*
- **CONTACT:** Glenwood/Pedlar Ranger District
  27 Ranger Lane
  Natural Bridge Station, VA 24579
  540-291-2188
  fs.usda.gov/gwj

The Hike at a Glance

- 0.2 Switchback left to rise to Whetstone Ridge
- 4.7 Traverse a cross ridge to begin walking on South Mountain
- 7.3 View of Shenandoah Valley
- 9.5 Switchback left to begin descent off mountain
- 11.8 Return to shuttled automobile

It was still a few hours before daylight when I unzipped my tent and stepped out into the 30-degree darkness. Once I became accustomed to the cold and my eyes wandered upward. Orion's distinctive belt was almost directly above, the Big Dipper was nearing the horizon, and so many stars were twinkling next to each other that it seemed as if there was little darkness between them. A couple of shooting stars with long tails reminded me that just a couple days before I had read about this being peak time for the Geminids meteor shower. Oh, how easy it is to forget what a grand show the night sky can be when you live within the brightly lit confines of a city.

I was on an overnight hike of the Whetstone Ridge Trail {FS 523} and hadn't really thought about how far away it was from any city of appreciable size. Staunton is about 20 miles to the north and Lexington is close to 20 miles to the south, while there are no cities for many miles to either the east or west.

The trail is the only pathway located off Virginia's portion of the Blue Ridge Parkway where it is possible to walk in just one direction (more or less) for close to 10 miles and not cross any kind of automobile-accessible road. Yes, the trail does follow an old woods road in places, but it has been many years since any kind of vehicle has driven on it. There are few vistas during the summer, yet when the leaves are off the trees, the views are almost continuous. It makes a nice overnight hike since the route is on forest service property where camping is permitted. Just be aware that water sources are practically nonexistent, so be sure to carry plenty of fluids. Also be aware that you'll encounter vigorous climbs over rocky knobs throughout much of the hike, with the most steep being located at about 3, 7, 8, and 9 miles into the journey.

DIRECTIONS It's a one-way hike, which means you'll be doing some car shuttling. The upper trailhead is at the ranger station parking area at Blue Ridge Parkway milepost 29, about 30 miles south of Waynesboro. The far end of the trail, where you will leave one car and drive back to the parkway, is reached by driving across the parkway from the ranger station onto Whetstone Ridge Road and, in 0.1 mile, turning right onto Irish Creek Road (VA 603) and following it 9.3 miles to the small trailhead parking area on the right.

Route Description

Begin the hike from the ranger station by paralleling the parkway northward for several hundred feet on a pathway that was a part of the original route of the Appalachian Trail (AT) during the late 1920s and early 1930s. Many miles of the AT had to be relocated after much

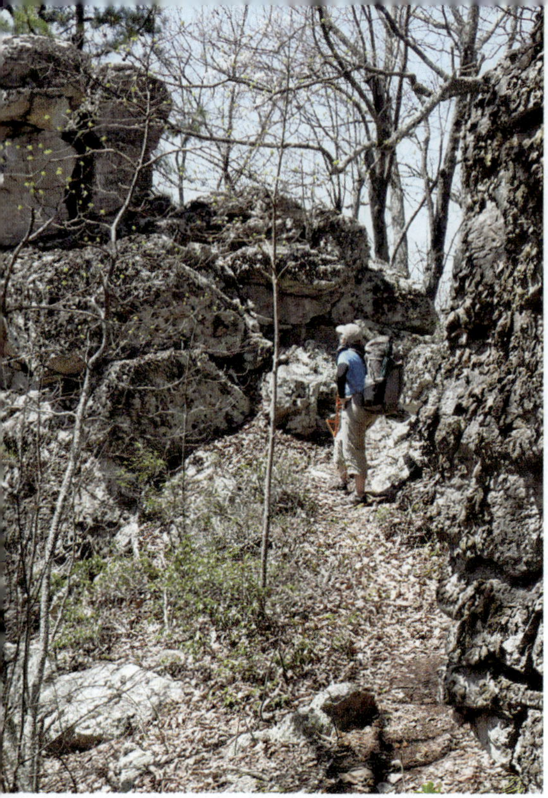

Whetstone Ridge Trail is often lightly used.

of the parkway in Virginia was constructed directly on top of the trail's route.

At 0.2 mile, switchback to the left and soon attain Whetstone Ridge (named for the fine-grained sharpening stones it provided early mountain settlers). The trail stays along the ridgeline for the next several miles, sometimes following an old woods road, sometimes leaving it to either avoid a knob or, incongruously, ascend a different one. At 4.0 miles, the trail begins a downward trend, and the ridgeline sometimes becomes wide enough to provide some room for a small tent site.

The trail reaches a low point at 4.7 miles as it traverses a cross ridge, taking the pathway off Whetstone Ridge and onto the South Mountain ridgeline. Both Whetstone and South Mountains are along the southern edge of the Adams Peak Roadless Area, 7,000 acres of land that have been de facto wilderness since the 2001 Roadless Conservation Area Rule that prohibits any logging or road building (except for firefighting). Because of this designation, views northward from South Mountain look upon peaks and valleys covered by an unbroken forest. The few farms and houses located within the Shenandoah Valley to the west add to the sense of remoteness.

The Virginia Wilderness Committee is working to have the area declared a National Scenic Area, a designation that would add another level of protection for the land. This is the same organization that you can thank for helping to secure the Omnibus Public Land Management Act in 2009, one of the largest pieces of environmental legislation to pass Congress in more than 25 years. The law designated more than 2 million acres of new wilderness in America.

Again, be ready for some steep ups and downs, but also take the time to enjoy the views (even in summer) of the Shenandoah Valley (at 7.3 miles) and the parkway twisting along the main crest of the Blue Ridge Mountains (at 8.2 miles).

There is another set of people you should also thank if you decide to undertake this journey. The farther you get from the trailhead, the more obvious it becomes that the Whetstone Ridge Trail is lightly used and would become harder to follow in places if not for the maintenance efforts of a group of mountain bikers from Harrisonburg, Virginia. Sometimes aided by riders from Charlottesville, these volunteers come out on an irregular basis to keep vegetation at bay and work on keeping erosion in check.

The trail is marked by plastic diamonds nailed to tree trunks, so be sure to watch for double diamonds at 9.5 miles that mark the turn to the left off the mountain. It'll take you to a descending pathway that crosses over a couple of spur ridges, goes by two possible, but not reliable, water sources, and returns you to your shuttled car at 11.8 miles.

Once you pick up your other car, you should consider driving northward on the Blue Ridge Parkway to hike the White Rock Falls Trail (see Hike 32), which begins at parkway milepost 18.5. It's a moderately easy walk of only 5.0 miles through abundant pine trees and mountain laurel bushes, with the reward of the falls cascading 40 feet down the steep hillside.

32 White Rock Falls and Slacks Overlook Trails

- **GPS:** N37.8962197 W79.0451205
- **TOTAL DISTANCE (circuit):** 5.0 miles
- **HIKING TIME:** 3.0 hours
- **VERTICAL RISE:** 1,050 feet
- **MAPS:** USGS *Big Levels; National Geographic Trails Illustrated #789 Lexington/Blue Ridge Mountains*
- **CONTACT:** Blue Ridge Parkway
  199 Hemphill Knob Road
  Asheville, NC 28803
  828-348-3400
  nps.gov/blri

The Hike at a Glance

1.6 Right onto trail leading to White Rock Falls; after falls, retrace steps to main trail and turn right

2.7 Turn left onto Blue Ridge Parkway, go a few yards, and turn into Slacks Overlook, taking trail just past picnic tables at north end of parking area. In 250 feet at trail intersection, turn left to come to Slacks Overlook Trail. Do not go left at that point, but rather right

4.5 Intersection with White Rock Trail; turn right and ascend

5.0 Return to parking area

Shenandoah and Great Smoky Mountains National Parks, two of America's most-visited and scenic national parks, are linked via another beautiful and popular component of the national park system, the Blue Ridge Parkway (BRP). Meandering along the crest of the mountains for more than 469 miles, the parkway provides an opportunity to become intimately associated with the natural and human histories of the southern Appalachian Mountains.

In 1933, President Franklin Roosevelt made an inspection tour of the first Civilian Conservation Corps camp, which was established in Virginia. Roosevelt not only enjoyed the beauty of Shenandoah National Park, but he was also well pleased with the progress and potential of the Skyline Drive. Prodded on by local politicians (who realized its economic benefits) and naturalists from Virginia, North Carolina, and Tennessee, Roosevelt approved the idea of the parkway, and development began on September 11, 1935. With the construction of the Linn Cove Viaduct on the eastern flank of Grandfather Mountain in North Carolina in 1983 and several more years of joining together "missing link" sections, the task was accomplished. On September 11, 1987, a ceremony on the viaduct officially declared the completion of the parkway, exactly 52 years after the project was started.

There are more than 100 park service trails along the parkway and dozens of forest service, state park, and private pathways that either connect or come in close contact with it—in other words, there exist ample occasions to experience and explore the mountains. In addition, the world-famous, 2,190-plus-mile Appalachian Trail parallels the parkway for more than 100 miles in Virginia. Also, the ambitious and soon-to-be famous Mountains-to-Sea Trail, which someday will stretch 1,000 miles from Clingman's Dome high atop the Great Smokies to the white sand and rolling surf of Nags Head on the Outer Banks, crisscrosses the parkway in western North Carolina numerous times. If you desire any more information, *Hiking and Traveling the Blue Ridge Parkway: The Only Guide You Will Ever Need, Including GPS, Detailed Maps, and More* contains detailed information on each and every trail along the full length of the parkway.

DIRECTIONS To reach the Blue Ridge Parkway, exit either US 250 or I-64 in Rockfish Gap a few miles east of Waynesboro. Follow highway signs for a very short distance and turn south onto the parkway. Before hiking the White Rock Falls and Slacks Overlook Trails, I suggest you walk two short pathways that will provide you with enough knowledge and insight to

White Rock Falls and Slacks Overlook Trails

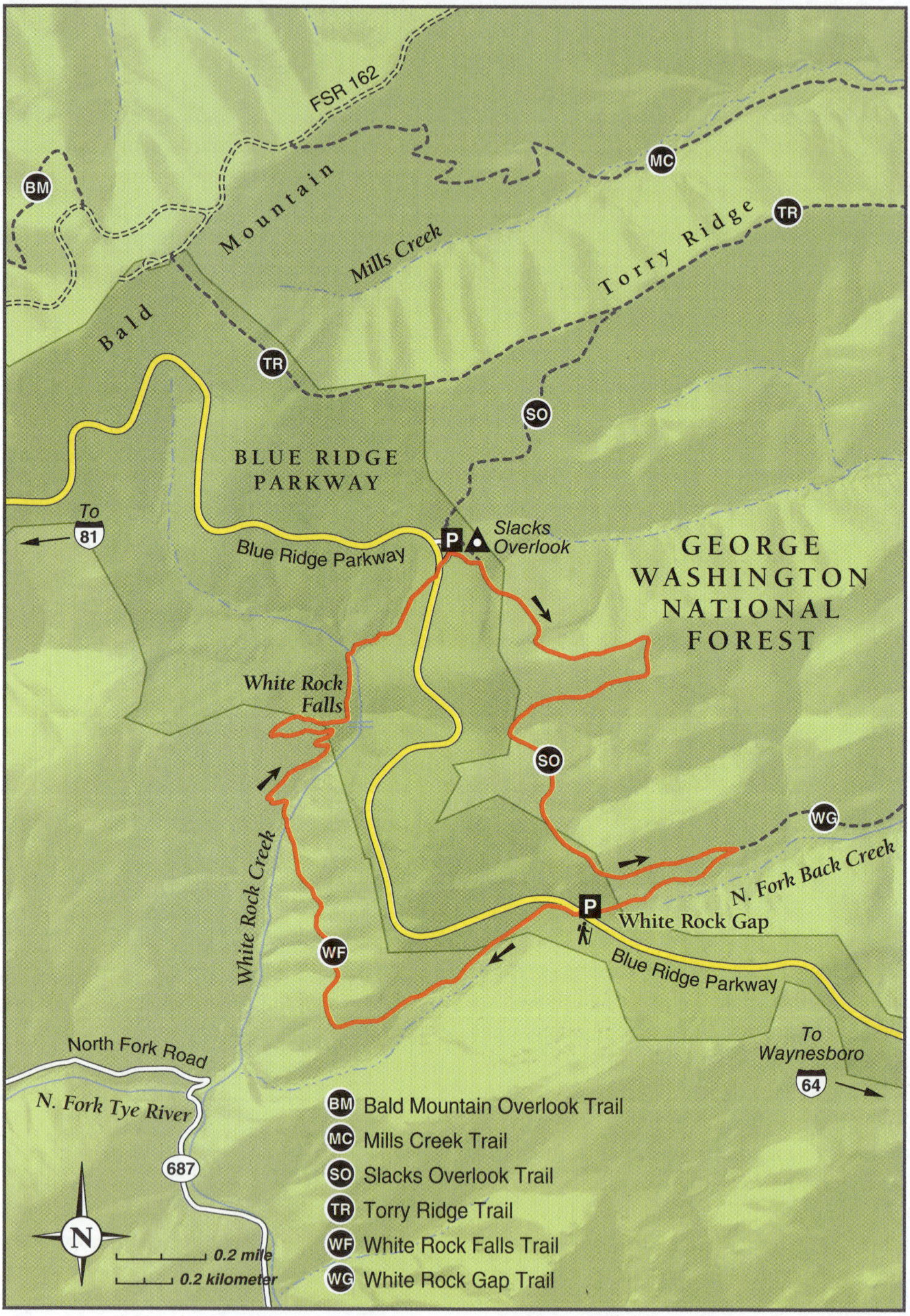

make your future ramblings in the Blue Ridge Mountains more enjoyable.

The Algonquin, Delaware, Iroquois, Catawba, Shawnee, and Cherokee Native Americans were living in, or making use of, the Blue Ridge Mountains when European explorers first arrived in the New World. Traveling southward from Pennsylvania or westward from the coast of North Carolina, settlers began arriving in the early 1700s. Their numbers gradually increased to the point that, by the end of the Revolutionary War, small communities were established throughout the mountains. Isolated from urban centers, these settlers became quite self-sufficient.

An excellent introduction to the lifestyle of these hardy folks is provided by the Mountain Farm Trail located at BRP milepost 5.9. The park service has reconstructed a typical mountain farm of the early 1900s along this 0.25-mile pathway. Signposts explain the uses of various structures, such as log cabins, gear lofts, and weasel-proof chicken houses. Here you will learn how a maul and frow, beatlin block, or ash hopper was used. A garden is planted for the growing season, and live demonstrations are presented during the spring, summer, and fall. Check at the visitor center for times and dates.

The 0.2-mile (circuit) Greenstone Trail is located at BRP milepost 8.8. Signs along the oak- and hickory-lined trail explain the volcanic origins of the northern Blue Ridge Mountains. Although this is a very short trail, the information learned on it will add greatly to your appreciation of the mountains as you drive and walk through them.

The White Rock Falls Trail {FS 482} is located at BRP milepost 18.5 in White Rock Gap, with a parking area on the western side of the parkway. White Rock Falls Trail was built by the Youth Conservation Corps in 1979 and is now excellently maintained by volunteers of the Tidewater Appalachian Trail Club, who have constructed a series of well-built switchbacks to eliminate the former steep climb up from the falls and back toward the parkway.

Route Description

To begin the hike, leave your car, cross the roadway, and gradually descend on the trail, which is lined with wintergreen. Farther on you may run across mayapple, trillium, and wild geranium in early to late spring. Within the first 0.2 mile you will cross three small footbridges above jumbles of large boulders in the valley below. Pass by old, crumbling stone walls that were probably, at one time, "hogwall" fences used by farmers to keep their razorback pigs from wandering too far. At 0.5 mile the pathway joins an old roadbed, but be alert because it soon makes an abrupt turn to the right, off the road, to gradually ascend through mountain laurel and pine. Sassafras is particularly abundant here.

Some of the older trees on this route bear the markings of successful feedings by, evidently, quite a number of woodpeckers. Continue with gradual ups and downs and at 1.2 miles cross a small stream. The spot is an ideal relaxation point. Ascend steeply at first, but then proceed on well-graded switchbacks.

Reach a trail intersection at 1.6 miles. The trail beside a rock wall to the right leads 300 feet to White Rock Falls—a most magical place. Admittedly, when compared to other falls, White Rock is not all that spectacular. However, the attractions here are that you have reached such a nicely isolated spot while expending such a little amount of energy to do so, and now you are able to enjoy the small but exceptional rocky gorge the water has carved out of the mountainside. The sun, beaming down on mountain laurel, creates shadows that dance about on the steep walls as the water cascades 30–40 feet through the boulders. After a stop at this enjoyable spot, return to the

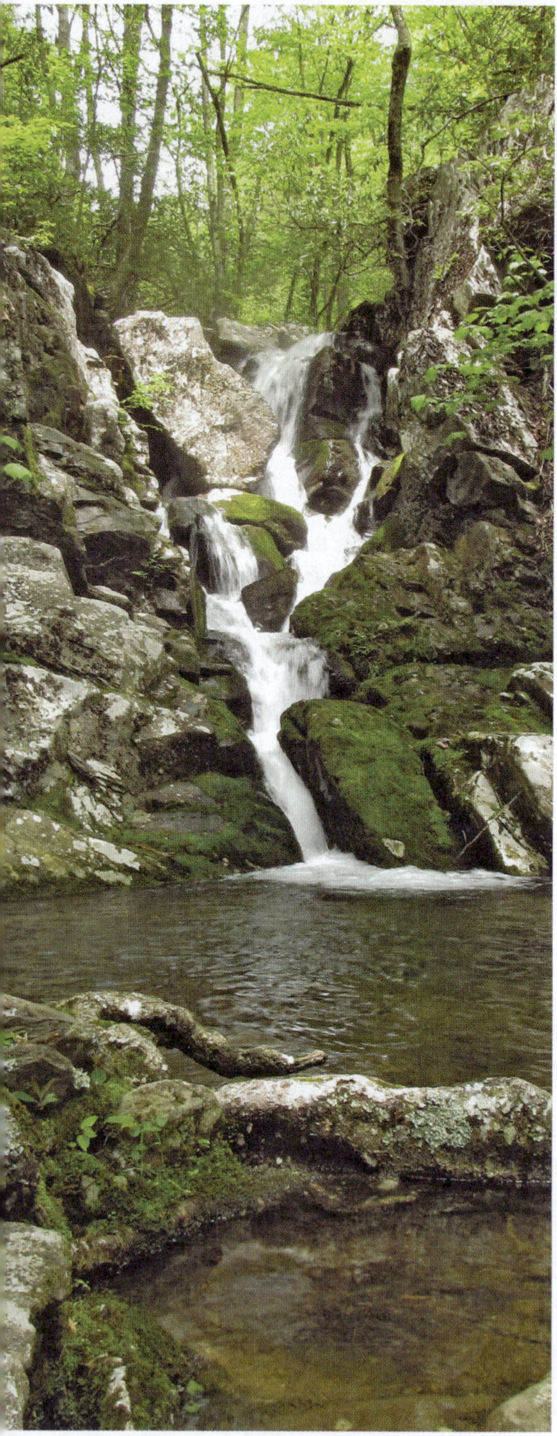

The glen of White Rock Falls can be a magical place.

photo: Johnny Molloy

intersection, turn right, and begin the climb back to the parkway.

At 1.9 miles, reach a sort of ridgeline and descend slightly. A few rocks to the right afford good views of the valley just before you cross a footbridge and gradually ascend. You must be alert at 2.2 miles, for no matter how inviting that shaded grove looks, the trail does not continue straight into it. Rather, make an abrupt right across the creek and ascend. Cross another footbridge and, at 2.7 miles, arrive on the parkway at milepost 20.

Continue by bearing left, crossing the parkway, and turning onto the trail past the picnic tables at the northern end of the Slacks Overlook parking area. In 250 feet, at the intersection of two trails, turn left downhill and intersect the Slacks Overlook Trail {FS 480A}, marked with blue diamonds. The Slacks Overlook Trail opens up a number of options for further hikes. A left turn onto the Slacks Overlook Trail would lead you to several paths descending into the Saint Mary's Wilderness (see Hike 34) or to other trails that drop down to the forest service's campground on Sherando Lake (see Hike 33). However, your present route does not go left, but rather right, and slabs the hillside. From here on out, it is a pleasant walk through a mountainside environment of hardwoods, mountain laurel, and berry bushes. In fact, it is more or less downhill from here until the last half mile.

Berry bushes are abundant as you walk onto and begin following a spur ridge at the 3.1-mile mark. Just 0.2 mile beyond, begin a gradual and then more rapid descent. Turn left onto an old roadbed at 4.3 miles. At 4.5 miles you reach the intersection with the orange-blazed White Rock Gap Trail {FS 480}, which drops to the left for about 2 miles to Sherando Lake. Turn right and ascend. Pass an old homestead site where raspberries should be plentiful (and delicious!) in season before coming to a sign identifying a spring as the headwaters of North Fork Back Creek. Continue to ascend. Arrive back in White Rock Gap on the parkway to complete the 5.0-mile circuit.

33 Sherando Lake

- **GPS:** N37.9201282 W79.0050024
- **TOTAL DISTANCE (circuit):** 1.6 miles
- **HIKING TIME:** 1.0 hour
- **VERTICAL RISE:** 280 feet
- **MAPS:** USGS *Big Levels; Sherando Recreation Area map; National Geographic Trails Illustrated #789 Lexington/Blue Ridge Mountains*
- **CONTACT:** Glenwood/Pedlar Ranger District
  27 Ranger Lane
  Natural Bridge Station, VA 24579
  540-291-2188
  fs.usda.gov/gwj

The Hike at a Glance

0.5 Left to cross dam, go to spillway; recross dam and turn left onto Cliff Trail

1.6 Return to parking area

Sherando Lake is one of George Washington and Jefferson National Forests' largest recreation areas. Attractions here include a sand beach, a visitor center with interpretive materials, a picnic area, and a campground; the recreation area can accommodate close to 900 people. The Civilian Conservation Corps built the 24-acre lower lake in the 1930s, while the upper lake of 7 acres was built in 1958 for flood control. Both lakes reportedly have good fishing for largemouth bass, bluegill, and catfish. Trout are stocked in the spring and fall.

With so much to offer, and because it is located within a few minutes' drive of the Blue Ridge Parkway, Shenandoah National Park, and the cities of Waynesboro and Staunton, the recreation area is exceedingly popular and is usually busy almost every summer weekend. The facilities are closed during the colder months, but you may still access the trails.

This hike is a fairly easy and pleasant stroll next to the lake and to an elevated viewpoint. The whole family should be able to enjoy the walk, which will help you escape the hustle and bustle of a noisy beach or crowded campground.

DIRECTIONS To reach the trailhead, take the I-64 Exit 96 at Waynesboro and follow VA 624 to Lyndhurst. After 2.5 miles bear left onto VA 664 for 7.5 miles to the entrance road, on the right.

Route Description

From the beach and picnic-area parking lot, take the paved trail to the right, walking to the front of the large bathhouse and visitor center. Make note of the chairs on the porched breezeway of the rustic but rather elegant stone-and-log structure. After your walk, this would make a nice spot to relax and enjoy the lake—framed by mountains in the distance—and the pleasingly manicured and landscaped lawn in front of the breezeway.

Continue on pavement around the beach and ascend stone steps onto a pathway (Lakeside Trail {FS 300}) entering the forest. The trail is more or less level as it continues just above the shore of the lake, passing abundant blueberry bushes, mountain laurel, and rhododendron.

The farther you get from the noisy beach area, the more likely you are to spot a belted kingfisher making a swooping dive into the lake in search of food. If successful, the bird will emerge a few moments later with a fish in its beak, sometimes emitting its distinctive dry rattle as it flies off to consume the meal.

An ancient Greek tale is the basis for a modern-day phrase and tells of the origin of kingfishers. Halcyone, daughter of the King of the Winds, threw herself into the sea to drown upon hearing of the death of her husband. She did not die; rather, she and the spirit of her husband were turned into kingfishers—birds

Sherando Lake

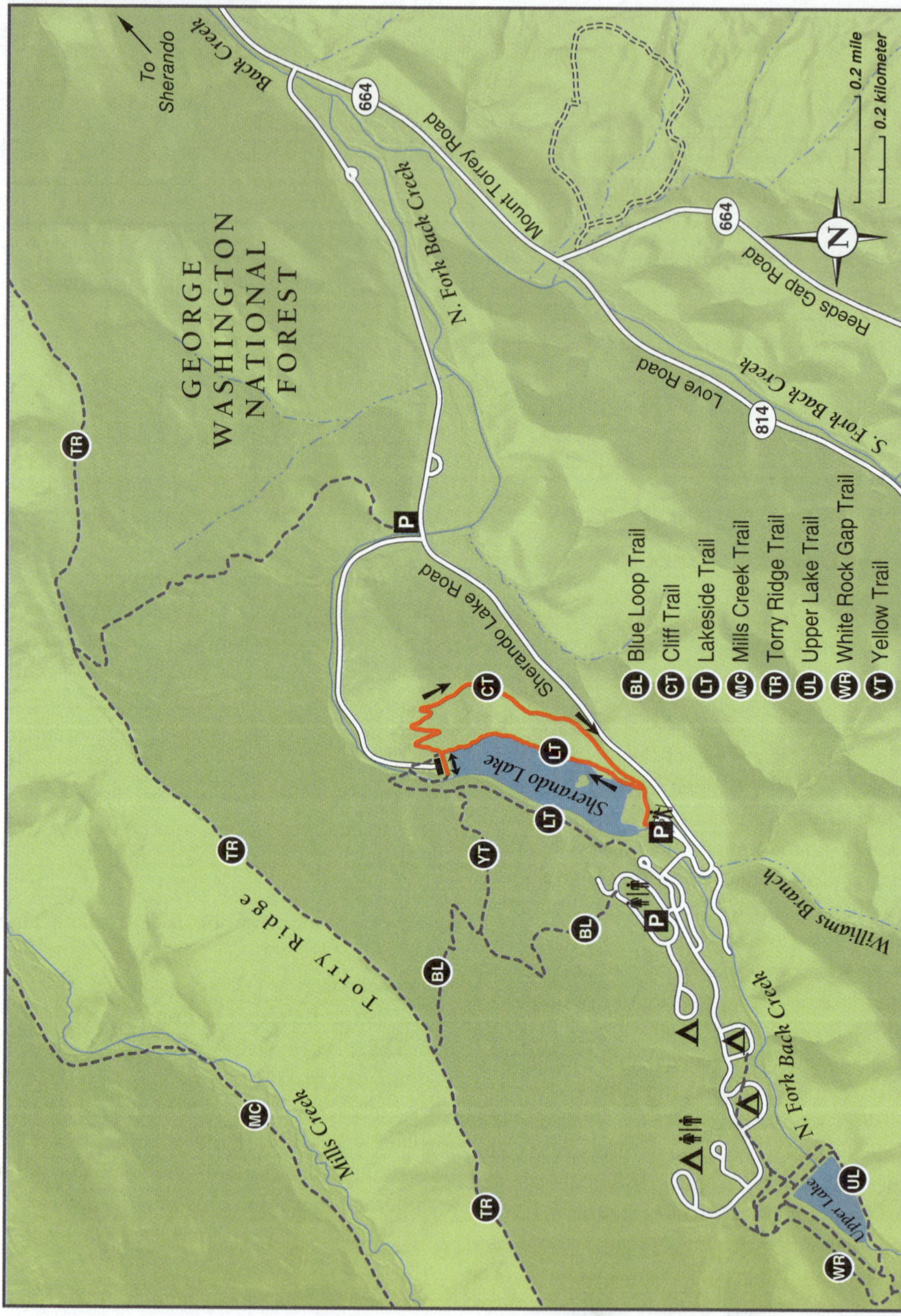

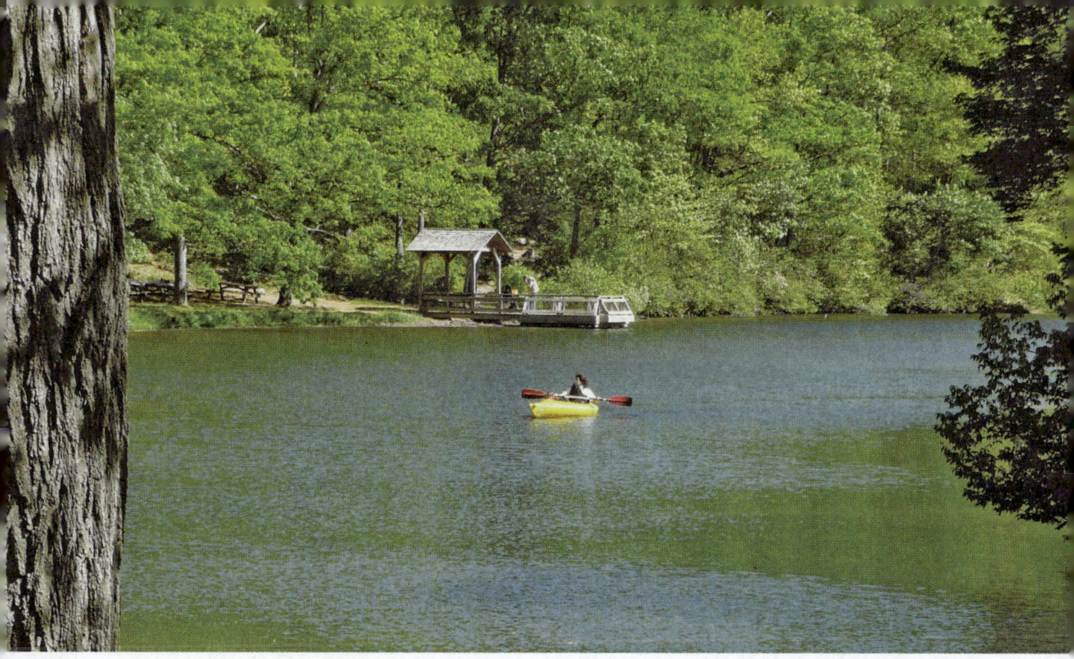

Sherando Lake is a popular recreational destination.

having the power to calm tumultuous waters. Thus, our use of the phrase "halcyon days."

Reach the far end of the lake at 0.5 mile and make a left across the earthen dam to a trail along the spillway. During times of heavy rain and high water, a descent on the short pathway (stay behind the fence for safety) can be exciting. Large volumes of water come rushing through the concrete canyon, loudly swishing and swirling, to make patterns and designs that exist momentarily, only to be replaced by others.

Retrace your steps to the other side of the dam and turn onto the Cliff Trail {FS 299}. Thanks to a series of switchbacks and the pathway's enterprising use of the natural lay of rock formations, the less-than-300-foot climb to the ridgeline is accomplished moderately easily.

Torry Ridge, the sloping valley formed by the north fork of Back Creek, and much of the lake can be seen from a viewpoint at 1.0 mile. The trail now begins a gentle descent along the ridgetop, where blueberries and sassafras are the dominant understory.

Identifying sassafras can be difficult at times. Its leaves may be one of three different shapes—three lobes, two lobes (resembling a mitten), or a single lobe. Just one type, or all three, may be present on any given tree. Sassafras bark can be used to make a delicious tea, and its dried and crushed leaf buds are used in gumbo filé. At one time, sassafras root is what gave root beer its distinctive taste. Today, of course, most root beers are flavored artificially.

A trail, which may not be discernible, comes in from the left at 1.4 miles; keep right and continue with the gradual descent. Walk past the beach and bathhouse and return to the parking lot at 1.6 miles. Better yet, get a cool drink, settle into one of the chairs on the bathhouse porch, read a good book, and look up occasionally to savor the scenery and the end of your halcyon day at the lake.

Myriad hiking opportunities fan out from the Sherando Lake campground. The Blue Loop Trail ascends to the Torry Ridge Trail, which, in turn, can be used to ascend Bald Mountain and connect with trails in the Saint Mary's Wilderness (see Hike 34). The White Rock Gap Trail goes upstream along the north fork of Back Creek to White Rock Gap on the Blue Ridge Parkway (see Hike 32). A handout map, available at the entrance station, shows the small network of trails located close to the lake and within the confines of the campground.

Saint Mary's Wilderness

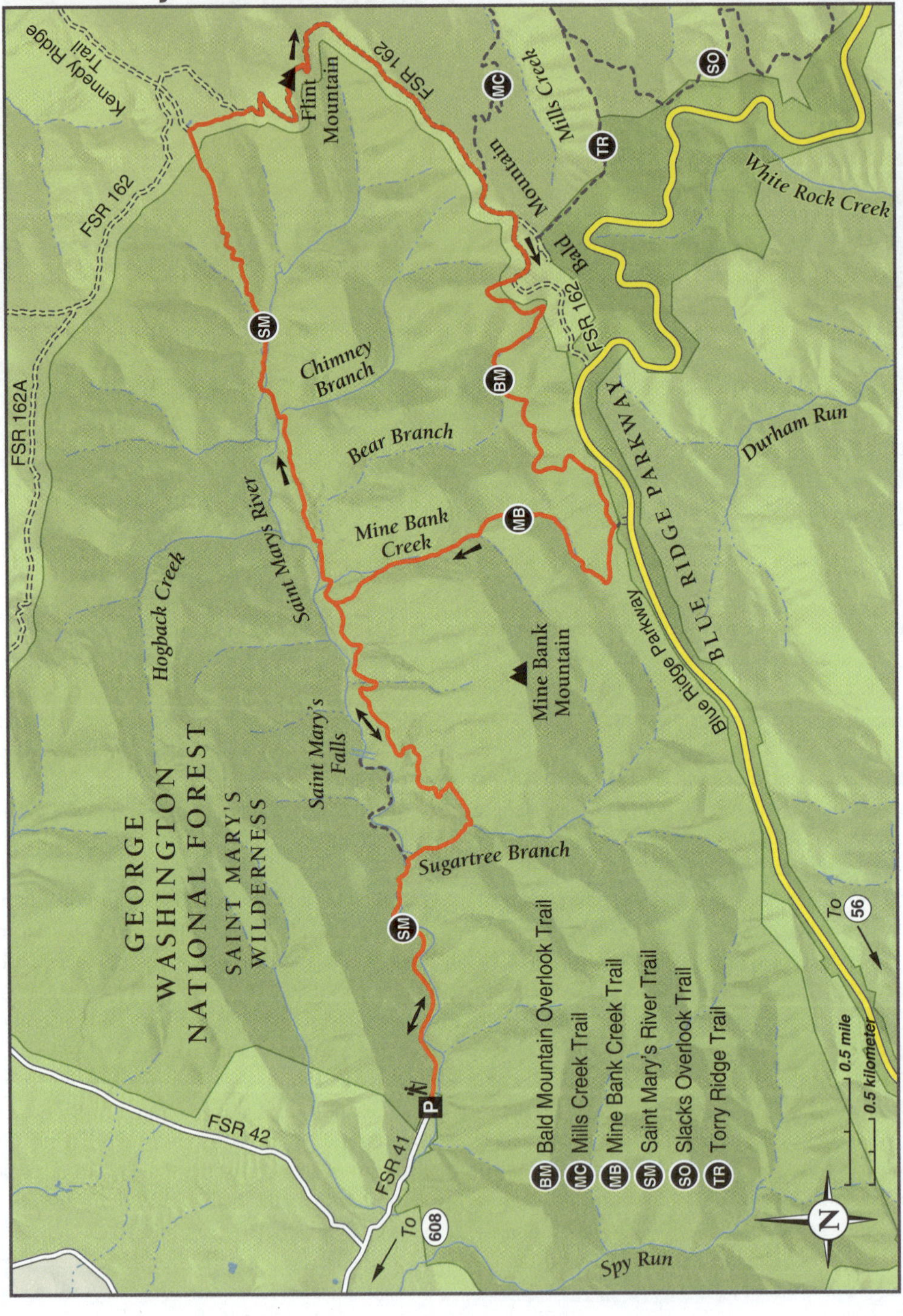

34 Saint Mary's Wilderness

- **GPS:** N37.9250949 W79.1374907
- **TOTAL DISTANCE (circuit):** 17.5 miles
- **HIKING TIME:** 10.0 hours; recommended as an overnight hike
- **VERTICAL RISE:** 2,400 feet
- **MAPS:** USGS *Vesuvius* and *Big Levels; National Geographic Trails Illustrated #789 Lexington/Blue Ridge Mountains*
- **CONTACT:** Glenwood/Pedlar Ranger District
  27 Ranger Lane
  Natural Bridge Station, VA 24579
  540-291-2188
  fs.usda.gov/gwj

The Hike at a Glance: First Day

1.4 Stay right on the Saint Mary's River Trail. (The trail to Saint Mary's Falls goes off to the left.)

3.6 Bypass Mine Bank Trail and stay left on Saint Mary's River Trail

6.2 After passing out of wilderness area, take pathway right and then turn right onto FSR 162

9.8 Right onto Bald Mountain Trail

10.8 Rise on old roadbed

11.7 Be alert when Bald Mountain Trail leaves old roadbed and turns right onto a pathway. Shortly thereafter, turn right on Mine Bank Trail

13.9 Left onto Saint Mary's River Trail

17.5 Return to parking area

In a farsighted move, the United States achieved permanent protection for certain tracts of public land with the passage of the Wilderness Act in 1964. Within a few years, more than 90 areas and more than 11 million acres had been brought into the National Wilderness Preservation System.

However, the system was not as far-reaching as its proponents had hoped—all but four of the wilderness areas were west of Wichita, Kansas. The law's definition of wilderness, with phrases such as "the area generally appears to have been affected primarily by the forces of nature, with the imprint of man's work substantially unnoticeable," prohibited almost any area east of the Mississippi River from being included in the system. Recognizing that the East, with its earlier settlement and heavier population concentration, had more disturbed land than the West, another law was passed in 1975. This one permitted places where the evidence of human activity was gradually being reclaimed by natural processes to fit within the definition of a wilderness. That law (and hard work by wilderness proponents) has given Virginia more than 200,000 acres of officially designated wilderness land.

Saint Mary's is a prime example of a spot that would have been excluded from the system before 1975. Railroads snaked into the river valley and onto some of the surrounding hills to transport the manganese ore and iron ore that was mined from the turn of the 20th century to about 1917. Activity, with much more elaborate methods of surface mining, began again during World War II and continued until the mid-1950s. Vegetation has begun to obscure some of the scars upon the land, yet, when explored with a historical mien, these reminders of bustling mining days can actually become a highlight of a hike.

The landscape this hike passes through is varied. The Saint Mary's River and some of its tributaries are brook trout streams, but due to several factors (one thought to be acid rain), the number of trout had been declining. Efforts by the forest service, such as liming the streams to neutralize the acid, seems to have helped remedy the situation somewhat.

At one time, the hike began rather gently by following one of the old mining roads along the environs of Saint Mary's River. It still follows that route, but hurricanes near the beginning of the 21st century, along with subsequent storms, have done some major damage. While there has been some work on the trail, you may find yourself sometimes searching for the correct route, scrambling up steep banks, fording the river several times, or walking along narrow ledges above the stream. *Please note:* In addition to all of this, the forest service is no longer blazing trails in the wilderness, and what blazes were there are long faded. Also, the trails may be overgrown in places, but their routes are usually discernible. Just be prepared to encounter such conditions before you consider doing this outing.

Less than 4 miles into the trip, the hike swings away from the river and into several areas of former mining activity. You leave the mines behind by making a stiff climb of about a mile to upland forests on Big Levels and Bald Mountain. From the high point, the hike descends into small stream valleys (providing secluded camping spots) before dropping back to Saint Mary's River for the return to the trailhead. If you hike it in two days, as suggested, even with the considerable change in elevation, it is a trip of only moderate difficulty.

DIRECTIONS Follow VA 606 east from the I-64/I-81 Raphine–Steeles Tavern Exit 205 for 1.5 miles to Steeles Tavern. Make a left onto US 11 for only 0.1 mile before making a right onto VA 56. In 1.1 miles is a left onto VA 608. Drive 2.2 miles from that intersection, watching for when VA 608 curves right to go through a railroad underpass. Just 0.3 mile from the underpass, turn right onto FSR 41 and continue 1.4 miles to its terminus at the trailhead parking area.

Route Description

Begin hiking at the far end of the parking lot where the Saint Mary's River Trail {FS 500} enters the wilderness area next to the river. Look up to your right to see the open talus slopes on the mountainside about 1,000 feet above you. Virginia creeper vines twist along the ground and onto tree trunks, as does a bountiful amount of poison ivy. Much of the time you will be walking on a rough and rocky pathway whose mud-caked stones reveal that it is actually a floodplain streambed. Depending on current conditions, you may have to cross the stream a couple of times or more. Periods of low water often permit rock-hopping, but high water sometimes makes for a nasty, and possibly dangerous, ford.

The Saint Mary's Falls Trail {FS 500B} goes off to the left at 1.4 miles. (A walk of less than 30 minutes, one-way, will bring you to the 20-foot falls.)

Keep right on Saint Mary's Trail and ascend into the hollow that the Sugartree Branch has created between Long Drive and Mine Bank Mountains. All too often, we hikers get caught up in the movement of the hike and fail to really see what we are walking through. You deserve a rest break, so stop for a while and gaze upon your surroundings. Don't look up, down, or even sideways. Look straight ahead and you will be amazed at how many things are located just at eye level. The angular twists and turns of a dogwood branch; the distinctive look of birch bark on the trunk of a tree; the two narrow, whitish strips highlighting the bottom of hemlock needles; shiny evergreen rhododendron leaves (which provide deer with nourishment in the winter); the sparkling water of the creek rolling over boulders in small cascades—all of these, and more, crowd your sight, almost demanding that you focus on them, that you take in all their various textures, shapes, and hues, so that this special little spot in the world will still be with you long after you leave the wilderness.

A wide, deep swimming hole beckons you to linger even longer at 1.6 miles, for soon you will cross the stream, ascend somewhat steeply, and be away from the sound of water for the first time on this hike.

While doing some off-trail exploring in the old mining area at 2.1 miles, you may find the remains of an old surface mine—concrete and steel blocks, pits dug deeply into the earth, scraps of sheet metal from former storage sheds, and bits of iron slag hidden in the underbrush. Small pathways head off in

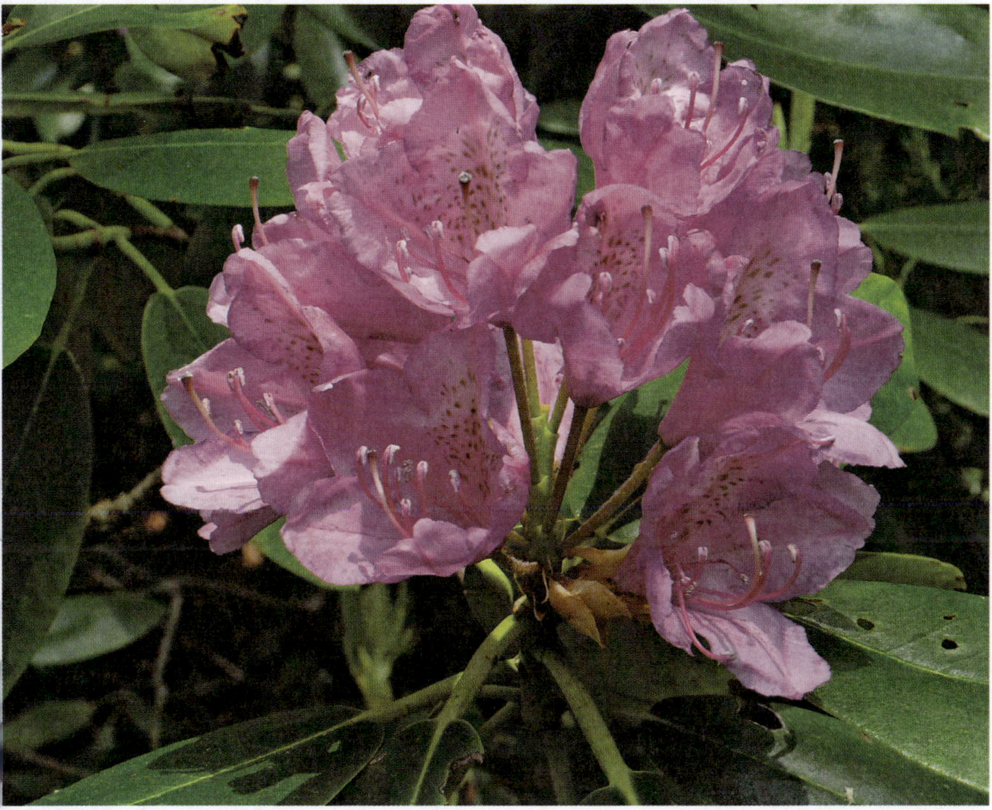

Rhododendron

many directions here, so you need to look for the main route in order to swing to the left and descend around a giant pit that opens up a view of Cellar Mountain to the north.

The rhododendron and mountain laurel become thicker where the route crosses a small stream on a culvert at 3.0 miles. Another water run is crossed before the Mine Bank Creek Trail {FS 500C} comes in from the right at 3.6 miles. Keep to the left, continuing on Saint Mary's River Trail.

Cross Bear Branch at 3.8 miles and come into another area bearing the scars of mining activities. Once more you can wander off the trail, closely inspecting crumbling foundations, large pits, and small mounds of dirt covering old equipment and mining waste products. When you are ready to continue, return to the main route, taking the trail around a number of pits and piles through numerous dogwood trees. Rhododendron has become noticeably more abundant. At 5.2 miles, the old roadway begins to rise steeply—so steeply that the route sometimes leaves the road for short switchbacks to make the ascent a little easier. Enter Big Levels at 5.9 miles—the name aptly describes the terrain you are now walking upon. The area was created hundreds of millions of years ago during the Paleozoic era when shifting continental plates caused the first uplifting of the Blue Ridge Mountains. Afterward, geologists believe, stream erosion carved out deep and narrow canyons into the uplift. As water wore away the ridges, they became more rounded and, as the streams deposited more silt into the ever-widening valleys, a gradual equalizing of ground elevations occurred, creating this high mountain plateau.

Arrive at the wilderness boundary at 6.15 miles. Directly ahead is Green Pond. Walk the few steps to observe this mountaintop swamp of boggy soil and water-inundated trees. Follow the grassy road from the boundary, swinging left around Green Pond. Pay attention at 6.2 miles because your route makes a sudden right off the road and onto a pathway. Follow the path to FSR 162. Turn right to soon begin ascending, by way of switchbacks, this four-wheel-drive roadway. (The Kennedy Ridge Trail {FS 479}, which goes about 3 miles to FSR 42, is the dirt road across FSR 162.)

During the month of June, FSR 162 is the place to be to see, possibly, the best display of rhododendron blossoms in the George Washington and Jefferson National Forests. Rounding each bend in the road, you are treated to different multitudes of flower petals ranging in color from pure white to bright pink to dark pink to rich shades of purple.

Descend after crossing the summit of Flint Mountain at 7.6 miles, but rise again in less than half a mile. The amount of rhododendron continues to delight the eyes, even when not in bloom, and 9.1 miles of walking delivers you to a clearing on the left for the only wide-open vista of the hike. Directly in front of you from the clearing is Torry Ridge, with the Blue Ridge Parkway and houses of Wintergreen Resort just behind it. To the east is Three Ridges with the Priest (see Hike 36) visible in the south to the right.

Continue along FSR 162, bypassing the road to the left at 9.5 miles (which leads 0.3 mile to the top of Bald Mountain). In order to turn onto the Bald Mountain Trail {FS 500E}, you need to watch for it coming in from the right at 9.8 miles. The path is somewhat obvious, but there may be no sign or blazes marking it.

The Bald Mountain Trail receives little foot traffic, so there is a good possibility of not seeing anyone while walking its full distance. Descend and, at 10.3 miles, switchback into the head of a small valley, which feels well isolated. Cross and begin paralleling a creek on a rocky, descending pathway. Cross the creek again as the valley opens up. You have reached your evening's destination. Find a good campsite somewhere within the next 0.4 mile, set up the tent, and watch, or at least listen, for wild turkey or ruffed grouse while enjoying your well-deserved dinner.

Begin the next day by leaving the creek and rising along the trail's old roadbed at 10.8 miles. You need to be alert once more because, at 11.7 miles, the route leaves the road to make an abrupt right turn onto a trail hedged by azalea and sassafras. Shortly, intersect and turn right onto the Mine Bank Creek Trail {FS 500C}. (The Blue Ridge Parkway, milepost 23, is about 300 feet to the left.)

Descend, sometimes somewhat steeply, through a forest of oak, maple, and black gum. Mountain laurel is at about eye level and Indian cucumber root, a member of the lily family, attains a height of 1–3 feet. It is an intriguing-looking plant that rises on a single stem to a whorl of leaves about halfway up its length to continue on to a second whorl on top. The uppermost leaves hide a small, dangling, yellow flower that blooms in May and June. The underground portion of the plant is edible.

In June, the beauty and plethora of rhododendron blossoms at and near the creek crossing make the 12.5 miles you have walked worthwhile. When you cross the stream again, appreciate the yellow birch, which provides browse for deer and whose catkins (flowers) are a favorite grouse food. Cross the creek several more times until the valley becomes a narrow gorge at 13.0 miles, where the stream drops quickly and your route now follows an old road.

You will negotiate delightfully green rhododendron tunnels before the terrain levels out for you to intersect the Saint Mary's River Trail at 13.9 miles. Turn left to descend along the trail you came up yesterday. Eventually you will cross the river again, return to FSR 42, and come to the end of your 17.5-mile hike in one of the largest national forest wildernesses in Virginia.

35 Crabtree Falls

- **GPS:** N37.8507979 W79.0791697
- **TOTAL DISTANCE (round-trip):** 5.8 miles
- **HIKING TIME:** 4.25 hours
- **VERTICAL RISE:** 1,520 feet
- **MAPS:** USGS *Massies Mill; Crabtree Falls Trail map; National Geographic Trails Illustrated #789 Lexington/Blue Ridge Mountains*
- **CONTACT:** Glenwood/Pedlar Ranger District
  27 Ranger Lane
  Natural Bridge Station, VA 24579
  540-291-2188
  fs.usda.gov/gwj

The Hike at a Glance

0.2 First overlook
0.4 Viewing platform
0.7 Another vantage point
1.5 Base of upper falls
1.7 Top of upper falls
2.9 Parking area on VA 826; retrace steps
5.8 Return to automobile

Amusingly, five different sources completely disagree on what makes the five cascades of Crabtree Falls, which drop from the northwestern face of Pinnacle Ridge, so special. One calls them the highest falls east of the Mississippi River. Another claims a total drop of 1,200 feet, while a third authority states the cascades have a combined descent of 1,080 feet. A book on the geology of Virginia gives the overall drop of the falls as only 500 feet. A fifth reference quotes no distance on the falls but proclaims them the highest cascading falls in Virginia.

For the hiker, there is no real need to be concerned with the exact distinction of Crabtree Falls. Suffice it to say that, often, you must go on an extended, arduous journey in order to reach and appreciate a waterfall of any significant or true scenic value, but not in the case of Crabtree Falls. In fact, you can reach the first of the impressive cascades by a relatively easy walk of less than 10 minutes from a trailhead located off a paved roadway. From there, the forest service's first-rate pathway of graded switchbacks and wooden staircases winding over and around giant boulders helps ease the burden of gaining about 1,000 feet in 1.5 miles to reach the top of the upper falls. Observation decks of native stone and timber, overlooking different portions of the falls, seem to appear at convenient spots—just at about the time you are looking for an excuse to pause and catch your breath.

DIRECTIONS To reach this moderately strenuous hike, take the I-81/I-64 Exit 205 at Raphine–Steeles Tavern and head east on VA 606 for 1.5 miles to US 11. Turn left onto US 11, but leave it in less than 0.1 mile by making a right onto VA 56. A 9.2-mile drive on this narrow, twisting road will bring you across the crest of the Blue Ridge Mountains and to VA 826, which comes in from the right. (If you have four-wheel-drive vehicles or ones with high clearance, you could take VA 826, which quickly becomes dirt, several miles to leave one of the vehicles at the Crabtree Meadows parking area and turn this into a one-way hike.) Continue on VA 56 2.8 miles beyond VA 826 to the Crabtree Falls Trail parking lot, on the right. Toilets (usually closed in the off-season) are located adjacent at the upper tier of the parking area.

Route Description

Due to the fragility of the area and the popularity of this hike, camping is not permitted within 100 feet of the south fork of the Tye River or within 500 feet of the trail. Because of the construction of the upper parking area near the turn of the 21st century, you no longer

Crabtree Falls

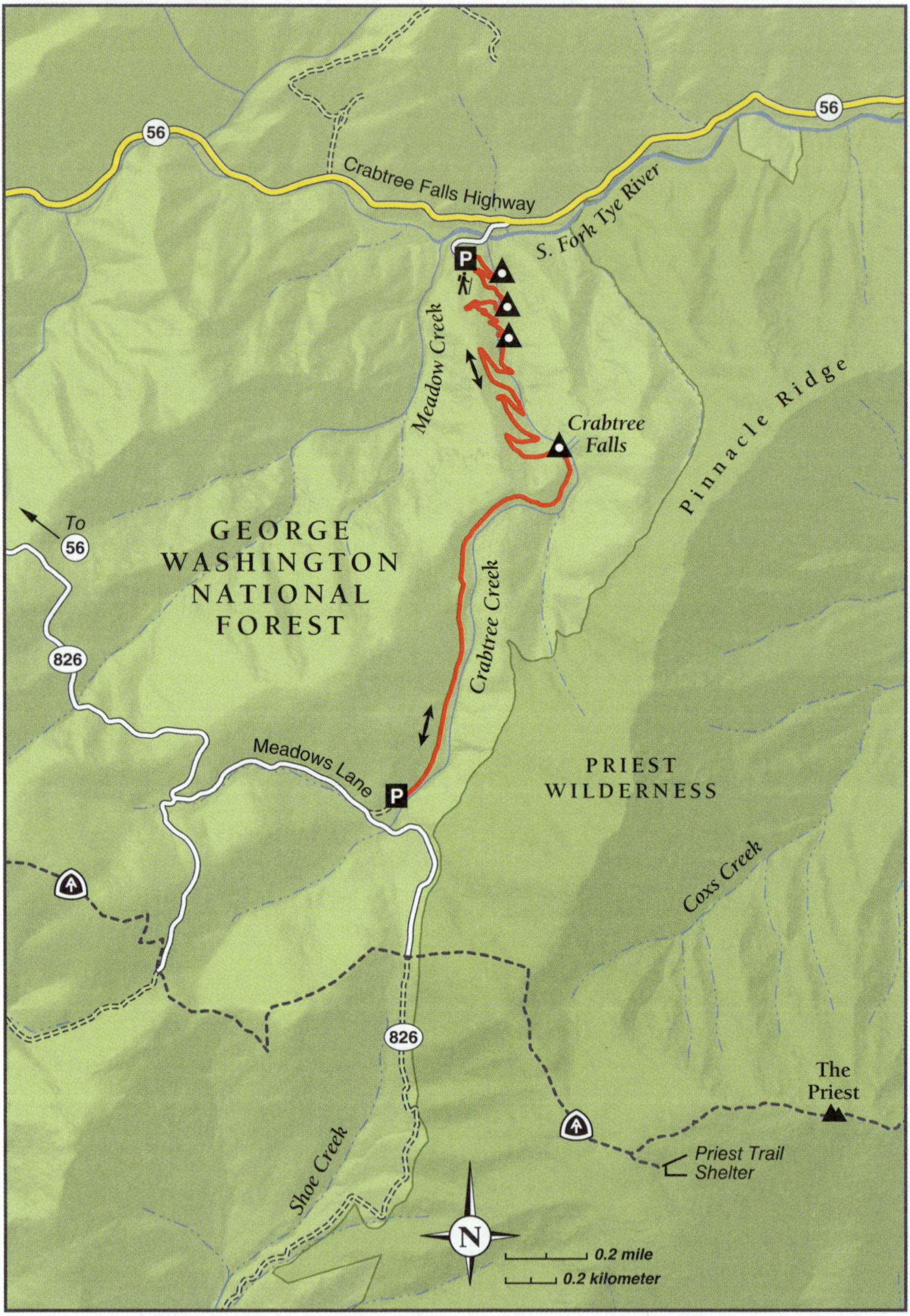

have to cross the south fork of the Tye River on a wooden bridge. Yet, it is still in place and you should stop for a moment or two to admire the effort, expense, and engineering expertise the forest service once expended. This is not an ordinary, built-on-site, rough, split-log trail bridge. It was constructed in one laminated arched span, transported by way of the narrow roadway you drove to reach here, and then lifted into place by cranes.

After admiring the handiwork of human beings, take a few more moments to "hear the river tearin' the mountain on down," as singer-songwriter Walkin' Jim Stoltz put it. Some geologists believe that at one time the Appalachians were at least as high as the present-day Himalayas, only to be eroded by wind and, especially, water. Most often, the rivers and creeks slowly wear away small bits of rock and soil. Sometimes, though, the erosion can take on cataclysmic proportions. In August 1969, Hurricane Camille, in combination with another stormfront, dropped somewhere between 2 and 3 feet of rain onto the Tye River Valley in less than 6 hours. The swollen streams—uprooting trees and sending house-size boulders crashing down the mountain sides—destroyed homes, bridges, and roadways and took a large toll in human life. Enough soil was stripped away to reveal granite rock that had been hidden for hundreds of millions of years.

Moisture-laden air coming from the creek, along with shade provided by the rich forest, should make you notice a slight drop in temperature as you come to the first falls overlook in 0.2 mile. The water dropping in front of you makes a picturesque scene, but be sure to look upward to appreciate the full length of the falls you are viewing. Moss-covered logs keep the area looking richly green throughout much of the year.

Indian cucumber root and wild bleeding heart grow along the trail as you switchback uphill. At 0.4 mile, you'll reach another platform, followed a short distance away by an excellent view of an approximately 70-foot cascade. Another vantage point, this one looking downstream, is reached at 0.7 mile. The falls and cascades seem to get taller and more impressive the farther you progress along the route. Violets, wild geranium, and jewelweed are now common.

Poplar trees line the creek where it drops down a smooth vertical rock face at 0.9 mile. You will soon get a short breather where the trail levels out onto a shelf and the stream descends over boulders in a series of small cascades. Ferns, the dominant green undergrowth, share the forest floor with jack-in-the-pulpits and false Solomon's seal. Distinguishing false Solomon's seal from Solomon's seal is best accomplished at either flowering or fruit-bearing time. The Solomon's seal's little bell-shaped flowers hang down from the stem, while the tiny, starred blossoms of false Solomon's seal extend from the end of the stem. Later in the year, Solomon's seal's fruit is a dark blue (almost black) berry, easily differentiated from the red berries of false Solomon's seal.

At 1.5 miles you reach the base of the upper, and certainly most impressive, falls. The water splits and takes many different paths down the rocks, so be sure to walk around as much as possible (remember to stay on the path, though) to gain various perspectives on the falls.

Come to the top of the upper falls at 1.7 miles. The water drops at such a precipitous angle that it is hard to really see any great portion of the falls. For safety reasons, don't be tempted to walk to, or on, slippery rocks in order to peer over the edge in hopes of obtaining a better look. (Keep pets on a leash as they, too, have fallen over the falls.) Rather, continue on a few feet and take the footbridge across Crabtree Creek to follow a side trail out to an observation platform. You still won't be able to see the falls from here, but you can tell how much elevation you have gained by gazing down into the narrow valley carved by the south fork of the Tye River. Fork Mountain is on the other side of the valley.

Retrace your steps, cross the creek, and continue upstream. Pay attention at 1.8 miles, where a trail on the left goes just a few feet to the side of the creek; you want to bear right

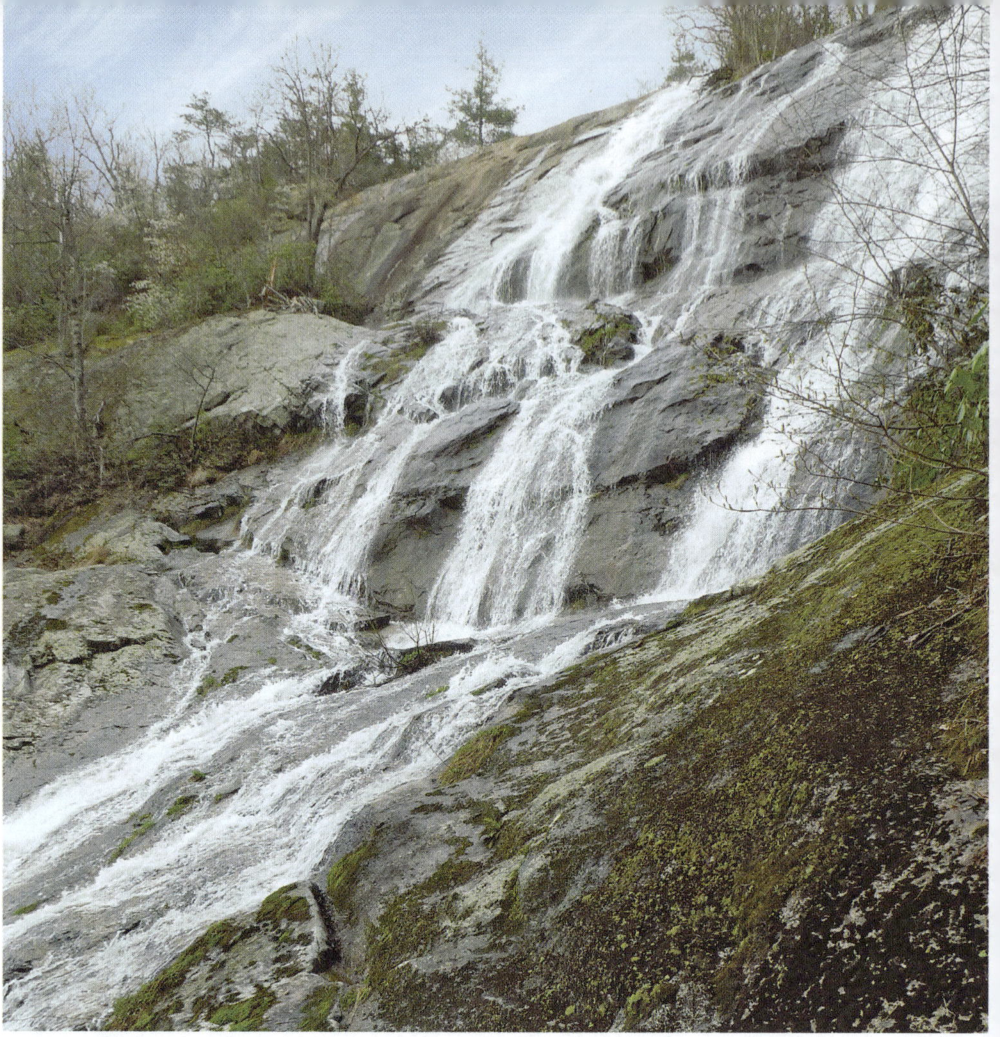

Crabtree Falls

onto the trail that ascends a short distance and then levels out. From here to the end of the hike, there is very little gain in elevation, so enjoy the easy walking beside mountain laurel bushes.

Make a mental note of how the pathway looks as your route intersects and turns right onto a woods road at 2.1 miles. Watch for this spot on your return trip, as it is easy to overlook and make the mistake of continuing to walk down the road. (If the road leads you to a crossing of the creek on your return hike, go back until you find the trail turning off the road.) Mayapple, violets, wild geranium, and cinquefoil add their touches of colors and shapes to the undergrowth near the road.

An old road comes in from the left at 2.7 miles; keep right. Arrive at the end of the trail and the parking area on VA 826 in 2.9 miles.

Across VA 826, gnarled old crabapple and apple trees grow in an area known as Crabtree Meadows. During the 1930s, a sawmill operated, and a number of people lived, on these acres of relatively flat land located between 4,040-foot Maintop Mountain and the 4,063-foot summit of the Priest. The Appalachian Trail (see Hike 36), which goes over both of these mountains, can be reached by following VA 826 uphill for about half a mile from the end of Crabtree Falls Trail. Unless you did a car shuttle, it is time to retrace your steps back to your car at the lower trailhead.

36 Appalachian and Mau-Har Trails

- **GPS:** N37.7596835 W79.1951835
- **TOTAL DISTANCE (one-way):** 26.1 miles
- **HIKING TIME:** 4 days, 3 nights
- **VERTICAL RISE:** Approximately 7,000 feet
- **MAPS:** USGS *Montebello, Massies Mill, Big Levels, Sherando,* and *Horseshoe Mountain; ATC Central Virginia Maps* 1 and 2; *National Geographic Trails Illustrated #789 Lexington/Blue Ridge Mountains*
- **CONTACT:** Appalachian Trail Conservancy
  PO Box 807
  Harpers Ferry, WV 25425
  304-535-6331
  appalachiantrail.org

The Appalachian Trail (AT) follows the crest of the Appalachian Mountains for more than 2,190 miles as it makes its way from Springer Mountain in Georgia to Mount Katahdin in Maine. Every year hundreds of hikers complete the full length in four–six months, but the majority of people make use of the trail for a few hours, a day, or a weekend. Benton MacKaye's 1921 proposal for a long-distance trail in the Appalachians resulted in volunteers constructing the first few miles in New York during 1922. Fifteen years later, the final link was completed in central Maine. One of the most beautiful aspects of the AT is that almost every mile of it was, and still is, built and maintained by volunteers, whose love of the outdoors leads them to invest their time and hard labor so that you and I can enjoy a walk along America's premier National Scenic Trail.

Virginia contains more than 500 miles of the AT, about one-quarter of its full length. This backpack trip along it and one of its side trails has almost everything that makes hiking worthwhile in central Virginia. The trek never drops below 3,200 feet for the first two days, and it crosses the 4,063-foot summit of the Priest on the third day out. From the Priest it plummets more than 3,000 feet, just to regain most of that elevation along a waterfall-studded creek. These up-and-down efforts are amply rewarded. There are magnificent views, rhododendron-lined native-trout streams, remote forest glens, open fields of green grass, wildflowers by the thousands, and ample opportunities for quiet, isolated, and scenic campsites.

This portion of the AT—well built, marked, and maintained by the Natural Bridge and Tidewater Appalachian Trail Clubs—is heavily traveled, especially in May and June when the bulk of thru-hikers (people hiking the AT's entire length) pass through. It is instructive and entertaining to be on the trail at this time, but no matter what month, carry a tent in the event a shelter becomes overcrowded. For a more solitary experience, hike at a different time of the year or camp at the numerous pretty little sites you will pass instead of staying in shelters. Water is available near the shelters and from several other sources. There are planned relocations for the AT, but the route will not be significantly altered, nor will any great distance be added or subtracted.

DIRECTIONS The easiest way to reach the two ends of the hike is to make use of the Blue Ridge Parkway. Take I-64 Exit 99 in Rockfish Gap, a few miles east of Waynesboro, and drive southward on the parkway to Reids Gap, BRP milepost 13.7. Parking for your ending trailhead is just to the left, off VA 664. Continue south on the parkway to exit at milepost 45.6. Follow US 60 east 4.0 miles to the left turn onto VA 634. Soon, make a right onto VA 755, which becomes dirt FSR 48. Along the way is wonderful Wiggins Spring; every day, gallons of water bubble up from its underground source. Past the

(continued on page 164)

Appalachian and Mau-Har Trails

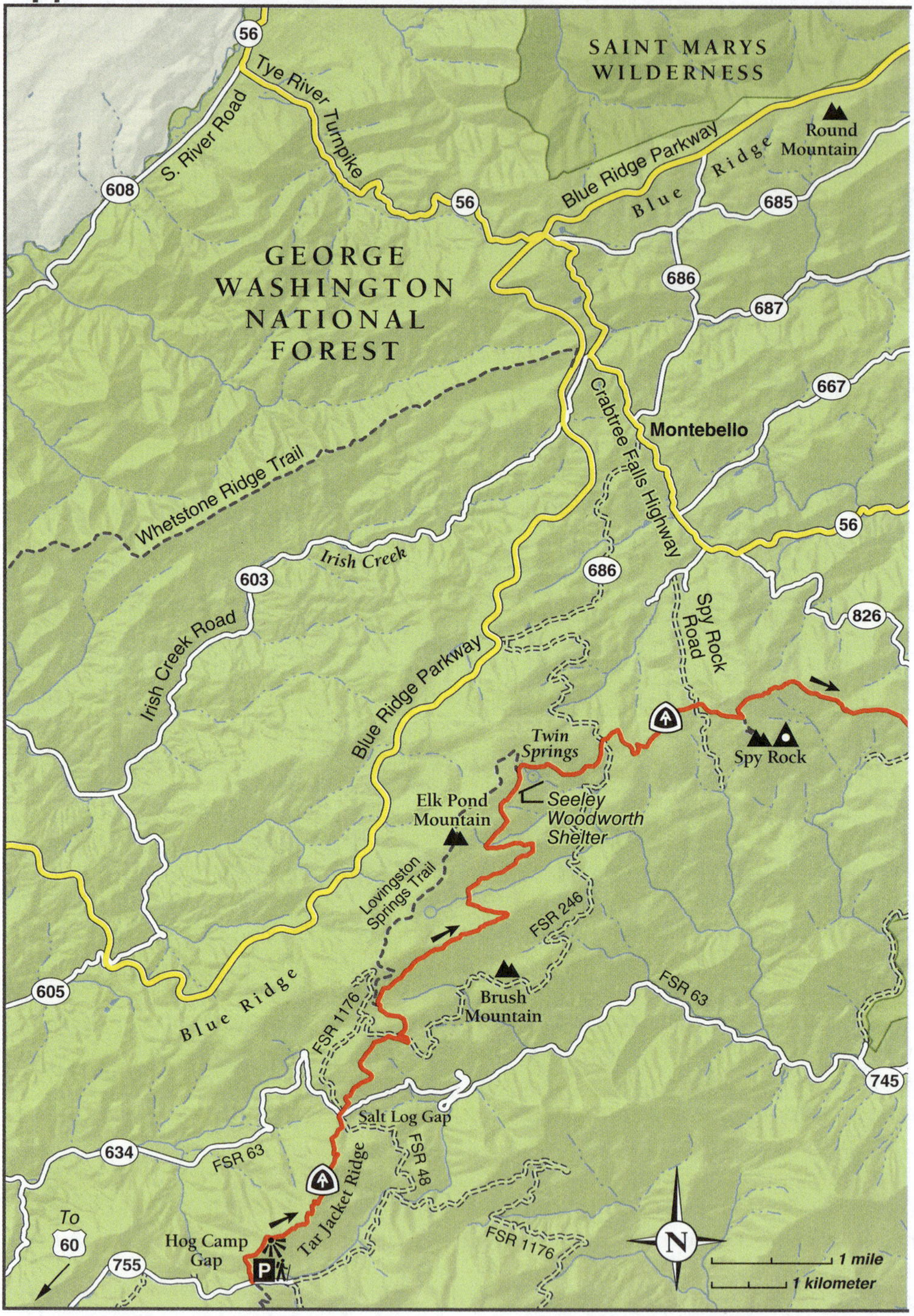

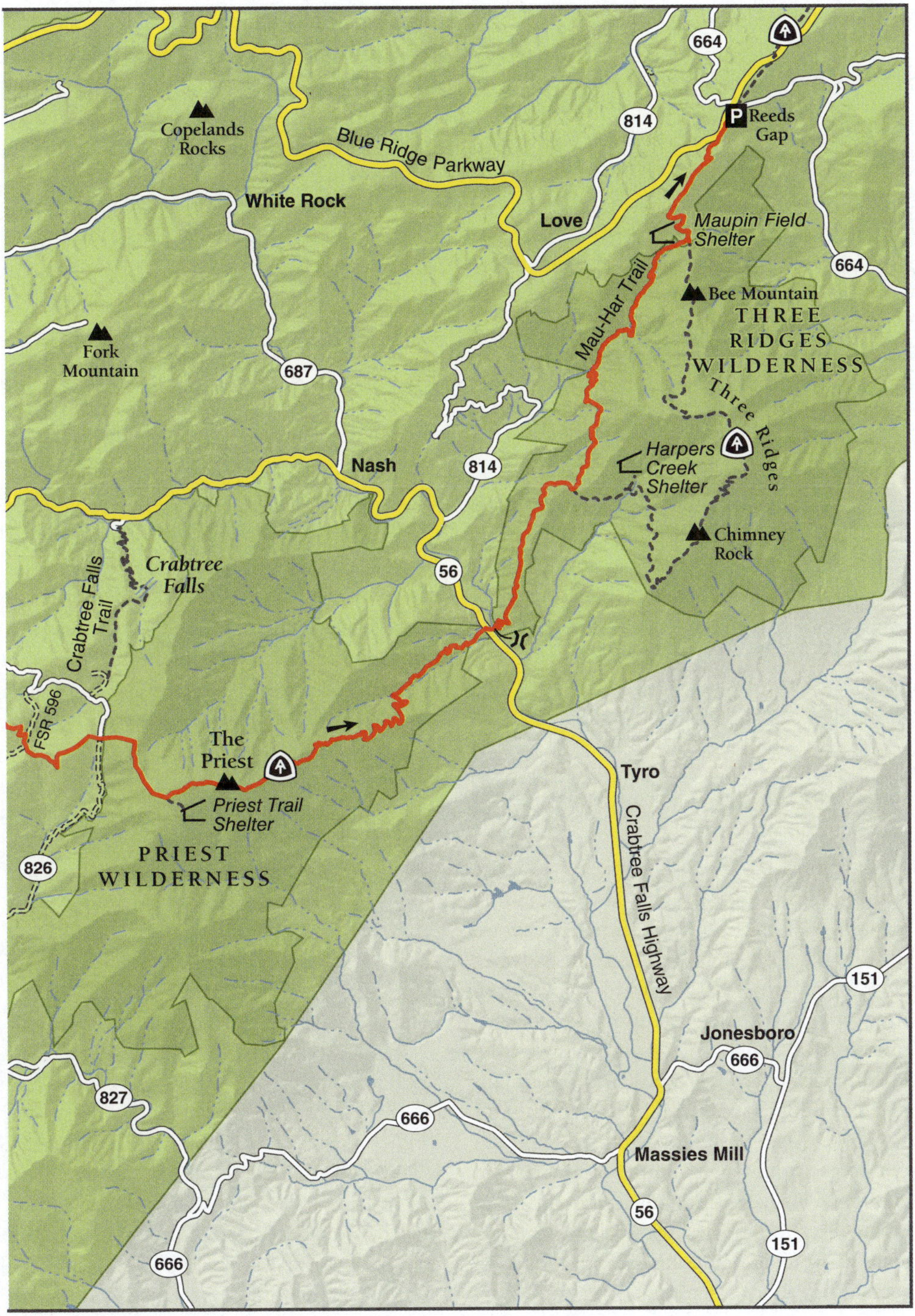

Copelands Rocks
Blue Ridge Parkway
White Rock
Love
Reeds Gap
Maupin Field Shelter
Mau-Har Trail
Bee Mountain
THREE RIDGES WILDERNESS
Three Ridges
Fork Mountain
Nash
Harpers Creek Shelter
Chimney Rock
Crabtree Falls
Crabtree Falls Trail
FSR 596
The Priest
Priest Trail Shelter
PRIEST WILDERNESS
Tyro
Crabtree Falls Highway
Jonesboro
Massies Mill
664
814
687
56
826
827
666
151

(continued from page 161)

spring in 0.5 mile is the trailhead parking for the AT in Hog Camp Gap. Hikes over Cole Mountain (see Hike 38) and Pompey Mountain and Mount Pleasant (see Hike 37) are nearby.

Route Description

First Day

- **TOTAL DISTANCE:** 7.7 miles
- **HIKING TIME:** 5.0 hours

The Hike at a Glance

FIRST DAY

0.5 Tar Jacket Ridge
2.2 Cross FSR 63
3.4 Cross FSR 246
3.9 Cross Greasy Spring Road
4.9 Wolf Rocks Overlook
5.8 Cross North Fork of Piney River
7.0 Cross Elk Pond Branch
7.7 Side trail to Seeley-Woodworth Shelter

Almost immediately you begin to reap the rewards of this hike by gradually ascending north from Hog Camp Gap in open meadows along the ridgeline of Tar Jacket Ridge. A better view unfolds with every upward step, culminating with the wide vista from Tar Jacket's summit at 0.5 mile. Turn around to see the AT working its way over open Cole Mountain and continuing southward into the forest of Bald Knob. East of Cole Mountain are the 4,000-foot summits of Pompey and Pleasant Mountains. The exciting thing, though, is to face the direction in which you are headed, for visible in front of you is the terrain you'll be traversing for the next couple of days. Closest is Rocky Mountain, and then Elk Pond Mountain. You will be coursing along their easterly facing slopes before ascending to the summit of Main Top Mountain. That large massif to the northeast is the Priest, the high point of your multiday trek.

Dropping from Tar Jacket Ridge, the AT enters the woods and crosses FSR 63 in Salt Log Gap at 2.2 miles. At 3,257 feet, this depression in the mountains is the lowest point you will hit until you drop into the Tye River Valley the day after tomorrow. The AT ascends and passes a viewpoint on the side of Rocky Mountain looking back at Tar Jacket Ridge; cross FSR 246 at 3.4 miles and Greasy Spring Road at 3.9 miles. (From Greasy Spring Road you have the option of leaving the AT to hike an alternate pathway for a while. You may even decide to camp somewhere along it. Blue-blazed Lovingston Spring Trail {FS 731}, a former route of the AT, goes left over the crest of Rocky Mountain to Lovingston Spring in 0.9 mile, an excellent water source and good campsite. From the spring it continues 2.6 miles to rejoin the AT at the Seeley-Woodworth Shelter.)

Continuing on the AT from Greasy Spring Road, you will walk through a woods representative of the typical forests of the southern Appalachians, with dozens of hardwood trees showing off their luxuriant summer foliage. Wolf Rocks Overlook provides a view of Spy Rock and the Priest at 4.9 miles. Wind in and out of small hollows and groves, crossing the headwaters of the North Fork of Piney River at 5.8 miles and one of its tributaries, Elk Pond Branch, at 7.0 miles. Your first day's walk is over after you turn right onto the blue-blazed side trail at 7.7 miles and arrive at Seeley-Woodworth Shelter in 500 feet. Drop the pack, unlace the boots, and kick back to enjoy the restful sounds of owls hooting in the forest.

Second Day

- **TOTAL DISTANCE:** 7.2 miles
- **HIKING TIME:** 5.0 hours

The Hike at a Glance

SECOND DAY

- **2.3** Cross Spy Rock Road
- **2.8** Turn right onto side trail to Spy Rock; ascend Spy Rock, then retrace steps to AT and continue northward
- **5.4** Cross Cash Hollow Road
- **6.2** Cross VA 826
- **7.1** Right onto side trail to the Priest Shelter
- **7.2** Arrive at the Priest Shelter

Because you don't have to invest any time in driving to a trailhead and have to do only a few hours' worth of walking, it's OK to be lazy and not get moving by the crack of dawn on your second day out. Use the early morning hours to sleep in, to cook a big breakfast, or to just watch the minutes of the day unfold in front of the shelter. The nocturnal activities of the shelter mice cease when the grainy, gray atmosphere of twilight retreats. New sun rays shine on the forest, bringing leaves, tree trunks, and underbrush into sharply defined, three-dimensional focus through the interplay of shadows with light.

Having finally packed up and walked back to the AT, make a right onto it. After descending and crossing a dirt road at Porters Field, you may huff and puff a little as you ascend, passing some good views to attain the high point of Porter's Ridge and dropping to Spy Rock Road at 2.3 miles.

Take the blue-blazed side trail to the right at 2.8 miles, following it about 0.1 mile to scramble up Spy Rock, which will unquestionably present you with the best vista of the hike. Main Top Mountain is to the north, while behind it and to the west, on the other side of the Blue Ridge Parkway, is Whetstone Ridge (see Hike 31). To the northeast, east, and south you are almost surrounded by the entire Religious Range—the Priest, Little Priest, the Friar, Little Friar, and the Cardinal. Southwestward are the miles you have walked since leaving your car yesterday—Elk Pond Mountain,

A view from Three Ridges

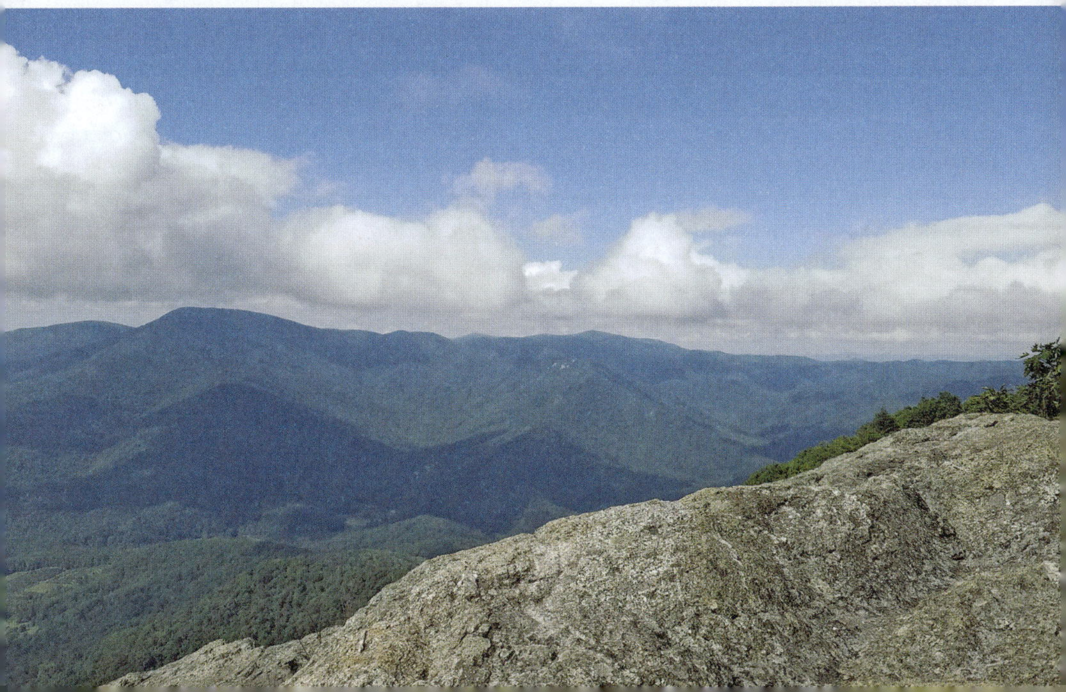

Rocky Mountain (the one with multiple towers on its ridgeline), and Tar Jacket Ridge. With less than 5 miles left to reach the evening's destination, you have time to dawdle; a good, long break is in order for the top of dome-shaped Spy Rock.

Return to the AT to continue northward and ascend to the summit of 4,040-foot Main Top Mountain (no view), soon passing into mountain laurel groves at 3.9 miles and using a trail relocation constructed by members of the Natural Bridge Appalachian Trail Club and volunteers of the Appalachian Trail Conservancy's Konnarock Crew. This relocation swings around a knob, adding a pleasant vista from Cash Hollow Rock of a number of ridgelines in the Religious Range. Continue with minor ups and downs over small ridges and into gaps where the twisted mountain laurel and rhododendron grow and cross dirt Cash Hollow Road at 5.4 miles.

After another up and down over a ridge, you will reach Crabtree Falls Road (VA 826) at 6.2 miles. If you did get an early start on the day and are feeling particularly energetic, you might want to take a side trip to Crabtree Falls. The Crabtree Falls Trail (see Hike 35) can be reached by following dirt VA 826 left for 0.5 mile.

Continuing on the AT, the climb from VA 826 is the final effort for the day, as the route gains about 600 feet of elevation to where you will turn right onto the blue-blazed pathway at 7.1 miles. Reach the Priest Shelter and a spring 0.1 mile beyond the intersection. This shelter, sitting nearly 4,000 feet above sea level, has a special feel to it. By now, thru-hikers, who started their journey 800 miles ago in Georgia, will have a few good memories and stories that they're willing to share—if not in person, then by their entries in the shelter's register. After dinner, when conversation is on the wane, places such as this are the best settings in which to read books recounting other people's adventures on the AT. David Brill's *As Far As the Eye Can See* and Cindy Ross's *A Woman's Journey* are two of the best.

Third Day

- **TOTAL DISTANCE:** 9.5 miles
- **HIKING TIME:** 7.5 hours

The Hike at a Glance

THIRD DAY

0.4 Left onto side trail to enjoy view; retrace steps to AT and continue northward

0.6 The Priest summit

2.2 Viewpoint

3.5 Cross Cripple Creek

4.8 Cross VA 56

6.6 Intersection; bear left onto Mau-Har Trail

7.2 Begin ascent of steep switchbacks

9.5 Maupin Field Shelter

Rise early today! You have an appointment with the sunrise to watch its alpenglow slowly spread pinkish gold tinges across the rugged slopes of Three Ridges. Reach the viewpoint from which you can observe this spectacle by retracing your steps to the AT and making a right. At 0.4 mile, turn left onto a 100-foot-long side trail. From the rock outcrop you can also see what you are going to spend the day doing—dropping thousands of feet into the Tye River Valley, only to regain most of the elevation before nightfall.

Continuing the northward journey on the AT, cross the 4,063-foot summit of the Priest (no views) at 0.6 mile and begin the long descent under the thick leaf canopy of a mixed hardwood forest. Your knees and ankles will probably demand a break when you come to the only view (on this descent) into the river valley at 2.2 miles. The cheeping calls of chipmunks, and their scampering antics, may accompany you as the trail spirals down on long switchbacks. Omnivorous, the chipmunks will eat snails, insects, small birds, and even mice and snakes. In the summer, their faces are often stained by raspberry and blackberry juice, while the fall sees them running toward burrows to cache the nuts they're transporting inside bulging cheeks.

After crossing Cripple Creek at 3.5 miles, the trail makes a more direct descent of the mountain by paralleling the creek and arriving at paved VA 56 at 4.8 miles. To the left it is almost 12 miles to milepost 27.2 on the Blue Ridge Parkway. At the AT crossing, a hiker parking lot is located on the near side of VA 56 for those who want to use this spot as a trailhead. (Be aware, though, that numerous cars have been vandalized here.)

Continue the hike on the AT by crossing VA 56. Members of the Tidewater Appalachian Trail Club, along with Konnarock Crew volunteers, have reconstructed the suspension bridge used to get you across the Tye River. The long ascent begins with switchbacks going by numerous poplar trees, but by the time you have topped a ridgeline at 5.4 miles, oak trees have become dominant. In winter it is possible to see a farm in the valley to the right with Three Ridges standing massively above it.

Soon the route ascends steeply on an old woods road to an intersection in a small gap at 6.6 miles. You now have the option of following the AT as it bears right, ascending approximately 2,000 feet to traverse Three Ridges and arrive at Maupin Field Shelter, having gone nearly 6 miles from this intersection. Instead, so that you can enjoy the waterfalls along Campbell Creek, and to make your day a little shorter, the following description has you bearing left along the old road and taking blue-blazed Mau-Har Trail.

Following nearly level contours, your route swings in and out of large bowls and draws on the side of the mountain, passing a couple of good springs. The roadbed fades at 7.2 miles as the trail ascends to the right on steep switchbacks. After topping the ridge and descending on a narrow, rocky pathway, you will be next to roaring Campbell Creek and its many rushing, gushing waterfalls and will begin an equally rocky and arduous ascent at 8.3 miles. Take a break at any spot that hits your fancy. A side creek, coming from a rock cleft in the hillside, is crossed at 8.8 miles, as the creek drops by way of some exceptionally pretty cascades down a rock facing.

Rhododendron tunnels lead the trail to a crossing of a side creek, and cancer root grows below birch trees where the trail thrice crosses Campbell Creek, now just a small water run. Switchbacks at 9.5 miles bring you to your home for the night, the Maupin Field Shelter.

Fourth Day

- **TOTAL DISTANCE:** 1.7 miles
- **HIKING TIME:** 1.0 hour

The Hike at a Glance

FOURTH DAY

0.1 Left onto AT

0.9 Begin switchbacking descent

1.7 End of journey

This last jaunt is short and easy, so, depending on what you want to do with the rest of the day, you can begin at whatever hour you wish. Take the trail in front of the shelter, turning left onto the AT at 0.1 mile. Star moss lines the ascending trail and grapevines entwine on the ridgeline at 0.6 mile. Wintertime views include Three Ridges to the east and Shenandoah Valley behind the mountains to the west. The switchbacking descent begins at 0.9 mile, passing through rhododendron before coming into an open field and the end of your journey at 1.7 miles.

Now that you have enjoyed 26.1 miles of the AT, it may be time to contemplate hiking the rest of the trail's more than 2,100 miles. My advice? Do it! Be forewarned, though: A thru-hike of the AT may change you and your outlook on life—forever. I had been on only one overnight backpack trip before I went to Georgia to hike the AT for the first time. During the ensuing years, I've been driven to walk more than 20,000 miles in the backcountry areas of the United States, Canada, the Caribbean, New Zealand, and Europe. There are thousands of AT thru-hiker stories, and mine is only one. Why not write your own?

Mount Pleasant

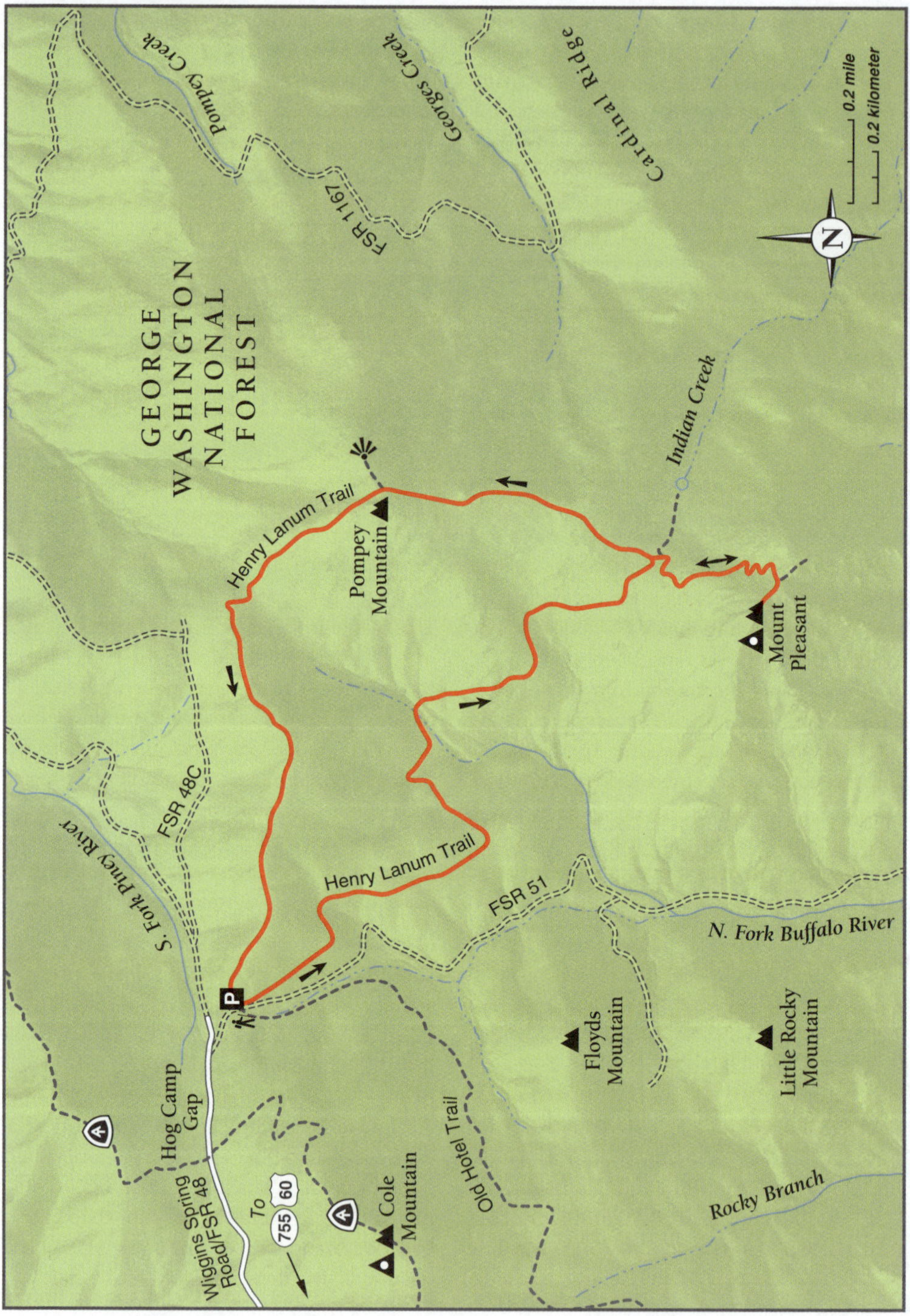

37 Mount Pleasant

- **GPS:** N37.7596835 W79.1951835
- **TOTAL DISTANCE (circuit):** 5.5 miles
- **HIKING TIME:** 3.75 hours
- **VERTICAL RISE:** 1,400 feet
- **MAPS:** USGS *Montebello* and *Forks of Buffalo; Henry Lanum Trail map; ATC Central Virginia Maps 1 and 2; National Geographic Trails Illustrated #789 Lexington/Blue Ridge Mountains*
- **CONTACT:** Glenwood/Pedlar Ranger District
27 Ranger Lane
Natural Bridge Station, VA 24579
540-291-2188
fs.usda.gov/gwj

The Hike at a Glance

2.3 Intersection; turn right and bypass other intersecting trails to arrive at the viewpoint; retrace steps

3.15 Bear right to continue journey on Henry Lanum Trail

5.5 Return to parking area

The 7,500-acre Mount Pleasant National Scenic Area was designated by Congress in 1994, protecting the region from commercial use. This makes it a place you will want to come back to time and again as the years go by. Freed from the changes humanity makes on the environment by farming, road building, and logging, nature will gradually make its own changes. Rocky roadways will become covered with leaves, moss, and new growth. Open fields will overgrow, eventually turning to forest. The trees you see today will die and decay, giving way to other trees that may not even be present now. These changes are already happening; be looking for them on this fairly easy circuit, which traverses the environs of two 4,000-foot mountains. As this is on national forest lands, camping is permitted.

DIRECTIONS Drive US 60 east from Buena Vista, crossing under the Blue Ridge Parkway. About 9.0 miles from Buena Vista (near the Long Mountain Wayside) turn left onto VA 634. Make a right onto VA 755, which becomes dirt FSR 48. Along the way is Wiggins Spring, a true joy as it churns forth gallons of cool, clear water every hour. Past the spring, at 0.5 mile, cross the Appalachian Trail and come to a parking area. You may need to park here; in some seasons, the road beyond may be gated or become too rough for most automobiles. Whether you are able to drive or walk, continue about another 0.4 mile and turn right onto an older dirt road (FSR 51), following it for a few hundred feet to a small parking area and the trailhead.

Route Description

Two old woods roads meet at the trailhead bulletin board. As you will be returning via the ascending road to the left, take the right one, pass through the fence stile, and gradually descend along the Henry Lanum Trail {FS #702}. (Some maps may identify this as the Pompey Mountain Trail. Its name was changed to honor the memory of a member of the Natural Bridge Appalachian Trail Club who was an ardent trail maintainer and instrumental in the protection of several areas throughout the United States. Trailhead signs reflect this name change.)

A matting of moss makes the walking soft and easy on the feet. From June to September you should search out and stop to study the unique ghost pipe, which appears in heavily shaded areas. A saprophytic plant, it gains nourishment from decaying matter through osmosis. This herb rises from the soil on translucent, waxy looking stems. The pinkish white flower nods back toward the ground, giving the whole plant the appearance of a fancily carved soapstone pipe.

Begin a short rise at 0.8 mile and pass an overgrown clearing with black locust trees. The black locust is actually a member of the legume family and is related to peas, beans, and peanuts. Once a black locust becomes established, it propagates itself by root sprouts. This could mean that many of the black locust trees you see in this clearing are not individuals, but clones of one another and connected by a giant root system.

The black locust is also a succession plant that will transform this clearing into a full-fledged forest. A bacterium in its roots allows it to "capture" nitrogen from the air and use it for its own purposes. Once the tree decays, it releases this nitrogen into the ground, adding a nutrient to the soil that was previously absent or in lower concentrations. Other trees needing a more nitrogen-rich soil can then establish themselves and, probably, crowd out most of the black locusts—a process that may have occurred by the time you hike here.

Resume the descent, steeper in places, as ferns line the trail and carpet the forest floor. Cross a small stream at 1.1 miles and pass by two small springs; these flow well in the rainy season, but they should not necessarily be counted on as water sources later in the summer or fall. Cross and begin to parallel a second water run in another 0.1 mile. A small camp could be made about 200 feet beyond the crossing. Take note of the exceptionally good job the forest service and volunteers of the Natural Bridge Appalachian Trail Club have done in designing and maintaining this trail. Waterbars and drainage systems are strategically placed and well built and should perform their function for a long time to come.

Be alert for double blazes at 1.5 miles as the trail turns to the left and begins to ascend. The route crosses a small stream at 1.6 miles, where the pathway becomes rougher and rockier. In 200 feet you must pay attention as the route leaves the old road, turns left onto a foot trail for 50 feet, and then right onto another roadbed.

Another turn, this one to the right, happens at 1.8 miles as the route leaves the road and passes by a well-flowing spring. Fringed phacelia put on a grand display during the spring. The flowers are so numerous that they make the ground look like someone has come along and cast bits of confetti throughout the forest. Close inspection of the plant reveals tiny, but deep, fringes (in botanical terms known as fimbriations) around the flowers' outer edges. The trail soon becomes steeper and rockier.

Come to a trail sign and intersection at 2.3 miles and bear to the right to continue on this hike (it may be identified as the Mount Pleasant Trail {FS #704}). In less than 0.1 mile you will pass by a shortcut trail that comes in from the left and, a little farther on, another trail to the left (often overgrown) leading to a spring. Ascend quite steeply.

Bear right at the intersection at 2.7 miles (the pathway to the left goes a few hundred yards to a viewpoint somewhat similar to that of Mount Pleasant, but with a more easterly exposure) and in 250 feet arrive at the rock outcrop on Mount Pleasant. Enjoy the nearly 360-degree view from your 4,070-foot vantage point. Behind you and to the north is Pompey Mountain, whose summit you will just miss crossing as you later continue the hike. To the northwest and west is the route of the Appalachian Trail, snaking its way across the open ridgelines of Tar Jacket Ridge and Cole Mountain (see Hike 38) and the wooded summit of Bald Knob. Chestnut Ridge is to the south. At your feet, Mount Pleasant drops quickly and steeply to the hollow created by the north fork of the Buffalo River.

Go back to the first intersection and turn left to continue retracing your steps. (Remember, right would lead to the other view.) Begin the descent of Mount Pleasant, and at 3.0 miles pass by the trail to your right leading to the spring. Again pass up the blue-blazed shortcut trail.

Return to the intersection with the trail sign at 3.15 miles and turn right toward Pompey Mountain. The blue-blazed shortcut trail comes in from the right at 3.3 miles. Bear left uphill

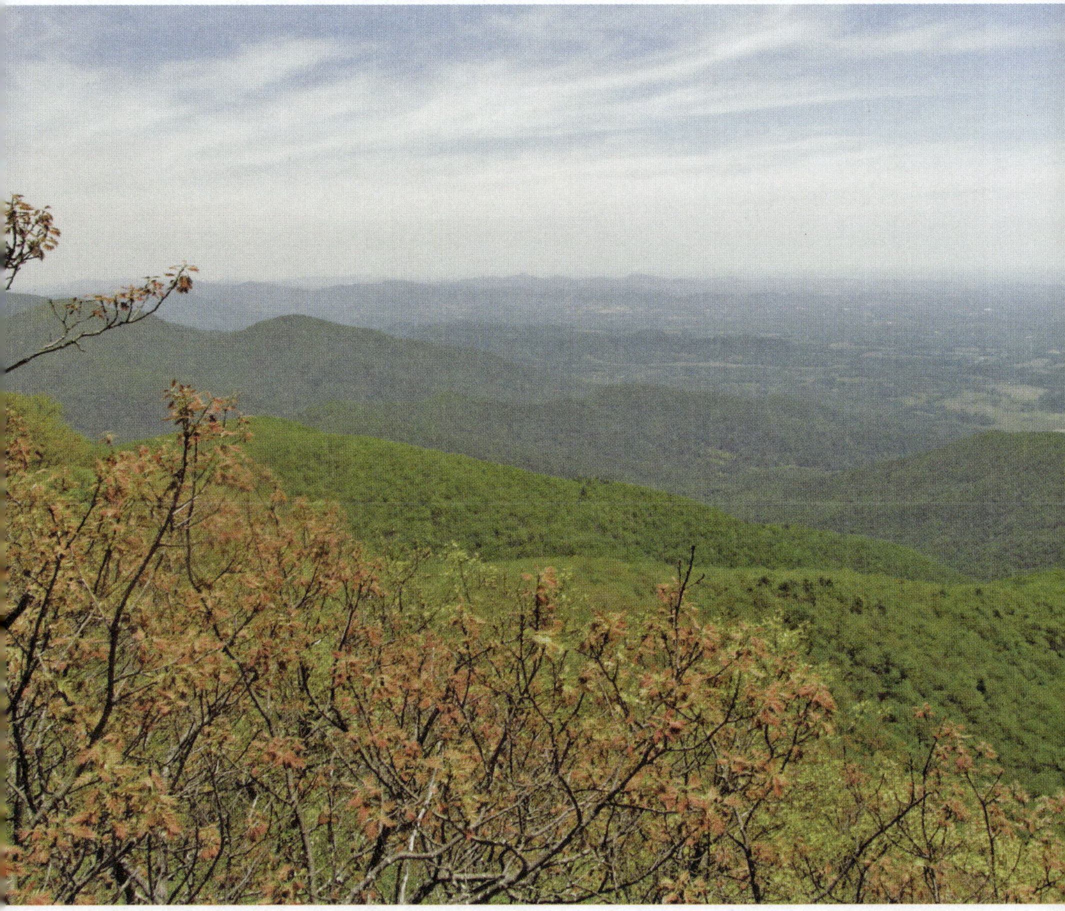

Take in panoramic views from Mount Pleasant.

photo: Johnny Molloy

toward the ridgeline. Begin descending, somewhat steeply at times, after reaching the high point of the ascent at 3.85 miles. The wooded, 4,032-foot summit of Pompey Mountain can be seen through the vegetation on your left.

After passing through a small patch of rhododendron, bear right onto an old road at 4.35 miles and gradually ascend via a switchback. You will soon begin a long, easy descent on a wide woods road. Cross through the fence stile and return to the bulletin board and parking area at 5.5 miles. An additional hiking opportunity, Cole Mountain (see Hike 38), can be reached by crossing the dirt road and following a blue-blazed trail 200 feet to a sign marking the beginning of that outing.

Cole Mountain

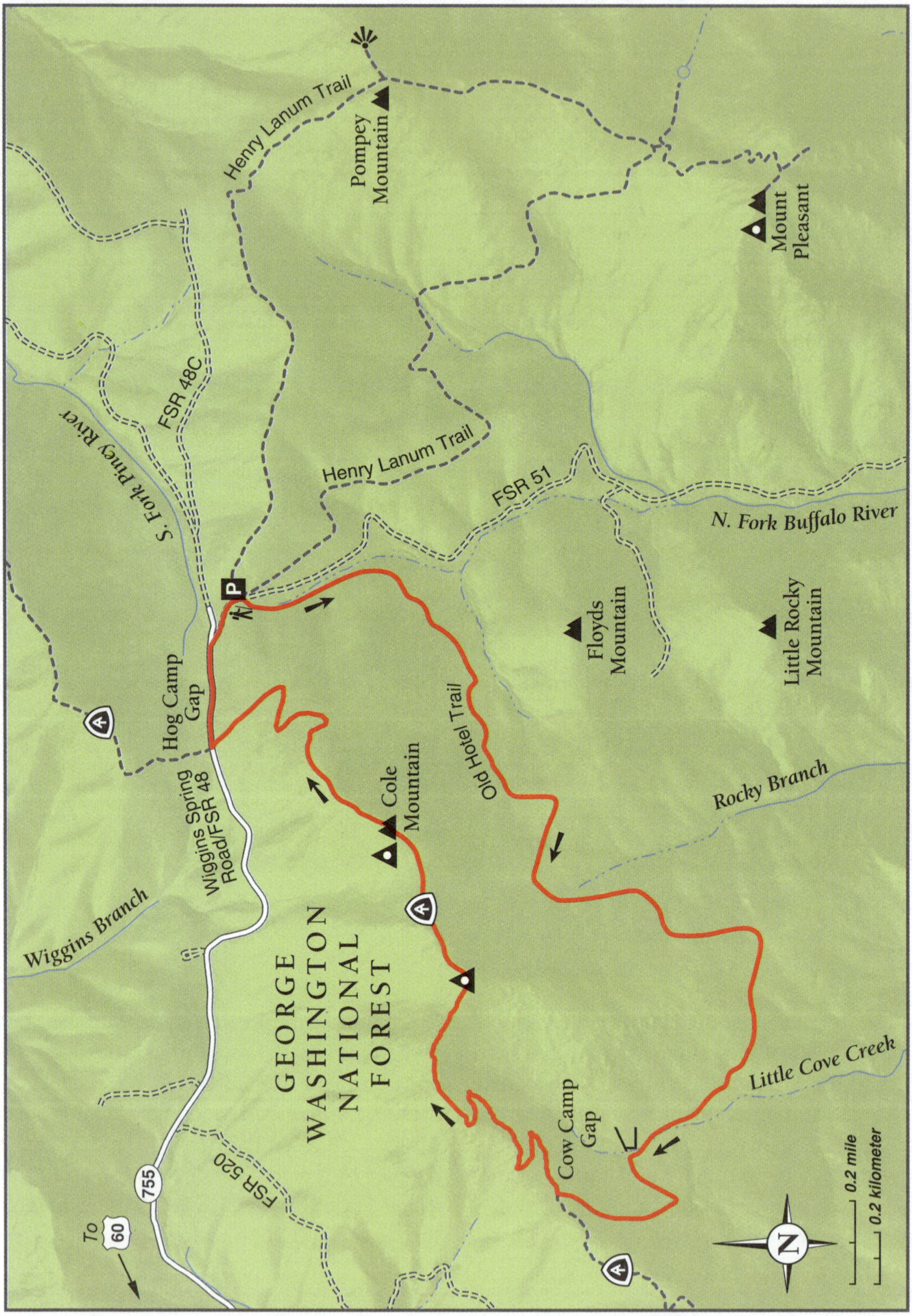

38 Cole Mountain

- **GPS:** N37.7596835 W79.1951835
- **TOTAL DISTANCE (circuit):** 5.75 miles
- **HIKING TIME:** 3.75 hours
- **VERTICAL RISE:** 1,320 feet
- **MAPS:** USGS *Montebello* and *Forks of Buffalo; ATC Central Virginia Maps* 1 and 2; *National Geographic Trails Illustrated #789 Lexington/ Blue Ridge Mountains*
- **CONTACT:** Glenwood/Pedlar Ranger District
27 Ranger Lane
Natural Bridge Station, VA 24579
540-291-2188
fs.usda.gov/gwj

The Hike at a Glance

0.8 This is near the site of the "Old Hotel"

2.0 Top ridgeline

2.75 Side trail to Cow Camp Gap Shelter

3.3 Right onto AT

4.0 Cole Mountain summit

4.8 Enter woods, cross dirt road twice, then turn right onto FSR 48. Soon turn right onto road to come to parking area

5.75 Return to parking area

As total public protection and domain over the entire Appalachian Trail draws ever closer to being a reality, a small but significant controversy has arisen among users and maintainers of the trail. Open mountaintop vistas are something of a rarity in the central and southern Appalachian Mountains. In bygone days, most of these fields and meadows were kept clear by grazing cattle or other stock. Sometimes the fields were mowed for hay or kept open by controlled burnings. Should these methods, or other human manipulations, be employed or should nature be allowed to have its way, eventually turning the meadows into forests and blocking the sweeping vistas? When I first hiked the Appalachian Trail, the summit and ridgeline of Cole Mountain (referred to by many as Cold Mountain) was a totally open, grassy meadow full of a variety of wildflowers. A decade later, many of the flowers were gone, having been replaced by knee-high scrub brush and young trees. A series of discussions among the forest service, local hiking clubs, and the Appalachian Trail Conservancy led to the conclusion that the rare scenic value of cleared ridgelines outweighed the desire to permit nature to take its course. Controlled burning and mechanical brush cutting are now being employed, and Cole Mountain has somewhat regained the open, grassy, flowered look it had when I first encountered it.

Gaining insight into this issue is only a small reason to take this hike. In addition to the views from the summit, you will hike through mountainside meadows, into a small stand of virgin timber, and along cascading Little Cove Creek. This hike is on national forest land, so camping is permitted. Cow Camp Gap Shelter, next to the creek, also provides a place to spend the night.

DIRECTIONS See Mount Pleasant (Hike 37) for automobile access to the beginning of this hike. (These two hikes could easily be combined for a long day trip or a leisurely weekend outing.)

Route Description

Begin by following the blue-blazed trail on the right side of the road from the parking area. In 200 feet come to the Old Hotel Trail {FS 515} sign, turn left, cross a fence stile, and begin following the trail, which at this point is an old roadbed. Abundant and sweet blackberries (in-season) add to the enjoyment of the hike. In 0.2 mile a road comes in from the left as your route enters a wooded area where copious ferns cover the ground with rich, deep shades of green. Several springs on the left flow together to form the beginning of the north fork of the Buffalo River. The route swings away from the stream, entering an open area at 0.5 mile. Virginia and white pine, thistle, and ironweed thrive in the bright sunshine of the meadow. Look to your left for a view of Mount Pleasant.

Pay attention at 0.8 mile as the trail makes a turn to the right. It was near this spot that a former landowner, a Dr. Richeson, had a dwelling to which he would frequently invite guests. It eventually came to be known as "The Hotel" (and thus the name for the trail). Foundations of the building are still there but are hard to find. There is a spring on your left a few hundred feet beyond the turn. The views continue to get better as you ascend through the open field. You must be alert once again at 1.0 mile. The trail turns off the road to the right, crosses a small water run, enters a wooded area, and reemerges back out into the field. The pathway may be indistinct, but follow the blazed posts and you'll be on the right track. Be sure to turn around every once in a while to appreciate the scenery. Spreading below are the meadows, pines, and flowers you have just ascended through. These drop down to the north fork of the Buffalo, where your eyes will be drawn upward to the wooded slope and craggy ridge on Mount Pleasant.

A grand camp could be made on the large, flat area underneath stately old oaks at 1.2 miles. Look for the trail to veer to the right immediately after entering the woods.

Descend on a pathway softened by Virginia pine needles dropped onto the trail over the course of many years. The route becomes a little faint at 1.5 miles; watch for blazes as you slab the side of the hill with slight ups and downs. Top the ridgeline at 2.0 miles in a slight

Cole Mountain

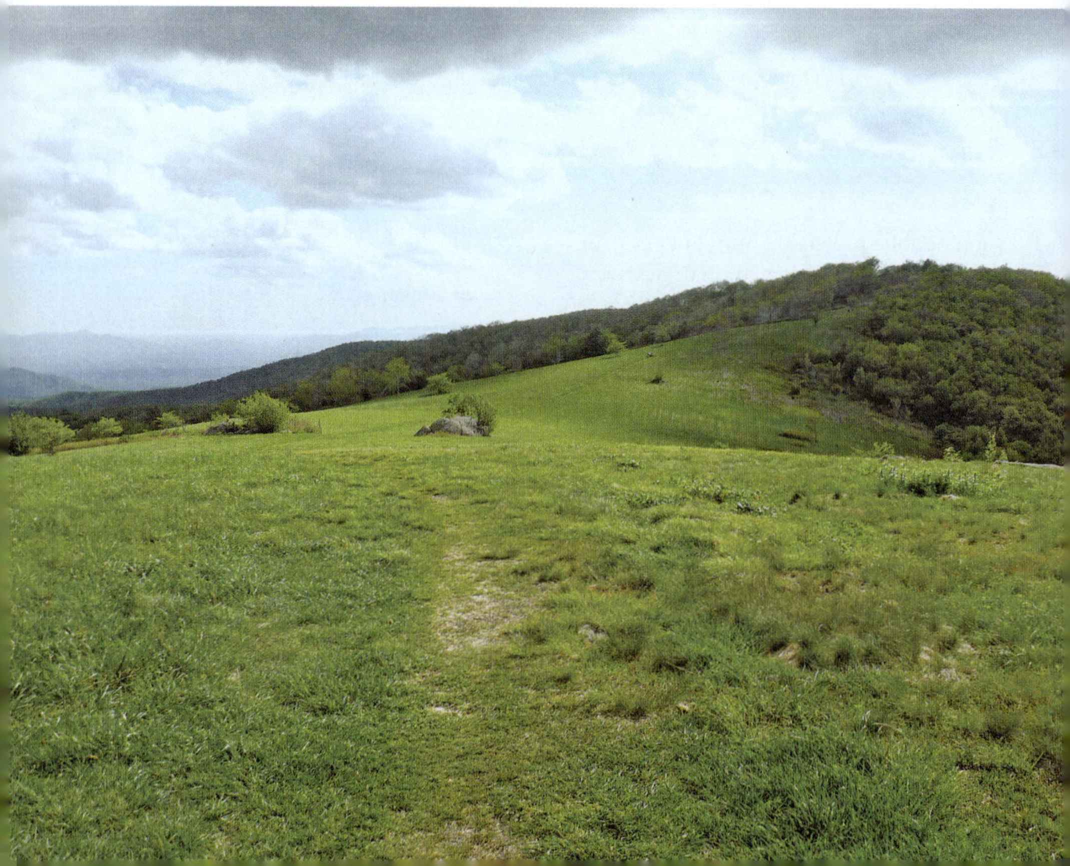

open area that could be used to set up a couple of small tents.

Descend to the right on a very old road lined by jewelweed (touch-me-not) and stinging nettle. If you look closely at both of these plants you will note that their tops may have been nipped off at almost a uniform height. Deer feed on these plants, and they will stop chewing at the point it becomes uncomfortable for them to bend any farther. This point is known as the "browse line." In years of scarce food the browse line may be lower than normal, as the deer continue to eat downward to obtain any nourishment they can.

Begin to rise and cross Little Cove Creek, which is lined with birch trees, at 2.5 miles. There is a small spring on the left, and soon a trail to the right, at 2.75 miles, crosses the creek to Cow Camp Gap Shelter. Turn uphill to the left and, in summer, make sure to have the camera out for this spot. Large patches of 4- to 5-foot-high touch-me-nots grow on both sides of the trail, peppering an otherwise green understory with a multitude of red-spotted orange flowers.

Switchback to the right, ascending the old road on an almost perfect grade made for easy walking. Intersect and turn right onto the white-blazed Appalachian Trail at 3.3 miles. Level out at 3.7 miles and cross over rock formations on the spine of the ridge.

Break out into the open at 4.0 miles and continue to the open summit of 4,022-foot Cole Mountain. To give you an idea of how spectacular this spot is, my notes from scouting this hike read, "Views! Strawberries, old apple trees, butter-and-eggs. Views! Views! Views!"

To the south is wooded Bald Knob (once as open as Cole Mountain), eastward are Pompey Mountain and Mount Pleasant, and northeastward is the Religious Range—the Priest, the Friar, Little Friar, and the Cardinal. In the far distance, Three Ridges is behind the Priest, while close at hand and almost due north you can see the Appalachian Trail winding its way across the bald expanse of Tar Jacket Ridge.

Descend the ridge to enter woods at 4.8 miles. Follow the white blazes as you cross a dirt road a couple of times.

Arrive in Hog Camp Gap and turn right, tracking blue blazes along unpaved FSR 48. Watch for the blazes to turn off the road to the right, go past the Old Hotel Trail sign, and return to the parking area at 5.75 miles.

Western Virginia

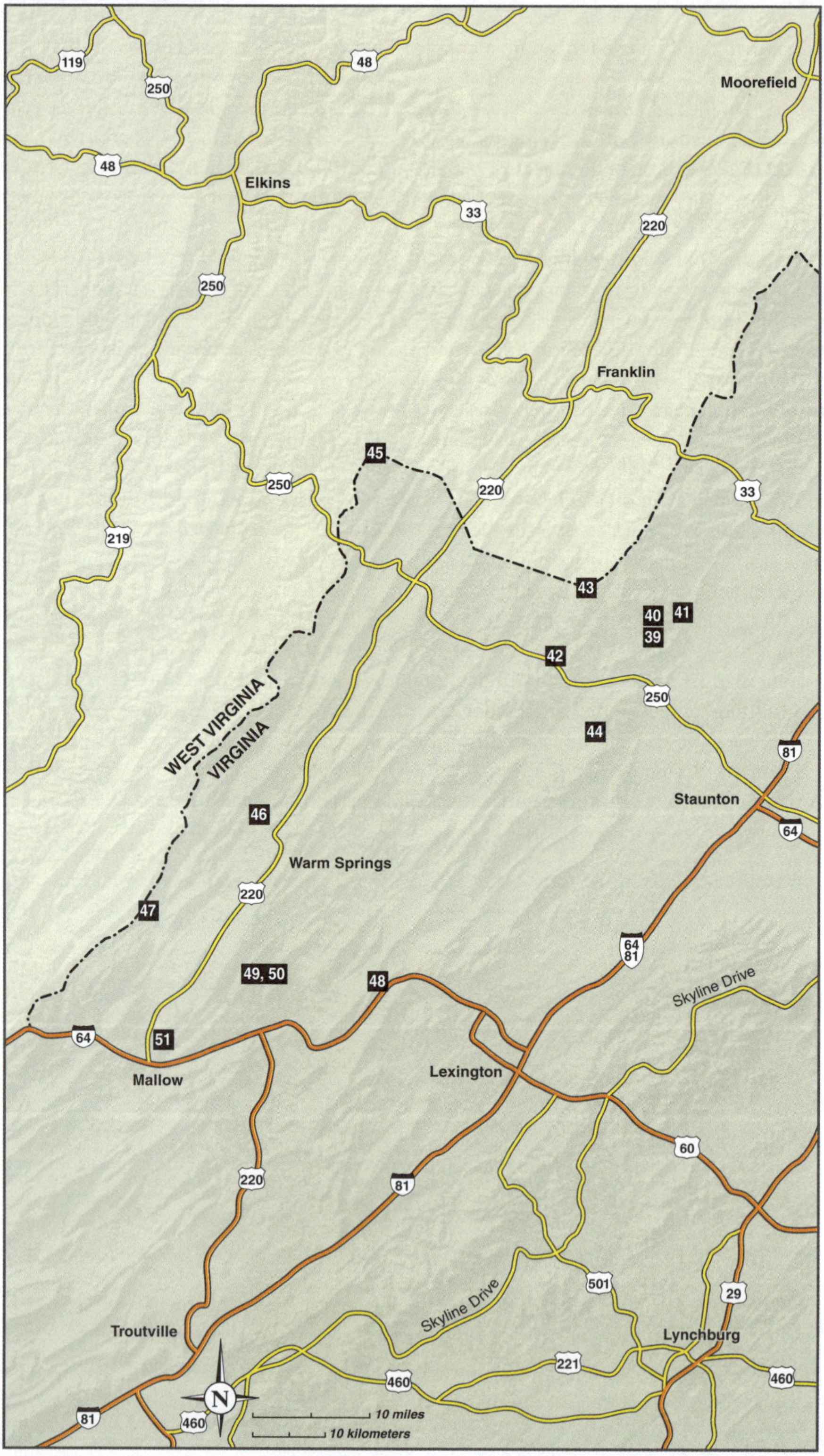

Western Virginia

North River Gorge

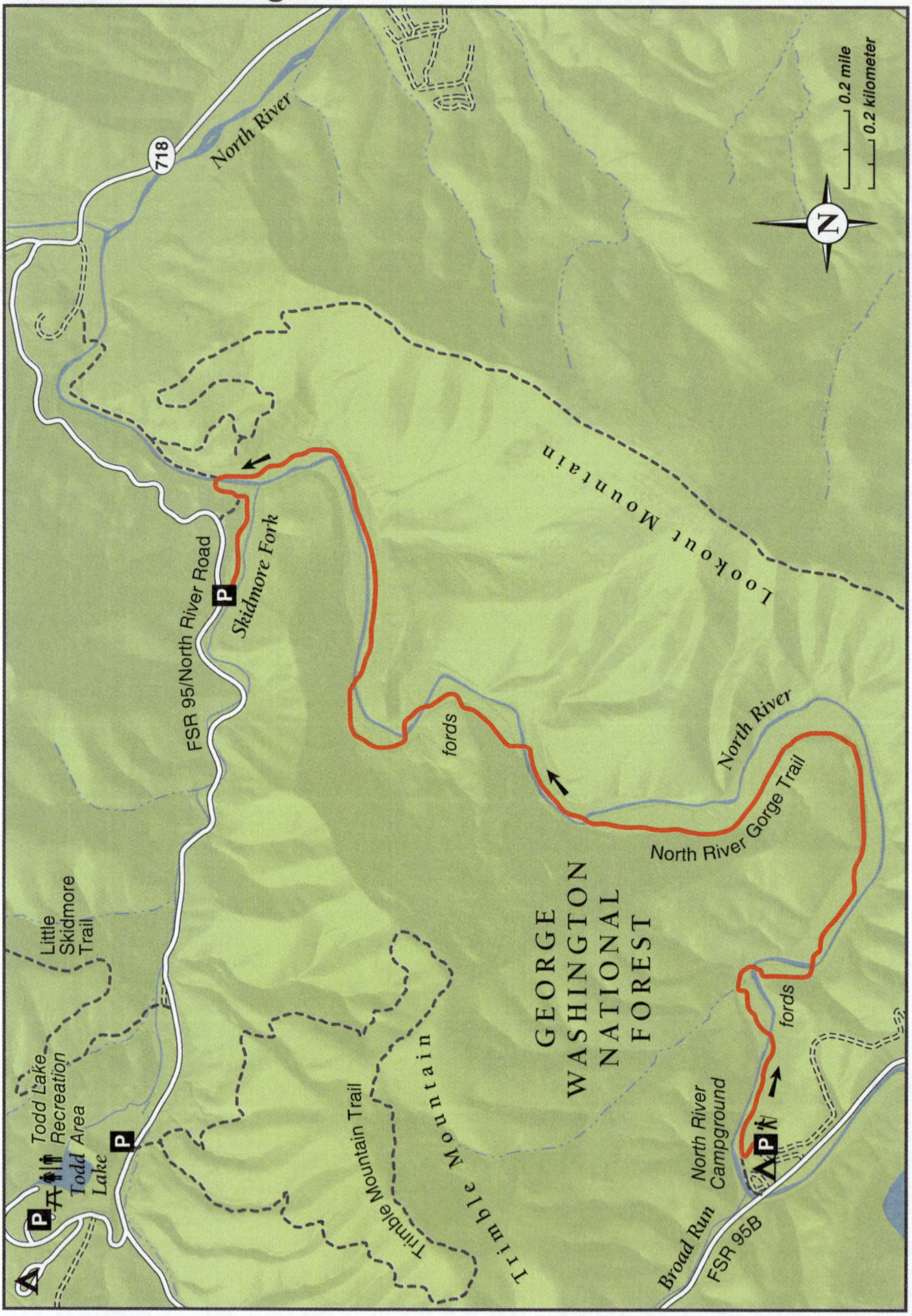

39 North River Gorge

- **GPS:** N38.3379811 W79.2065375
- **TOTAL DISTANCE (one-way):** 4.5 miles
- **HIKING TIME:** 3.5 hours
- **VERTICAL RISE:** 40 feet
- **MAPS:** USGS *Stokesville; North River Gorge Trail* map; *National Geographic Trails Illustrated Map #791 Staunton/Shenandoah Mountain*
- **CONTACT:** North River Ranger District
  401 Oakwood Road
  Harrisonburg, VA 22801
  540-432-0187; fs.usda.gov/gwj

The Hike at a Glance

0.4 First ford
0.7 Third ford
2.5 Fifth ford
2.8 Sixth ford
2.9 Seventh ford
3.1 Eighth ford
4.0 Ninth ford
4.5 End of hike at FSR 95

A thousand feet below the 2,800-foot summits of Lookout and Trimble Mountains, the serpentine North River Gorge Trail {FS 538} twists and turns on a nearly level route of exuberantly full, vibrant, and green foliage. This is a hike for those who don't need far-off vistas to feel that they are having a worthwhile woodlands experience. The lack of views is more than offset by the freedom to saunter down the gorge with almost no rise in elevation and to wander around its broad floor, searching out hidden burrows of beavers on the riverbanks or standing in far-reaching gardens of wispy ferns.

The best time to visit the gorge is in late spring and early summer, when literally hundreds of opulent pink lady's slippers will accompany you on almost every mile of the hike. This time of year also permits you to negotiate the nine fords of the river when there is still enough water flowing in the stream to make the crossings exciting and challenging. It's best to avoid the hike during the spring runoff season, and don't ever attempt to cross North River (or any stream) after heavy rains. The fords will slow your progress and you will certainly be walking in wet boots, but think of the crossings as a chance to rest for a few moments and refresh tired feet. Consider bringing along fishing gear; North River is stocked with trout by the Virginia Commission of Wildlife Resources.

DIRECTIONS You will need a car shuttle, so follow the directions for reaching the Segment A trailhead of the Wild Oak National Recreation Trail (see Hike 41). From that trailhead, continue driving on FSR 95 for about 1 mile to a paved parking area on the left side of the road. You can leave one car here. Continue with the second car, passing Todd Lake in another 1.6 miles. At 1.3 miles from the lake, turn left onto FSR 95B, following it for 1.0 mile to the North River Campground. The campground was once a base of operations for the Civilian Conservation Corps. It is now open seasonally and has vault toilets, fireplace grills, and picnic tables. If you are not staying in the campground, leave your car in the parking area at the North River Gorge Trailhead {FS 538}, 0.2 mile beyond the campground entrance.

Route Description

Begin hiking by passing through the gate, and in less than 200 feet keep left on the purple-blazed dirt roadbed. Tiny, pale bluets hugging the ground next to the roadway are hovered over by the light purple of wild geranium petals. Because all parts of the wild geranium contain tannin, it was once used as an astringent, and its leaves were brewed into a tea to treat diarrhea and bleeding ulcers.

Ford North River for the first time at 0.4 mile, passing a wildlife clearing and crossing a side stream. The second ford is trickier, with large, slippery boulders causing your feet and ankles to twist and turn. You will make good use of your walking stick as a brace for the third ford at 0.7 mile. Because the riverbed is made of large, flat, smooth, slippery slabs of rock, there are very few cracks in which to wedge your feet to keep them, and you, from being pushed downstream by the current. Probably the best place to cross is a few feet upstream from where the trail actually comes into contact with the river. Use caution and common sense!

After that ford, the roadway becomes soft and grassy, passing a wildlife clearing at 1.0 mile. From May to July, the forest floor erupts in a riot of 6- to 14-inch-tall pink lady's slippers.

Lady's slipper

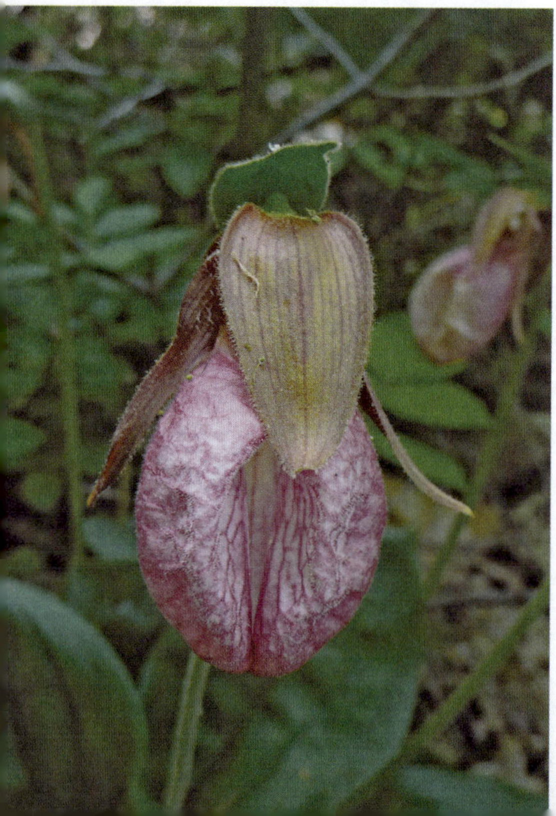

They are next to the road, spread throughout the woods, and on the other side of the river. Like other orchids, the pink lady's slipper has an exotic structure that is designed to attract certain pollinators. After insects work their way through the slit in the red-veined pouch, they deposit pollen from other plants by brushing against the stigma—the tip of the pistil, or female organ. Exiting the flower by way of the two openings at the rear of the slipper, the insects then pick up that plant's pollen by grazing the anthers—the pollen-producing part of the stamen, or male organ. It appears that at one time or another almost every plant has been used for medicinal purposes, and the lady's slipper is no exception. Native Americans made a tea from its dried leaves as a cure for insomnia, and physicians, up until the 1930s, used its roots as a nerve medication. Don't, however, be tempted to touch the lady's slipper. Some people report having experienced a mild to severe skin inflammation after doing so.

At about the same time of year that the pink lady's slippers are in bloom, the vanilla-sweet smell of autumn olive, planted in the wildlife clearing at 2.2 miles, can be almost overpowering just before you ford the river for the fourth time. You will ford it again at 2.5 miles, and a sixth time at 2.8 miles.

The seventh crossing, at 2.9 miles, is a little more interesting because the trail traverses a small island that formed after the great flood of 1985. There are also a number of side streams you'll cross in order to continue to the eighth ford at 3.1 miles.

Scores of additional pink lady's slippers may keep you from being alert when coming to the far end of the Adirondack shelter camping area (used by Girl Scouts from Camp May Flather). The roadway continues straight, but your route makes an abrupt turn to the left to ford the river for the final time at 4.0 miles. It may be a little confusing after crossing the river. Do not make a turn to the right or follow the pathway going uphill. Instead, turn left, crossing two small streams in quick succession, and emerge onto FSR 95 at 4.5 miles.

40 Todd Lake Recreation Area and Trimble Mountain

- **GPS:** N38.3625126 W79.2056331
- **TOTAL DISTANCE (circuit):** 3.8 miles
- **HIKING TIME:** 2.75 hours
- **VERTICAL RISE:** 1,120 feet
- **MAPS:** USGS *Stokesville; Trimble Mountain Trail map; National Geographic Trails Illustrated Map #791 Staunton/Shenandoah Mountain*
- **CONTACT:** North River Ranger District
401 Oakwood Road
Harrisonburg, VA 22801
540-432-0187
fs.usda.gov/gwj

The Hike at a Glance

1.2 View of Elkhorn Lake
2.2 Trimble Mountain summit
2.8 Spring
3.8 Hike ends back at FSR 95

Todd Lake Recreation Area can be a comfortable base from which to explore the Allegheny Mountains west of the Shenandoah Valley. Facilities in the 20-acre area include a campground with running water, hot showers, flush toilets, and huge picnic grounds. A sandy beach borders the 7.5-acre lake. Canoeists, and anyone else willing to power their boat with muscles and not motors, are permitted in the nonswimming areas of the water. Among the many trailheads within an hour's drive of Todd Lake are the North River Gorge (Hike 39), Wild Oak National Recreation Trail (Hike 41), Ramseys Draft (Hike 42), and Shenandoah Mountain (Hike 43).

Passing by several good views (wintertime views are the best) of Todd Lake, Shenandoah Mountain, and soaring Reddish Knob, and following deer trails through thickets of mountain laurel, the Trimble Mountain Trail {FS 375} makes it possible to take a hike right from the campground and not have to drive anywhere. Fossils found at some of the rock outcrops show the outlines of plants that grew on the mountain as it was formed about 300 million years ago during the Paleozoic era.

DIRECTIONS See the Wild Oak National Recreation Trail (Hike 41) for directions to the Todd Lake Recreation Area and Campground. To reach the trailhead from the campground entrance, you can either walk the roadway back to FSR 95, turn left, and continue for a few hundred feet or simply cut downhill past the dam. If you are not staying in the campground, you can leave an automobile at either side of the road near the RV dump station on FSR 95, directly across from the trailhead, but be very aware: Do not park at the dump station or risk getting a ticket—which has happened to many hikers!

Route Description

From the dump station, walk across FSR 95 and follow the yellow-blazed Trimble Mountain Trail {FS 375} into the woods, coming to an open area in 300 feet. This clearing, beginning to overgrow, was created when soil was removed to build the dam for Todd Lake. Turn right at the loop-trail intersection and ascend along an old road. Pay attention 0.2 mile from FSR 95; the route leaves the old roadway you've been following and bears right to ascend on a narrow pathway. In the fall, you are likely to see squirrels busily harvesting the hundreds of acorns dropped by oak trees as the trail switchbacks to the right for a limited view of Todd Lake at 0.5 mile. Incredibly, all those nuts they gather are buried and concealed in individual shallow holes. The gray squirrels live in nests of leaves and twigs located in tree forks high

Todd Lake Recreation Area and Trimble Mountain

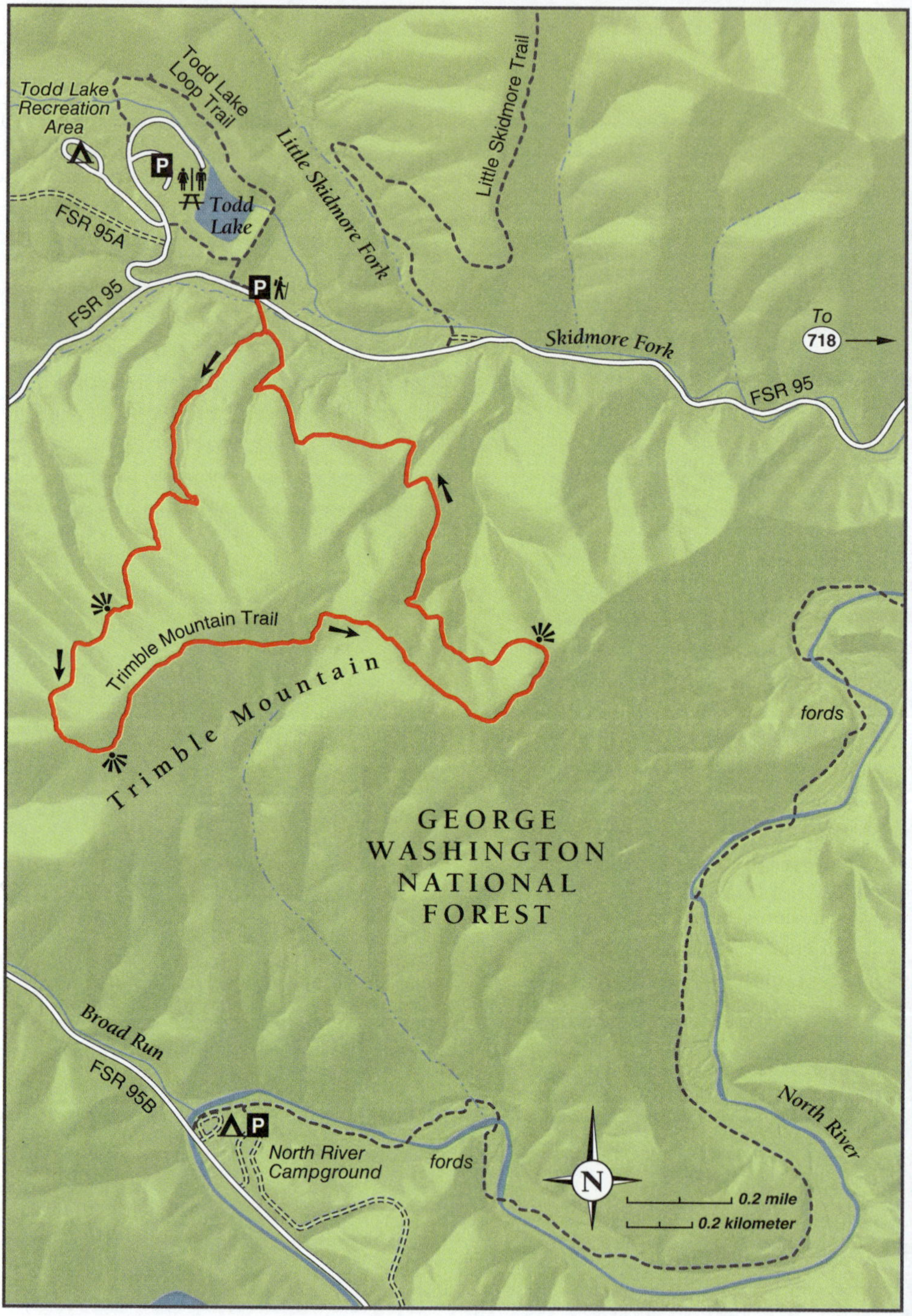

above the ground, or in tree cavities, which they line with soft vegetation.

The trail swings around the ridge for a view to the northwest of 4,397-foot Reddish Knob, a high point on Shenandoah Mountain. Stretching for more than 50 miles, the southern section of Shenandoah Mountain's prominent ridgeline marks the border of Highland and Augusta counties, while its northern section delineates Virginia from West Virginia. Notice that the land directly below you at this viewpoint was also used to obtain fill dirt for the dam.

The focus of the vistas changes when the trail curves to the southern side of the mountain. The rocks at 1.2 miles overlook Elkhorn Lake (a popular fishing spot), which is surrounded by Elkhorn, Hankey, and Lookout Mountains. From 1.4 miles, the broad ridgeline the trail follows could provide nice tent sites as you descend to mountain laurel thickets in a saddle and ascend to attain the 2,740-foot wooded summit of Trimble Mountain at 2.2 miles. The trail crosses the ridge and swings around to another view of Reddish Knob at 2.5 miles.

Water has been nonexistent on the trail thus far, so on hot summer days you may be happy to drop steeply to a spring at 2.8 miles; then resume a more gradual descent past mountain laurel to a wintertime view of Todd Lake. Mountain laurel can develop into such heavy thickets because, besides the usual cross-pollination of flowers to produce seeds, the laurel reproduces by sending up new shoots from its spreading root system. In addition, branches that touch the ground grow new roots, radiating outward and sending up shoots of their own.

You will pass water sources three more times before arriving back at the loop-trail intersection and making a right to return to FSR 95 at 3.8 miles.

You never know when you might see a deer on the Trimble Mountain Trail.

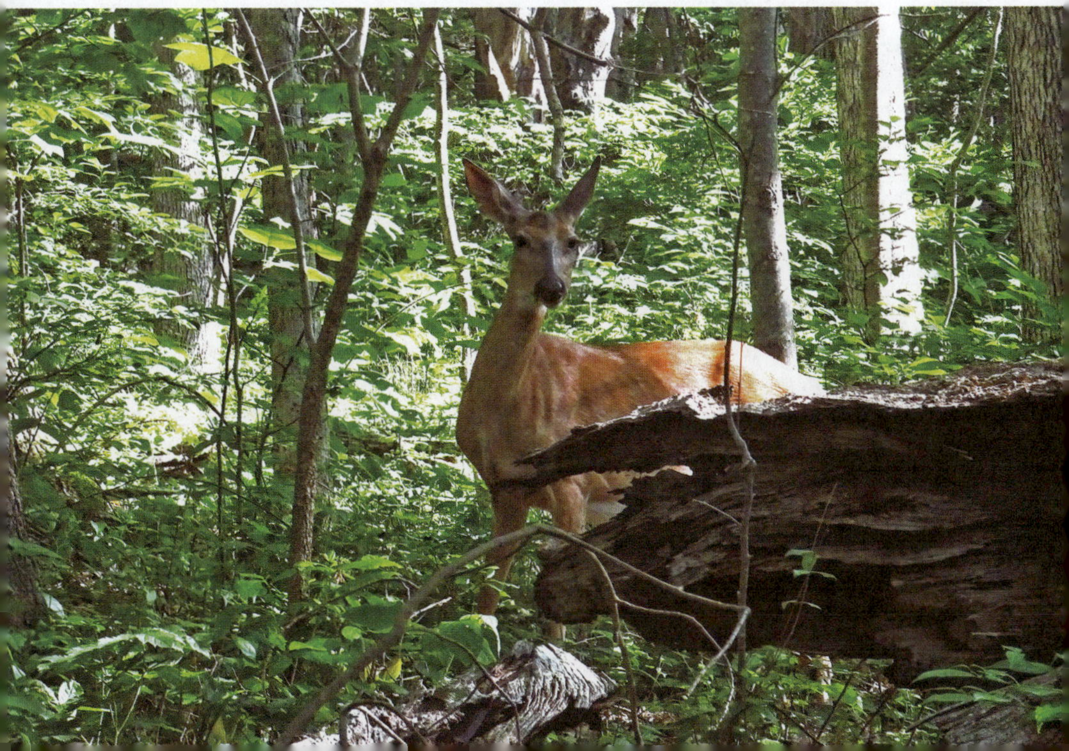

41 Wild Oak National Recreation Trail

- **GPS:** N38.3669897 W79.1644445
- **TOTAL DISTANCE (circuit):** 27.2 miles
- **HIKING TIME:** 3 days, 2 nights
- **VERTICAL RISE:** Approximately 7,550 feet
- **MAPS:** USGS *Stokesville, Reddish Knob, Palo Alto (VA and WV),* and *West Augusta; Wild Oak Trail map; National Geographic Trails Illustrated Map #791 Staunton/Shenandoah Mountain*
- **CONTACT:** North River Ranger District
  401 Oakwood Road
  Harrisonburg, VA 22801
  540-432-0187; fs.usda.gov/gwj

Exceptionally steep ascents, miles of trail at high elevation, good water sources few and far between, a major river ford, and a rough and rocky treadway in many places—descriptions such as this may scare off timid hikers. But if you are in good shape and view these challenges as reasons to hike, the Wild Oak National Recreation Trail (WONRT) {FS 716} can be a great escape from the crowds.

Just a few words of advice: An abundance of wildlife makes the entire route a favorite of hunters, so take the proper precautions if hiking during the season. In addition, the WONRT has become popular with mountain bikers; be prepared to have one whiz by you at any moment. Last bit of advice: Water is scarce, especially on the second half of the hike. Fill up with water whenever you can, and carry lots of it!

DIRECTIONS Since this is a circuit hike, you won't need a shuttle, but because the trail comes into contact with drivable roadways at three points, you could use two automobiles to split the hike into day trips—designated Segments A, B, and C by the forest service.

To reach Segment A, and the beginning and ending point of the circuit, follow US 250 west from Staunton. Passing through Churchville in about 10 miles, make a right onto VA 42. In 1.3 miles, turn left onto VA 760 for 3.4 miles to a left onto VA 747. Another 1.1 miles brings you to a right onto VA 730. Don't follow VA 730 when it makes an abrupt turn in 1.3 miles; keep straight, following VA 718 and making a left onto FSR 95 in an additional 1.3 miles. You will find the Segment A parking area in 0.1 mile, on the right.

For access to the other segments' trailheads, continue following FSR 95, passing by parking for the North River Gorge Trail (see Hike 39) in 1.1 miles, the Trimble Mountain Trail in 2.8 miles, and the Todd Lake Recreation Area (see Hike 40) in 3.0 miles. Continue on (now) dirt FSR 95, keeping right when you come to a T-intersection 1.3 miles from Todd Lake. (The North River Gorge trailhead and campground are about 1 mile to the left on FSR 95B.) Keep right in another 1.6 miles, passing by FSR 533 to Elkhorn Lake. In an additional 0.4 mile, you'll come to the next intersection, where the trailhead for Segment B is about 3 miles to the right on FSR 95, and Segment C's trailhead is approximately 2 miles to the left on FSR 96.

Route Description

From the Segment A parking area, take the "spur" trail into the woods. This pathway was constructed so hikers could avoid having to use an old woods road that had some of the largest tank traps I've ever seen. Built to discourage off-road vehicle use, one of the pits was so deep that it had developed into a permanent little pond. In about 0.2 mile, arrive and turn right onto the white blazes of the WONRT. The ridgeline narrows at about 0.7 mile as the

First Day

- **TOTAL DISTANCE:** 11.5 miles
- **HIKING TIME:** 8.0 hours

The Hike at a Glance

FIRST DAY

1.4 Grindstone Mountain summit

2.2 Little Skidmore Trail comes in from left; stay right

4.1 Groom's Ridge Trail comes in from right; stay left

6.2 Switchback left

6.6 Keep left when old road comes in from right. Soon come to FSR 427 (Little Bald Knob Road), turn right on it for a few feet to good viewpoint; then retrace steps to resume hike on WONRT

9.8 Trail to right is option to miss ford of North River. Continue on WONRT to follow this description and ford North River

10.0 Cross FSR 95

11.5 Campsite for the night

route steepens, coming to a view of Lookout Mountain. You will be traversing its ridgeline on the last day of this hike. The trail begins an immediate descent after crossing the 2,702-foot summit of Grindstone Mountain, at 1.4 miles.

Passing through a wildlife clearing, resume the ascent, coming to an intersection at 2.2 miles. The Little Skidmore Trail {FS 715}, actually a logging access road, descends left for more than 2 miles to Little Skidmore Fork, eventually emerging onto FSR 95. Your route continues to follow the WONRT uphill, going through a wildlife clearing surrounded by oak, maple, hickory, black locust, and dogwood at 2.3 miles. Despite its name, dogwood was not named for man's best friend. The tree was originally called dagwood, as its timber is so strong it was once carved into daggers. Studies of ancient civilizations show that the dogwood was as highly prized as horns for making such weapons; hence the tree's Latin generic name, *Cornus*.

The trail makes a couple of small ups and downs, ascending by patches of star moss to the main crest of Chestnut Ridge. A broad, flat knob at 4.1 miles would provide a good tenting site. From here, Groom's Ridge Trail {FS 424} descends 4.0 miles to FSR 101. Your route bears left, where thickets of mountain laurel close in on the trail and mosses cover the pathway like padded carpeting. Switchback to the left at 6.2 miles, and keep to the left when an old road comes in from the right at 6.6 miles. Soon after this, when you come to dirt Little Bald Knob Road {FSR 427}, be sure to turn right for 100 yards to the most spectacular view you are going to have on the hike. Far off to the northeast is Massanutten Mountain and, on very clear days, behind it are the Blue Ridge Mountains of Shenandoah National Park. Closest to you, to the west and northwest, is the knobby ridgeline of Shenandoah Mountain, while beyond are wave after wave of Allegheny Mountain summits in West Virginia. This is such a lofty site from which to watch the sun set and rise that you may want to search out a sheltered spot along the edge of the meadow to pitch your tent and spend the evening.

Return to and continue on the WONRT, crossing the very summit of 4,351-foot Little Bald Knob. Immediately begin the long descent, passing a limited view of Elkhorn Lake at 7.2 miles. Switchbacking off the ridgeline, follow a sidehill trail through fields of rock, entering a mountain laurel and pine tunnel at 8.0 miles and soon emerging into a mixed hardwood forest.

(You will need to make a decision when you come to a trail going off to the right at 9.8 miles. This trail description continues straight ahead and fords North River. To avoid the ford, you could turn right onto the intersecting trail, follow it for a distance to make a left turn onto the forest road, cross the river on a road bridge, and follow the road for 0.4 mile to meet back up with the WONRT at the 10.0-mile point in the description below. This alternative will save the ford of the river but increase the overall mileage of the hike by a little less than a mile.)

(continued on page 188)

Wild Oak National Recreation Trail

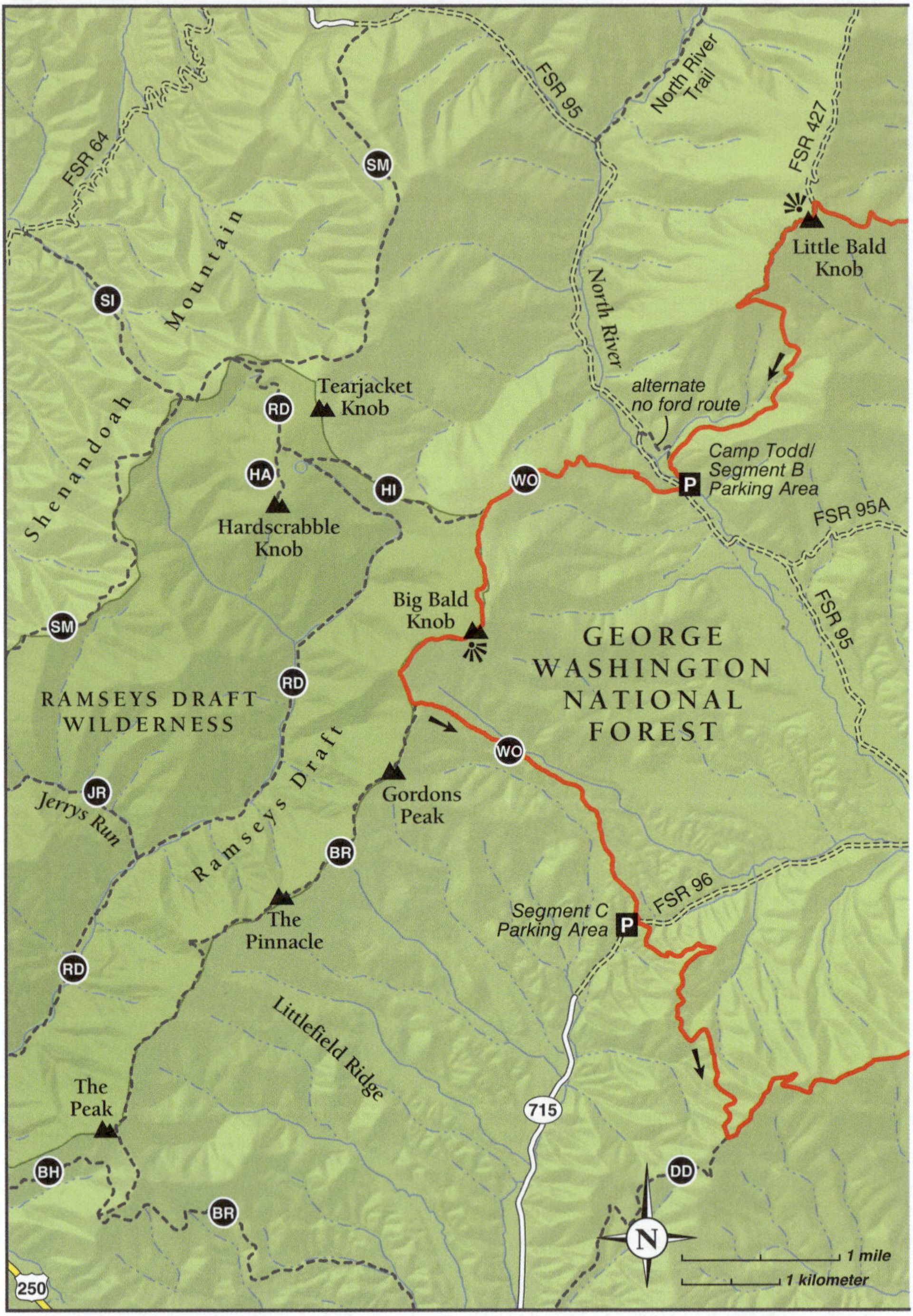

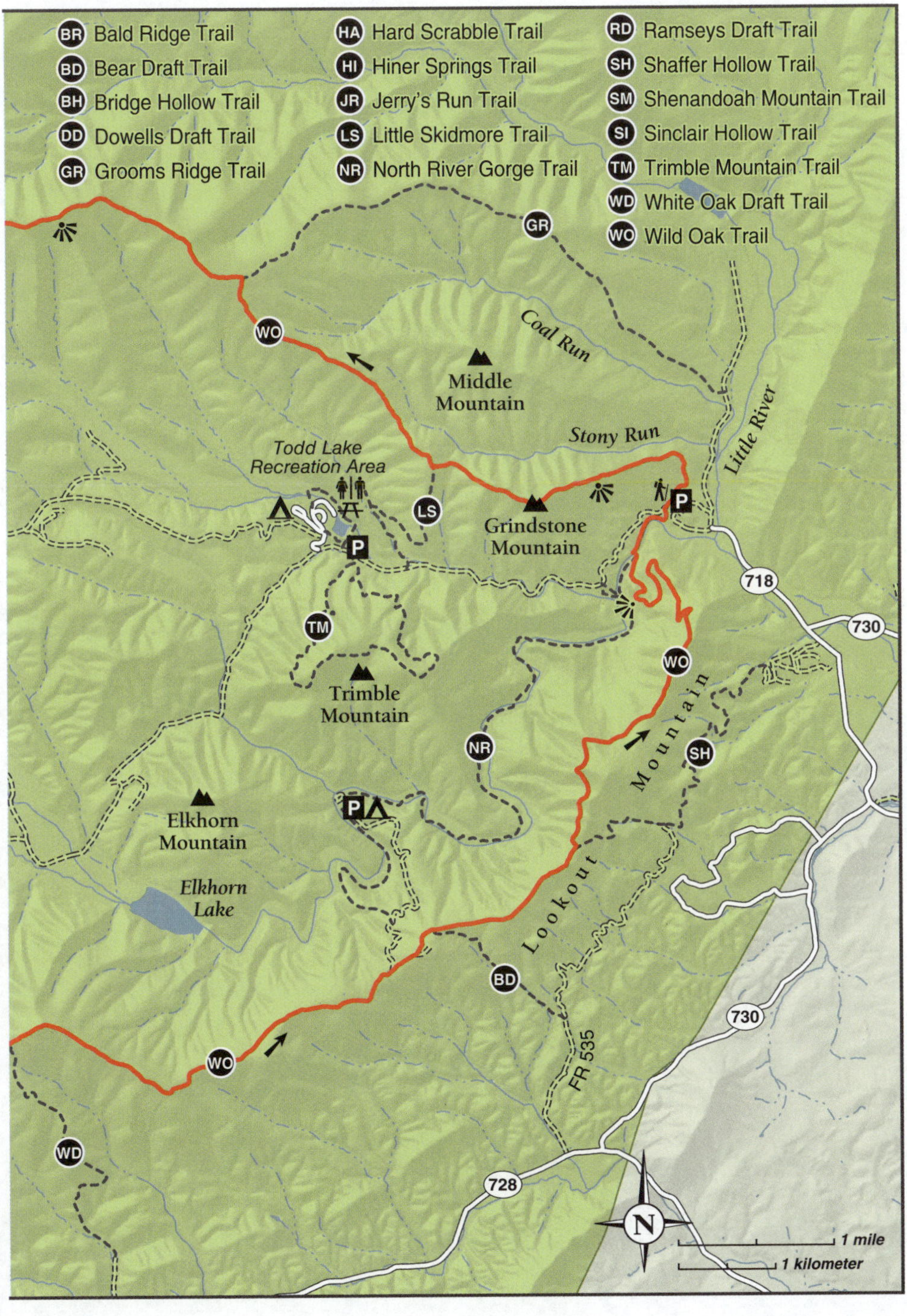
BR Bald Ridge Trail
BD Bear Draft Trail
BH Bridge Hollow Trail
DD Dowells Draft Trail
GR Grooms Ridge Trail
HA Hard Scrabble Trail
HI Hiner Springs Trail
JR Jerry's Run Trail
LS Little Skidmore Trail
NR North River Gorge Trail
RD Ramseys Draft Trail
SH Shaffer Hollow Trail
SM Shenandoah Mountain Trail
SI Sinclair Hollow Trail
TM Trimble Mountain Trail
WD White Oak Draft Trail
WO Wild Oak Trail
Coal Run
Middle Mountain
Stony Run
Little River
Todd Lake Recreation Area
Grindstone Mountain
Trimble Mountain
Elkhorn Mountain
Elkhorn Lake
Lookout Mountain
FR 535
718
730
728
N
1 mile
1 kilometer

(continued from page 185)

To continue on the WONRT from the intersection, stay to the left, soon coming to the river. (Consider getting water here, as the sources at the suggested campsite described below may be dry.) There might be a fallen tree over North River to help you get across, but use caution if you must ford it before arriving at FSR 95, the Camp Todd site, and the end of Segment A at 10.0 miles. There are a few campsites along the road, but for quieter and more pleasant surroundings for the night, you are going to continue into Segment B, following the white blazes as they leave Camp Todd and ascending steeply along a stream.

At 10.4 miles, the trail switchbacks right to gain the ridge, passing an area recovering from a fire from several decades ago at 10.7 miles. If you're hiking when the leaves are off the trees, you will see Elkhorn Lake to the southeast at 11.0 miles. In addition, almost in front of you is Big Bald, which you'll be crossing early tomorrow morning. You have hit your evening's destination when the trail comes to two springs at 11.5 miles (the second one is usually flowing best). Please practice no-trace camping and use your stove to cook. There have been few signs of camping on the entire WONRT, but they are increasing; it would be nice to do your part to keep the area as pristine as possible.

Take in the view near Big Bald Knob.

photo: Johnny Molloy

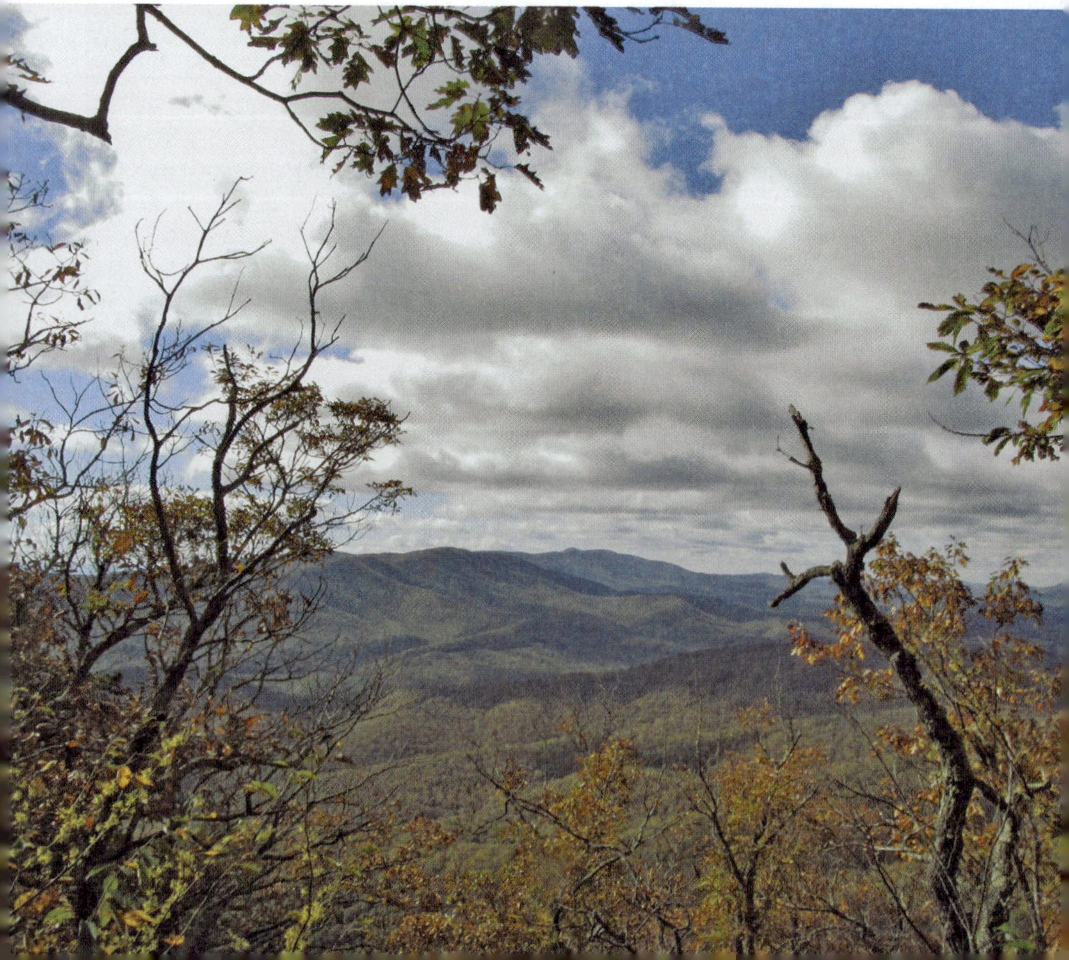

Second Day

- **TOTAL DISTANCE:** 9.9 miles
- **HIKING TIME:** 6.0 hours

The Hike at a Glance

SECOND DAY

0.9 Big Bald Knob summit

1.8 Pond. At far end of pond, Bald Ridge Trail comes in from the right; keep left

4.2 Cross FSR 96

5.9 Dowell's Draft Trail comes in from right; keep left

7.0 White Oak Draft Trail comes in from right; keep left

9.9 Campsite for the night

In wandering around last night, you might have found, about 0.1 mile from your campsite, that the Hiner Spring Trail {FS 446} goes right to descend into Ramseys Draft Wilderness. This morning you should keep to the left at that intersection, following the white blazes along the border of the wilderness area. Ascending through mountain laurel and evergreens, the treadway is softened by the accumulation of pine needles. Big Bald Knob, at 0.9 mile, was evidently an open wildlife clearing at one time, but it has become overgrown. Near the summit, there is a short path to the left, leading to a good view of Elkhorn Lake with the Shenandoah Valley and Blue Ridge Mountains visible beyond Lookout and Crawford Mountains.

Descending, the WONRT passes a couple of open areas of maples and ferns, which would make good campsites. The trail continues with quick ups and downs, passing several other possible camps, and arrives at an overgrown wildlife clearing and pond (many deer prints in the soft mud) at 1.8 miles. Swing left of the pond and bear left, descending steeply away from Ramseys Draft Wilderness on the white-blazed pathway. (The trail ascending from the far end of the pond is the Bald Ridge Trail {FS 496}, which runs along the eastern border of the wilderness area.)

Make a short side excursion off your wintergreen-lined pathway at 2.4 miles. Mitchell Branch to the left is the last sure water you will come across for the rest of the hike. After taking proper precautions in treating the water, drink your fill and be sure to carry enough to get you through the rest of today, tonight's dinner, and the long, dry walk along Hankey and Lookout Mountains tomorrow.

The WONRT now descends gradually on an old road along Dividing Ridge, arriving at FSR 96 and the end of Segment B at 4.2 miles. Continue on into Segment C, climbing steeply by blueberries and wintergreen. Wintergreen's evergreen leaves and bright-red berries add a welcome splash of color to an otherwise brown and gray forest in the colder months. Its fruit is an important food source for many animals in the winter. Mice and chipmunks nibble away at the fleshy berry; deer, grouse, and bears swallow the fruit whole, and, after their bodies absorb the digestible part, they drop the seeds somewhere else—a classic example of how animals help disperse seeds.

The climb becomes even steeper at 4.6 miles before you attain the ridgeline. This hard labor continues with several ups and downs (and passing Betsy Trail {FS 651}) to a knob at 5.9 miles, where Dowell's Draft Trail {FS 650} drops for about 3.5 miles to US 250 near West Augusta. Your route swings left into a gap before climbing to attain a grassy area surrounded by oak and hickory at 6.2 miles—the first peak of Hankey Mountain, 3,407 feet above sea level. When you come into the wildlife clearing at 6.6 miles, the trail begins to follow a woods road. You could camp just about anywhere you wish along the broad crest of the mountain, but as the walking is now fairly effortless, it is easy to put in a couple more miles before stopping for the night.

At 7.0 miles, White Oak Draft Trail {FS 486} drops to the right for about 2.5 miles to US 250 near Whites Store. Continue on the WONRT, topping the second peak of Hankey Mountain (3,450') at 7.2 miles. There is a dazzling display of wild azalea next to the road as it descends along the mountain crest. Dogwood adds bits of white when the route enters a clearing and the roadway becomes well surfaced. The trail makes use of this road, open to motorized traffic during the hunting season (usually mid-October to the end of December), for the next few miles.

You will pass by five more clearings. If you can keep count, make it to the fifth and largest clearing, at 9.9 miles, before setting up camp, although any one of these open areas would provide a fairly good tent site.

Third Day

- **TOTAL DISTANCE:** 5.8 miles
- **HIKING TIME:** 3.5 hours

The Hike at a Glance

THIRD DAY

0.5 Bear Draft Trail comes in from the right; stay left

1.7 Shaffer Hollow Trail comes in from the right; stay left

5.0 Side trail right to viewpoint

5.8 Return to your automobile

After shouldering your pack and heading out for the day, pay attention when the main road descends to the left. You want to keep right on a less-traveled roadway, following the white blazes. The road splits again at 0.2 mile; keep right, passing through a field and descending on a steep, grassy woods road. Join up with another road at 0.5 mile, staying right and bypassing Bear Draft Trail {FS 535} when it goes off to the right. (Bear Draft descends for approximately 3 miles to arrive at VA 728 near Stribling Springs.) Keep left at 1.0 mile, when another roadway joins up with your route.

Shaffer Hollow Trail {FS 513} comes in from the right at 1.7 miles; stay left, soon swinging around, but not attaining the summit of Lookout Mountain. The side trail to the right at 5.0 miles leads to a small viewpoint. Soon begin the final descent, paying close attention to take the switchback to the left (avoiding a pathway straight ahead). From here, continue downhill (avoiding the trail to the left that leads to the North River Gorge Trail—see Hike 39) to a footbridge that enables you to cross the North River with dry feet. At one time hikers faced a somewhat dangerous and tricky ford of the river, having to choose their own route through the rippling waters.

Soon after crossing the river, step over FSR 95 and quickly come to the spur trail where a right turn will bring your three-day excursion away from the world of motor vehicle travel to an end as you return to the Segment A parking area, at 5.8 miles.

42 Ramseys Draft

- **GPS:** N38.3081430 W79.3610703
- **TOTAL DISTANCE (circuit):** 8.5 miles
- **HIKING TIME:** 6.0 hours
- **VERTICAL RISE:** 1,080 feet
- **MAPS:** USGS *West Augusta; U.S. Forest Service Ramseys Draft Wilderness* map; *National Geographic Trails Illustrated Map #791 Staunton/Shenandoah Mountain*
- **CONTACT:** North River Ranger District
  401 Oakwood Road
  Harrisonburg, VA 22801
  540-432-0187
  fs.usda.gov/gwj

The Hike at a Glance

0.1 Left onto Road Hollow Trail
2.6 Right onto Shenandoah Mountain Trail
3.6 Right onto Jerry's Run Trail
4.2 Old chimney
6.0 Right onto Ramseys Draft Trail
8.5 End of hike

In 1912, a team of U.S. Forest Service employees who were headquartered at an inn named the Mountain House walked, drove, and otherwise surveyed the mountains, hills, and valleys of Highland, Bath, and Augusta Counties. The recommendations contained in their reports led to the 1913 purchase of more than 38,000 acres on and around Shenandoah Mountain—some of the first property to be acquired for the Shenandoah National Forest, which eventually grew to become the present-day, 1.8-million-acre George Washington and Jefferson National Forests. Recognizing that much of the land still existed in its pristine state—never having been logged—the area has been managed essentially as a wilderness by the forest service since 1935. The Virginia Wilderness Act of 1984 ensured that lands around Ramseys Draft will remain this way for generations to come.

Framed by Shenandoah Mountain, Tearjacket Knob, and Bald Ridge, Ramseys Draft flows freely through these high Allegheny Mountains. From its headwaters of spewing springs at nearly 4,000 feet in elevation, the stream drains the wilderness's 6,500 acres. Up until the 1960s, it was possible to drive more than 3 miles upstream from US 250 on a road made passable by the construction of 11 fords by the Civilian Conservation Corps in the 1930s. Automobile traffic came to an abrupt halt in 1969, when rainwater from Hurricane Camille—the same storm that did so much damage to the Tye River Valley (see Hike 35)—wiped out most of the man-made enhancements at the stream crossings. While not downplaying the need to negotiate the numerous fords, post-hurricane forest service literature spoke of the joys of using the flat surface of the old road to hike along the draft. That information had to be updated when the great flood of November 1985 not only caused the roadbed to deteriorate and, at some spots, completely disappear, but even changed the course of the stream in several places. In February 1996, Hurricane Fran caused more changes in the stream channel and blew over scores of trees, making travel along the drainage system even more difficult. Today's visitors definitely have to be more determined than those of the past.

Don't let flood-damaged terrain deter you from taking this hike to explore the wilderness. The quiet, isolated hillsides of Road Hollow, a mile of gentle, nearly level walking in the deciduous forest on Shenandoah Mountain, and an easy descent next to Jerry's Run are all things that will help you forget the stresses and strains of modern life. And besides, you will have a chance to see firsthand the effects of hurricanes and floods on a mountain river valley. Just remember, this is a wilderness area and trails will not be well maintained. You will most likely encounter numerous blowdowns

Ramseys Draft

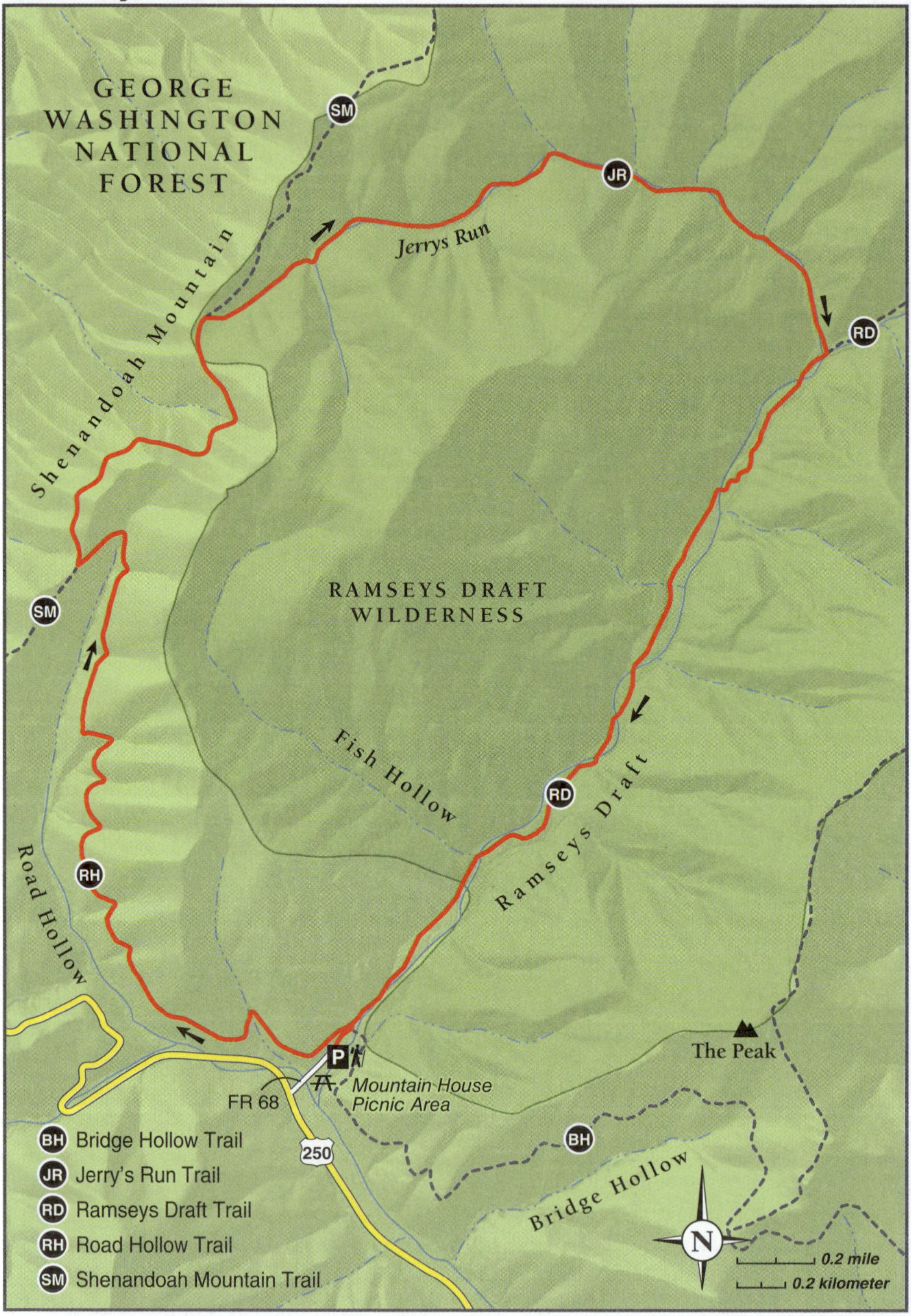

and have stinging nettle, poison ivy, and other vegetation crowding in on the trails (it might be wise to wear long pants). Be prepared for these obstacles—and the many river fords—to slow your forward progress.

DIRECTIONS Take US 250 west from Staunton, passing through Churchville. About 14 miles from the small hamlet, turn right onto FSR 68 and into the forest service's Mountain House Picnic Area. (The area was named for a tollhouse on the Staunton-to-Parkersburg turnpike constructed before the Civil War. Being approximately 20 miles from Staunton, Mountain House was about as far as a team of horses could comfortably pull a wagon in a day, and the station became a popular overnight destination. It was a place to let the horses rest prior to making the long haul over Shenandoah Mountain and for travelers to enjoy indoor lodging and an evening meal for all of 35¢. A local legend maintains that, during the Civil War, an inebriated Confederate soldier, patronizing the house while on break from his duties at the breastworks on top of the mountain, made advances toward Mrs. Rogers, the proprietor. More than annoyed by his attentions, she dispatched the soldier to an early grave by using a rolling pin to deliver a number of blows to his head.) From the picnic area, which has seasonal toilet facilities, continue on FSR 68 for a few hundred feet to the trailhead parking area.

Route Description

Begin the hike on Ramseys Draft Trail {FS 440}, bypassing the Bridge Hollow Trail {FS 442} as it goes to the right and ascends about 2 miles to connect with the Bald Ridge Trail {FS 496}, which runs along the eastern border of the wilderness. At 0.1 mile, make a left onto the Road Hollow Trail {FS 448}. Bridge Hollow and Road Hollow Trails were constructed during the summers of 1988 through 1992 by members of the Student Conservation Association. The nonprofit, educational organization provides high-school and college students the opportunity to volunteer their services and work for public lands throughout the country. You should thank these young folks for their hard labor because this circuit hike used to be longer, and you once had to walk several miles along heavily traveled US 250 to complete it.

Road Hollow Trail leaves Ramseys Draft and ascends in a forest of mountain laurel, blueberries, and pines. At 0.5 mile, cross over a small water run after having swung into the first of eight draws that you walk into during the ascent. The highway sounds of US 250 finally begin to fade at about 1.0 mile, when the trail makes a wide arc to the north and the road makes a horseshoe bend to the southwest. With the gain in elevation, the evergreens become less common, replaced more and more by deciduous trees; in the spring, the draw at 1.75 miles is adorned by dozens of dogwood trees in bloom. Commonly mistaken for the flower, the pink and white that you see on the trees are actually leaf bracts encircling the petals of the dogwood's small blossom. Look inside the bracts to see the true beauty of the state flower of Virginia. The tree's green berries appear around the first of September, about the same time its leaves are changing to a deep, dark crimson. As the leaves drop off, the fruit turns a shiny red, providing the forest with some color for the cooler months ahead.

Road Hollow Trail ends when it tops the ridge and meets the Shenandoah Mountain Trail {FS 447} at 2.6 miles. To the left, it is 1.4 miles to the Confederate Breastworks Overlook on US 250. You, however, want to make a right to walk along this wonderfully built and nearly level pathway as it swings around a hollow at 3.0 miles, where there are some limited views to the west. Although the mountainside drops off steeply, the trail continues at a level contour and is almost wide enough for two people to walk abreast. The broadly flat ridgeline at 3.5 miles may make you wish you had brought a tent so that you could camp amid the hemlocks, hardwoods, and pines.

At 3.6 miles, not far from the wilderness boundary, leave Shenandoah Mountain Trail (see Hike 43 if you want to keep following that route) to make a right and descend on Jerry's Run Trail {FS 441}. Cross the run a couple of times before coming to an open area at 4.2 miles and an old chimney marking the site of the Potomac Appalachian Trail Club's Sexton Cabin, which was dismantled in keeping with the spirit of returning Ramseys Draft to wilderness status. Beyond this good campsite, the trail swings left, continuing downhill to cross the stream again as the valley becomes narrower. Be careful on an eroded section of trail at 5.1 miles—in times of high water you may have to follow a scrambling trail around fallen trees, taking care not to tumble into the creek. The route crosses Jerry's Run twice more and enters a wide valley where jack-in-the-pulpits are unusually abundant. The trail makes a faint, abrupt turn at 5.8 miles to recross the run and end as it meets Ramseys Draft Trail, at 6.0 miles.

Turn downstream to follow the old roadbed and cross Jerry's Run for the final time before fording Ramseys Draft for the first of many times. In fact, allow plenty of time from here to the end of the hike because, for the next 2.0 miles, you are more or less on your own. The roadbed disappears in many places, and you will have to make your own decisions as to what route to take around blowdowns, giant boulders, and logs carried down the mountainsides by raging waters. The draft is a native-trout stream, but since the flood of 1985 changed their habitat, the fish are reported to be less abundant and no longer reaching the size of their ancestors. The beaver population must also have diminished because I did not see any evidence of them the last time I was here.

Passing by the Road Hollow and Bridge Hollow Trails, arrive back at the parking area at 8.5 miles, possibly exhausted, but certainly richer in spirit from the experience.

This old chimney marks the site of the Potomac Appalachian Trail Club's Sexton Cabin.

photo: Johnny Molloy

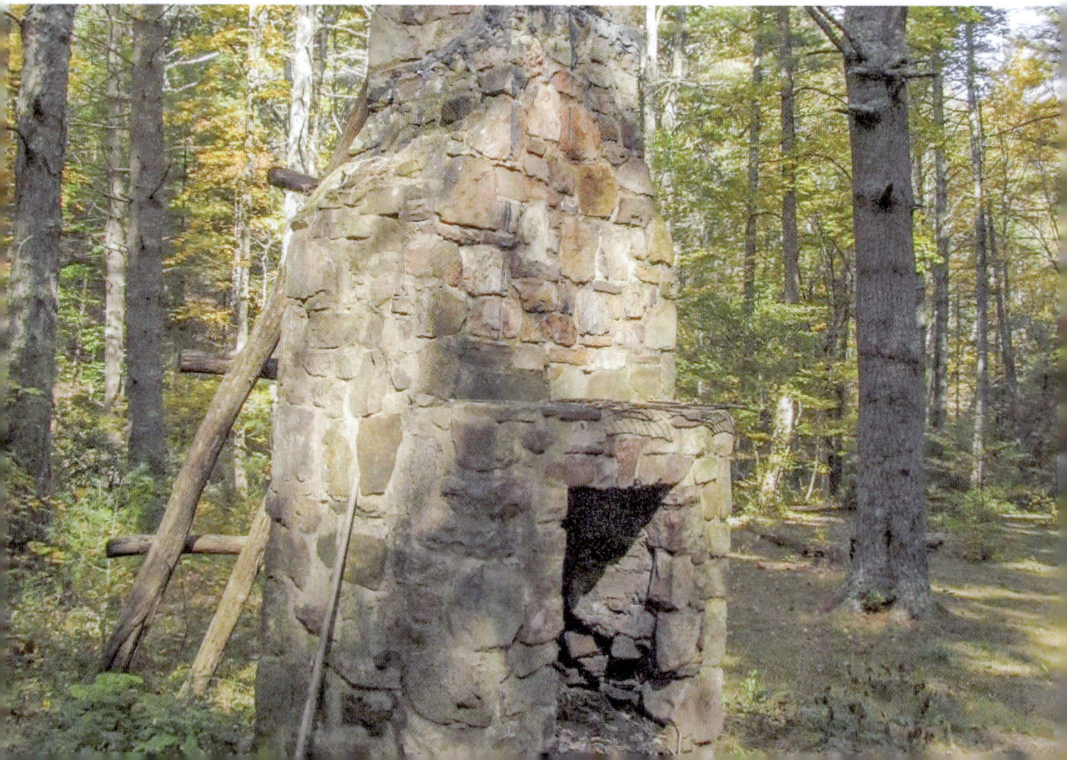

43 Shenandoah Mountain

- **GPS:** N38.4117820 W79.3099057
- **TOTAL DISTANCE (one-way):** 10.6 miles
- **HIKING TIME:** 6.0 hours
- **VERTICAL RISE:** 1,400 feet
- **MAPS:** USGS *McDowell, West Augusta,* and *Palo Alto (VA and WV); U.S. Forest Service Ramseys Draft Wilderness* map; *National Geographic Trails Illustrated Map #791 Staunton/Shenandoah Mountain*
- **CONTACT:** North River Ranger District
401 Oakwood Road
Harrisonburg, VA 22801
540-432-0187
fs.usda.gov/gwj

The Hike at a Glance

- 0.2 Right onto Shenandoah Mountain Trail
- 1.4 Road Hollow Trail comes in from the right; stay left
- 2.3 Enter Ramseys Draft Wilderness; a few hundred yards later stay left where Jerry's Run Trail comes in from the right
- 6.4 Ramseys Draft can be heard below the ridgeline. Shortly thereafter Sinclair Hollow Trail comes in from left; keep right
- 7.2 Ramseys Draft Trail comes in from the right; keep left
- 9.1 Begin gradual descent
- 10.6 End of hike at FSR 95

The Shenandoah Mountain Trail may well be the easiest long-distance excursion you can take in the mountains of western Virginia. Following a route first dug by the Civilian Conservation Corps during the Great Depression, the route, sometimes wide enough to invoke visions of a carriage road, traverses the spine of Shenandoah Mountain for more than 10 miles. Along its entire distance there are no places where your calf muscles will begin to ache from having to work hard to get you up steep inclines, nor will there be any pressure on your knees or jolts to your ankles from making long, rapid descents. Unlike other ridgeline trails, which seem to go up and over every knob and knoll, this pathway skirts these natural fluctuations, negotiating what little bits of elevation changes it does have by means of gradual grades or gentle switchbacks. Because of this ease of travel and the fact that good, level campsites can be found every few miles, the Shenandoah Mountain Trail is the perfect place to bring the kids for an overnight hike or to break friends into the pleasures of backpacking in some extremely isolated backcountry (Highland County is one of the least populated in the state) without introducing them to the rigors of a more rugged terrain. Be sure to carry enough water; it is not readily available right on the route.

The trail has so many good things going for it that it's a worthwhile hike any time of the year. In spring there are thousands of azaleas and other wildflowers in bloom; the green leaves of maple, birch, oak, beech, poplar, and other deciduous trees provide deep shade to keep hikers cool on hot summer days; and, because the forest has such a variety of vegetation, walks during the fall leaf season are more colorful than in many other parts of the state. The wide pathway, gentle grade, and quite frequent heavy snowfalls of winter make the trail a good proving ground for novice snowshoers.

DIRECTIONS Since this is a one-way hike, a car shuttle will be necessary. The shuttle involves many miles of dirt-road travel, so allow ample time. Drive US 250 west from Staunton, and in about 20 miles—immediately after crossing the Calfpasture River—make a right onto VA 715. Stay on this route (which eventually becomes dirt FSR 96) for 6.4 miles to make a left turn onto FSR 95. In 3.2 miles you will pass a sign identifying Camp Todd, and 4.1 miles beyond that, stay left on FSR 95 at the junction with FSR 85.

Shenandoah Mountain

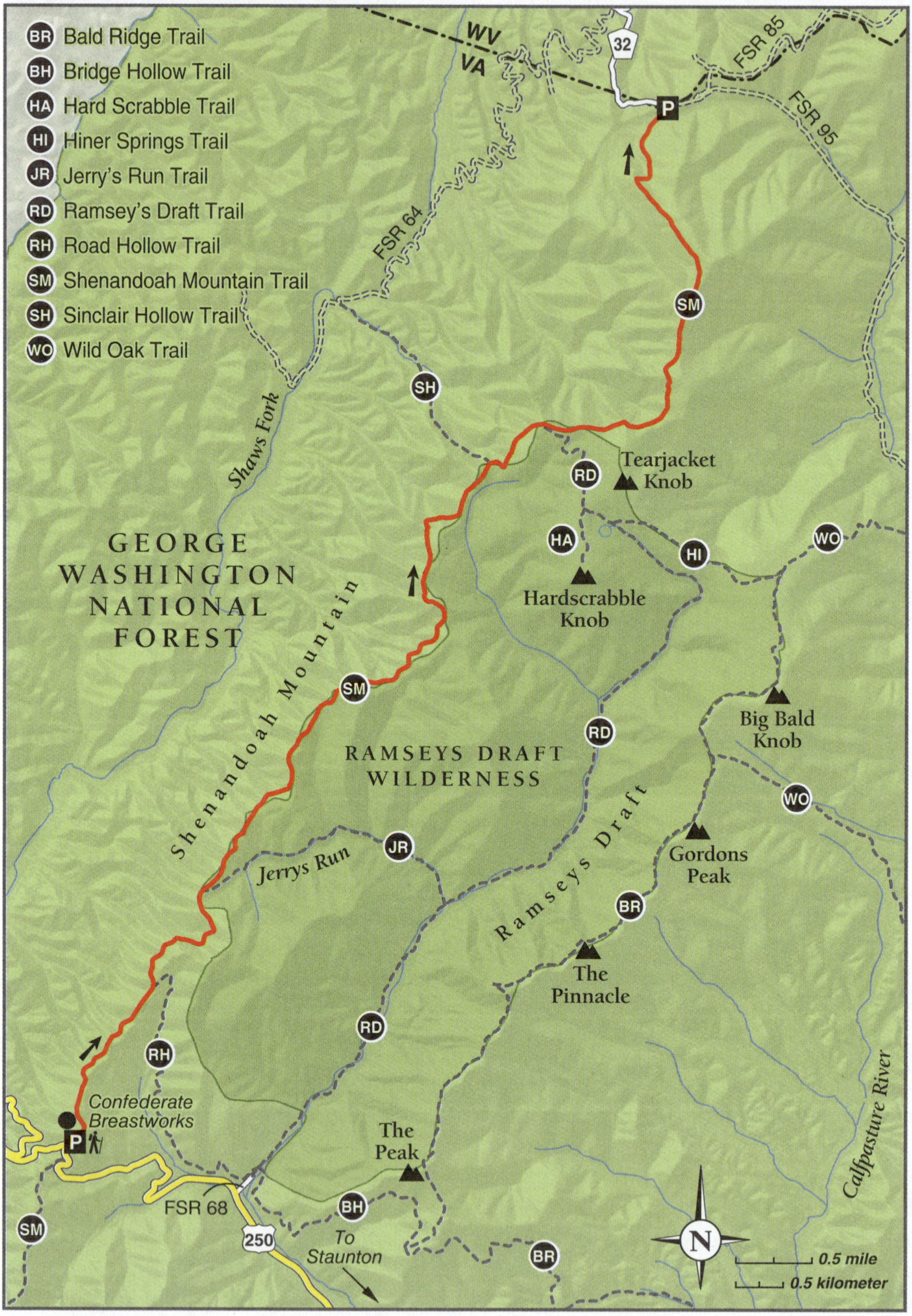

In 0.4 mile more you must be paying close attention, as the trailhead for the Shenandoah Trail may be marked only by a faint blaze on the left side of the road. If you find yourself in West Virginia, turn around and look again for the trailhead—eventually you will find it located about halfway between the West Virginia border and the FSR 85 and FSR 95 junction. Leave one car here (there's not much room, so make sure it is well off the road) and retrace your route all the way back to US 250. Make a right onto US 250, pass by the Mountain House Picnic Area and Ramseys Draft trailhead (see Hike 42), and in 7.3 miles park at the overlook on top of Shenandoah Mountain.

Route Description

Before you "officially" begin your hike of the Shenandoah Mountain Trail, take the 20-minute interpretive trail looping through trenches remaining from the days of the Civil War. To prevent Union forces from using the Staunton-to-Parkersburg turnpike (now US 250) to gain access to the Shenandoah Valley from the west, Confederate soldiers under the command of General Edward Johnson constructed a network of breastworks on the western side of Shenandoah Mountain in March 1862. On April 18, despite the strategically placed fortifications, Union general Robert Milroy's superior forces caused the Southern men to abandon what had become known as Fort Edward Johnson. The occupying army subsequently built additional breastworks on the eastern side of the ridge to check the flow of Confederates to the west. Yet on May 5, the combined armies of Stonewall Jackson and General Johnson were enough of a threat to make Milroy retreat and give the mountain back to the Confederacy.

Once back at the parking lot, start your longer hike by taking the right branch of the breastworks loop trail, staying more or less level to swing around the knob; do not follow the unauthorized trail going uphill. At 0.2 mile, turn right off the interpretive trail to begin following the Shenandoah Mountain Trail {FS 447}. Hikers are surprised to see wild turkeys this close to the road, but they are often spotted here because the oak and hickory trees provide plenty of mast for the healthy flocks inhabiting the Allegheny highlands. The golden yellow flame azalea can be seen throughout much of George Washington and Jefferson National Forests, but notice that it is the pink azalea thriving here on Shenandoah Mountain.

At 1.4 miles, the Road Hollow Trail {FS 448} (see Hike 42) heads off to the right, descending to the Ramseys Draft trailhead off US 250. Stay left, slabbing the western side of the ridgeline. The green fields along Shaws Fork can be seen through breaks in the vegetation at 1.8 miles. The hillside drops off steeply, but the trail remains level and almost wide enough for two hiking partners to walk side by side. At 2.3 miles, come onto a broad flat area of hardwoods and pines, where you may be tempted to set up camp. Here you may pass a sign letting you know you've entered the Ramseys Draft Wilderness, and a few hundred feet beyond the sign you'll see Jerry's Run Trail {FS 441}, which descends right 0.2 mile to a water source and continues about 2 more miles to reach the lower elevations of the wilderness area.

Staying left, it becomes evident that most people use the Shenandoah Mountain Trail for access to the wilderness area because the pathway is now very obviously less used. As you continue along the ridge with minor ups and downs, the decline in human foot travel is accompanied by a corresponding increase in the signs of wildlife—deer tracks, bear scat, and turkey scratchings. In the spring and early summer, as you pass through a small gap at 4.7 miles you may hear the water of Al's Run, a tributary of Jerry's Run, dropping down the mountain to the right. If you are hard up for water, you could bushwhack down to it; just remember it'll be a steep climb back to the trail. Of course, you could enjoy the jack-in-the-pulpits on the way down and back up.

A grassy area at 5.2 miles is another inviting campsite, and those who wander around this small mountain lawn may have their hearts skip a beat when a grouse suddenly comes flying out of the underbrush, flapping noisily just a few feet in front of startled faces. Diminutive bluets, whose pale color replicates that of an early morning sky, line the trail at 6.4 miles, where the left prong of Ramseys Draft becomes audible below the ridgeline. Shortly beyond this, another broad, flat area would provide additional, nicely situated tenting spots. From here, the Sinclair Hollow Trail {FS 4470} drops to the left about 2 miles to reach FSR 64 next to Shaws Fork. Keeping to the right, the Shenandoah Mountain Trail makes one of its rare climbs by switchback to gain a few hundred feet and arrives at the intersection with Ramseys Draft Trail {FS 440}, which comes in from the right at 7.2 miles. Once again, it may be tempting to set up camp in the flat gap, especially when the wet-weather spring is flowing well. It is located about 100 feet down the west side of the mountain, directly opposite the trail junction.

Continue on the Shenandoah Mountain Trail, leaving the wilderness area at 7.5 miles, where the route is high above the Brushy Fork Valley to the northwest.

Soon the Shenandoah Mountain Trail, now sometimes a little overgrown, makes a short ascent through azaleas, whose delightful fragrance is so strong that it eclipses any other smells that may be present. Swinging around the ridge at 8.4 miles, there is a limited view of Little Bald Knob (see Hike 41) to the east. When the trail begins its long, gradual descent at 9.1 miles, your eyes will be drawn beyond ridge after ridge to some of the loftiest mountains of West Virginia, rising along the northwestern horizon. The large leaves of the striped maple give the woods a lush-green, almost rainforest look just before the trail makes its final drop to cross the Little River and comes to an end at 10.6 miles, on FSR 95.

FSR 95 is a gateway to a multitude of hikes in this part of George Washington and Jefferson National Forests. Looking at the descriptions for North River Gorge (Hike 39), Todd Lake Recreation Area and Trimble Mountain (Hike 40), and the Wild Oak National Recreation Trail (Hike 41) may make you wish you had brought enough supplies to stay out here for at least another week. And, if you want more hiking on Shenandoah Mountain, the Shenandoah Mountain Trail has another section of about 20 miles that heads southward from the Confederate Breastworks, on US 250.

Keep your eye out for grouse here.

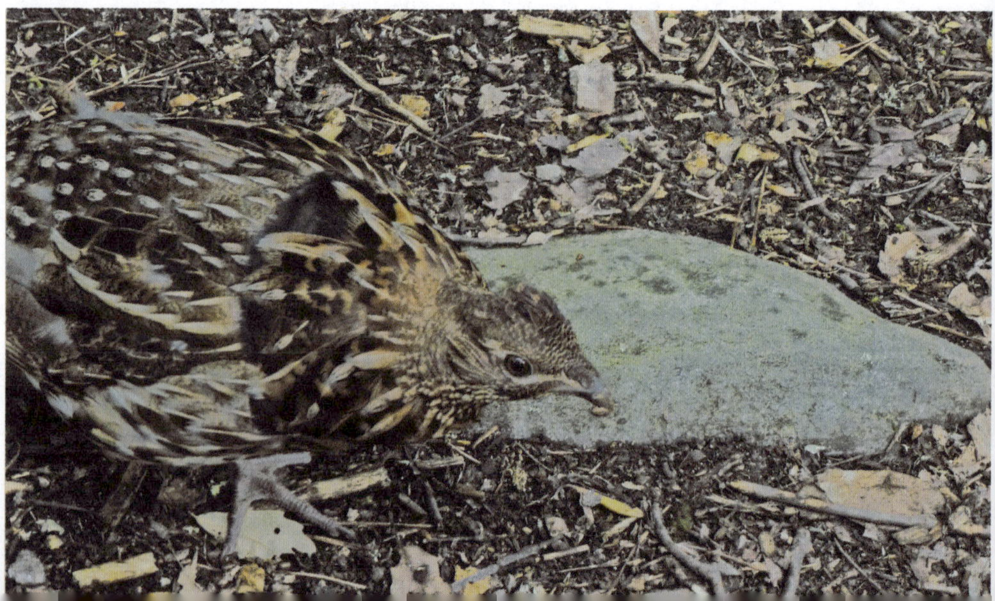

44 Elliott Knob and Falls Hollow

- **GPS:** N38.2132683 W79.2958696
- **TOTAL DISTANCE (one-way):** 9.0 miles
- **HIKING TIME:** 6.0 hours
- **VERTICAL RISE:** 2,060 feet
- **MAPS:** USGS *Elliott Knob; National Geographic Trails Illustrated Map #791 Staunton/Shenandoah Mountain*
- **CONTACT:** North River Ranger District
  401 Oakwood Road
  Harrisonburg, VA 22801
  540-432-0187
  fs.usda.gov/gwj

The Hike at a Glance

1.8 Side trail to Buffalo Spring comes in from the right; keep left

4.4 Turn right onto Elliot Knob Road. Soon after this the road swings left to communications installation and North Mountain Trail turns left to descend knob, but you keep straight toward summit

4.7 Elliot Knob summit and fire tower. After enjoying view, retrace steps, go past the two segments North Mountain Trail, and begin steep descent on Elliot Knob Road

6.2 Left onto Falls Hollow Trail

7.7 Swing away from creek and begin following road

9.0 Return to shuttled car

Elliott Knob, the summit of Great North Mountain, is the highest point in Augusta ounty. Although this hike involves a verti-al rise of more than 2,000 feet to reach the ummit, the elevation is gained gradually over he course of almost 5 miles. Enjoyment and nspections of assorted spring and summer vildflowers can make the ascent seem even asier, and the downhill portion of the journey as charms of its own, providing a forest and nvironment quite different from that found n the mountain's ridgeline. A stream drops hrough the narrow canyon of Falls Hollow in n extensive series of cascades, best appreciated in the spring and early summer when the flow is at its highest volume.

DIRECTIONS To do the complete hike as a one-way trip will require a car shuttle. Take I-81/I-64 Exit 220 at Staunton and follow VA 262 northward 4.2 miles, take the VA 254 (Parkersburg Pike) exit and follow VA 254 westward, and in about 7 miles, in Buffalo Gap, continue straight onto VA 42. In just a short distance, VA 688 comes in from the right. Stay on VA 42 but pay close attention to the odometer because 2.4 miles from this intersection you need to pull into the possibly unmarked Falls Hollow trailhead parking area, on the right side of the road. Leave one car in the large turnaround next to the gated road. Take the second car and backtrack to make a left onto VA 688, ascending almost 4 miles to the top of the ridge. Look for a small, possibly unmarked parking area on the left side of the road in Dry Branch Gap.

Route Description

Walk through the gate and follow yellow-blazed North Mountain Trail {FS 443}, gradually rising on an old road along the ridge. At 0.2 mile, the route becomes a pathway on the west side of the mountain. When you swing around a spur ridge, Elliott Knob looms high on the horizon to the south. Because forest service history shows that North Mountain never had any great number of inhabitants living on it, the old fruit trees you pass by once the trail gains the top of the ridge hold an air of mystery. Did the trees sprout from some hiker's discarded lunch half a century ago? Were the seeds secreted away by a squirrel and then forgotten? Or did some valley dweller use the mountaintop as an orchard?

Elliott Knob and Falls Hollow

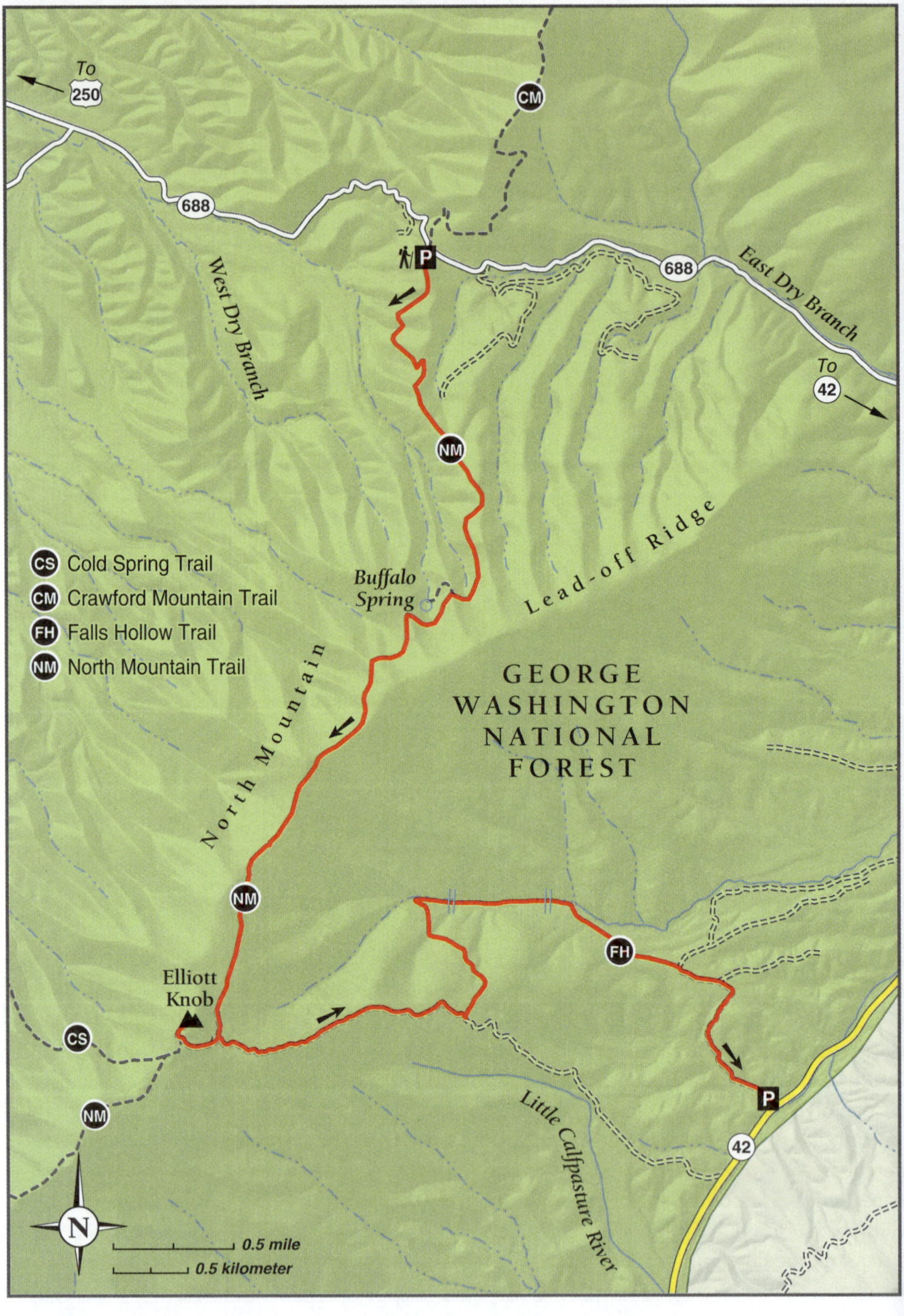

Next to the trail and growing 1–2 feet tall is wild geranium, with its pink and purplish flowers of five petals. After the petals drop off, an elongated ovary becomes part of the seedpod, which resembles a bird's head with a long beak rising up from the stem. Europeans hundreds of years ago named the plant cranesbill, and even the word *geranium* comes from the Greek *geranos,* which means "crane."

Learning to "read" a forest as you walk through it can tell you of past events. When you level out a bit at 1.0 mile, note how the trees on the left side of the trail are thinner and younger looking, while to the right the trees have broader trunks. This pretty much leads to the conclusion that this high up on the mountain, loggers only timbered the eastern slope. If, however, you were to drop down to the west, where the mountainside is not so steep, you would find ample evidence of logging.)

Rounding the side of a knob, look to the west for views into the Calfpasture Valley and out to Shenandoah Mountain (see Hike 43) on the Highland–Augusta County line. Along the trail, wild azalea grows just about at eye level, and crow's foot, a club moss resembling running cedar, is at your feet. Jack-in-the-pulpit pops up between the boulders, which are covered in a soft, 3-inch layer of moss. Many people think that the green, white, or purple sheath with a hood—the pulpit—which surrounds and covers "Jack" is the plant's flower. Actually, the sheath is just a leaf bract, and in order to see the diminutive flowers you need to lift up the hood and look inside to find them clustered around Jack's base. When you come back here in the fall, the pulpit will have fallen away and red berries will have replaced the flowers. After putting the plant's roots through an elaborate cooking process, early Native Americans pounded them into powder to be used as a type of flour. Hence, jack-in-the-pulpit's other name, Indian turnip. Don't try eating a raw root, though—it's quite poisonous.

If you have worked up a thirst by the time you've gone 1.8 miles, you are in luck because a side trail {FS 443A} to the right leads to the somewhat-dependable Buffalo Spring in less than 500 yards.

Birch trees are a part of the forest now, and gooseberries are abundant in the understory in late summer. It is possible to eat this half-inch, round, translucent green relative of the currant right off the shrub, but they will taste better when cooked into a jam or jelly with sweeteners added. As you traverse the east side of the mountain, the fire tower on Elliott Knob comes into view. By mid-spring, pink lady's slippers will have popped up trailside here. At 4.4 miles, turn right and ascend on graveled Elliott Knob Road, but pay attention when what appears to be the main dirt road swings right to a communications installation. The North Mountain Trail turns left to descend off the knob, but you want to keep straight, walking amid bleeding heart and climbing on a different roadbed.

At 4.7 miles, spread out the picnic blanket and enjoy lunch in the clearing on top of 4,463-foot Elliott Knob. Luckily, you don't have to climb the fenced-off fire tower—built in 1958 but abandoned when aircraft took over the job of fire detection in the 1960s—to enjoy the fine panorama. The ridgeline of Great North Mountain courses northeast and southwest. Shenandoah Mountain is to the west, and to the east, across Little Calfpasture Valley, is the Virginia Department of Wildlife Resources' Wildlife Management Area on Little North Mountain. (Consider visiting the area someday to wander around its 17,500 nearly trailless and roadless acres. Except during hunting season, you could most likely be the only person on all of that acreage.) If, during lunch and maybe a subsequent nap, the sunshine beaming down on Elliott Knob becomes too warm, it is possible to retreat to cool shade in the stands of spruce planted by the Civilian Conservation Corps in the 1930s.

When you're ready for the next phase of this excursion, retrace your steps back down the road, walking past the two segments of the North Mountain Trail and coming to multiple springs (a couple of which are boxed and piped) gushing out of the mountain on the left side of the road, 5.1 miles after beginning the hike. There are some nice campsites beneath larch and spruce around the wildlife pond and across the road. After descending on the steep roadway, your knees and ankles are going to be thankful when you can turn left onto the gently sloping Falls Hollow Trail {FS 657} at 6.2 miles. Pay attention because there will most likely not be a sign identifying the trail, only blaze marking.

For a small burst of refreshing flavor, chew on a leaf of wintergreen. Also known as teaberry, it is the ground cover next to the trail growing on creeping stems and erect branches of 2–6 inches with shiny, oval, evergreen leaves. Native Americans used extracts from the plant to lessen the pain of a headache or discomforts of a fever, and they obviously knew what they were doing because wintergreen contains a concentration of methyl salicylate—or, as most of us call it, aspirin.

At 7.0 miles, come into a forest of hemlocks and plush green moss. Go upstream a couple of hundred feet to see the first of many falls you're going to enjoy while in Falls Hollow. After a snack break, follow the route downstream, passing numerous falls and, in some places where the gorge becomes steep and narrow, rising high above the stream. The cascades of these narrow stretches are some of the most impressive in Falls Hollow, but be extremely cautious if you decide to drop off the trail to get a closer look—forest service records show that more people are injured from slips and falls at waterfalls than at any other type of site. If you're hiking during spring runoff season, be prepared for high water when fording the stream at 7.4 miles and then again a few feet beyond that.

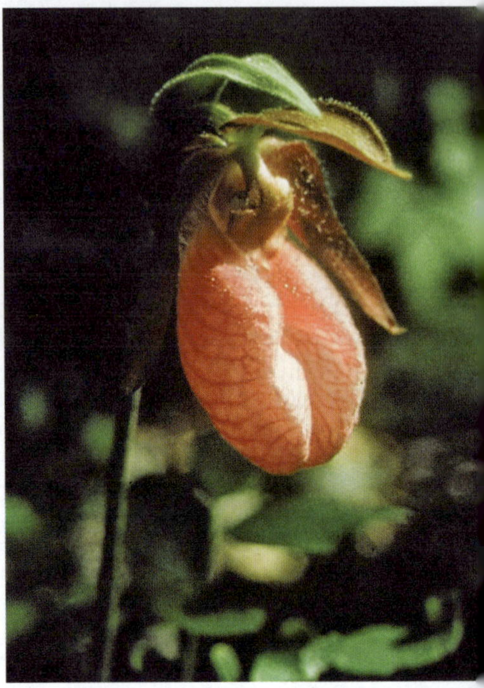

Pink lady's slipper

At 7.7 miles, the route begins to swing away from the creek and soon becomes a major dirt road. It could be easy to become confused in the maze of roads passed within the next mile, but the roadway to stay on is the one that is the best maintained and is obviously the main route through the series of areas that have been clear-cut in the past. At a turn in the road, at 8.5 miles, Elliott Knob can be seen to the west, soaring high above and dramatically illustrating the more than 2,000 feet you have dropped since being on its summit. Passing through a gate, find your shuttled automobile awaiting your return from hiking 9.0 miles in the more than 1.8 million acres that make up the George Washington and Jefferson National Forests.

45 Laurel Fork

- **GPS:** N38.5854594 W79.6422967
- **TOTAL DISTANCE (circuit):** 14.0 miles
- **HIKING TIME:** 8.5 hours, or an overnight backpack trip
- **VERTICAL RISE:** 2,300 feet
- **MAPS:** USGS *Thornwood (VA and WV)* and *Snowy Mountain; National Geographic Trails Illustrated Map #791 Staunton/Shenandoah Mountain*
- **CONTACT:** Warm Springs Ranger District
  422 Forestry Road
  Hot Springs, VA 24425
  540-839-2521
  fs.usda.gov/gwj

The Hike at a Glance

- **1.1** Buck Run Spur Trail comes in from left; keep right
- **1.6** Right onto Locust Springs Run Spur Trail
- **2.8** Arrive at FSR 106 and descend on Slabcamp Run Trail
- **5.5** Ford Laurel Fork and turn right onto Laurel Fork Trail
- **5.8** Left on Christian Run Trail
- **7.2** Trail may be hard to find in meadow; soon turn left onto Cold Springs Run Trail
- **9.9** Turn left to follow Laurel Fork upstream
- **10.4** Ford Laurel Fork; begin following Buck Run Trail
- **14.0** Arrive back at parking area

Laurel Fork, a tributary in the headwaters of the Potomac River, flows through a high-altitude region on the Virginia–West Virginia border that more closely resembles the forest lands of New England and Canada than the central or southern Appalachians. Red spruce, red pine, and birch thrive here, interspersed between tall sugar maples and oaks. Beaver ponds may flood the mountain valleys, creating the tannin-darkened bogs that are so well associated with natural areas in Maine, New Hampshire, and Vermont. In addition to the usual assortment of Appalachian Mountain wildlife—turkeys, black bears, deer, mink, and raccoons—the area is home to snowshoe hares and is one of the few places in Virginia to have a known population of northern flying squirrels.

Old railroad grades, abandoned since logging operations ceased around the turn of the 20th century, provide ready-made and gently sloping access routes to the region's inner reaches. Although the forest service reports somewhat heavy hiker use, the area's nearly 11,000 acres provide plenty of elbow room. I have never run into more than a handful of people each time I've hiked here; in fact, on a Fourth of July weekend, I saw only two other hikers the entire time I was on this 14-mile excursion.

Be aware: One of the reasons I have run into so few people may be that, although this is not an officially designated wilderness area (although that designation has been proposed), it is pretty much operated like one. You may be lucky to get here at a time when there has been a concerted effort to work on the pathways and things may be in good shape. However, for the most part, the trails may receive little, if any, maintenance. Although trails are blazed, it may sometimes be spotty. Routes could be overgrown with stinging nettle and other scratching vegetation (best to wear long sleeves and pants), and there may be some places where a trail has washed out and you will need to walk in a stream for some distance. This hike may test your navigation skills and tolerance for "bucking the brush," as a hiking acquaintance calls such conditions. Yet, there is absolutely no other place in Virginia (once you get a bit of distance from the parking area and forest service roads) that will provide you with a better sense of isolation and being truly away from civilization.

DIRECTIONS From the US 220–US 250 junction in Monterey, travel on US 250 west for about 20 miles to reach the

Laurel Fork

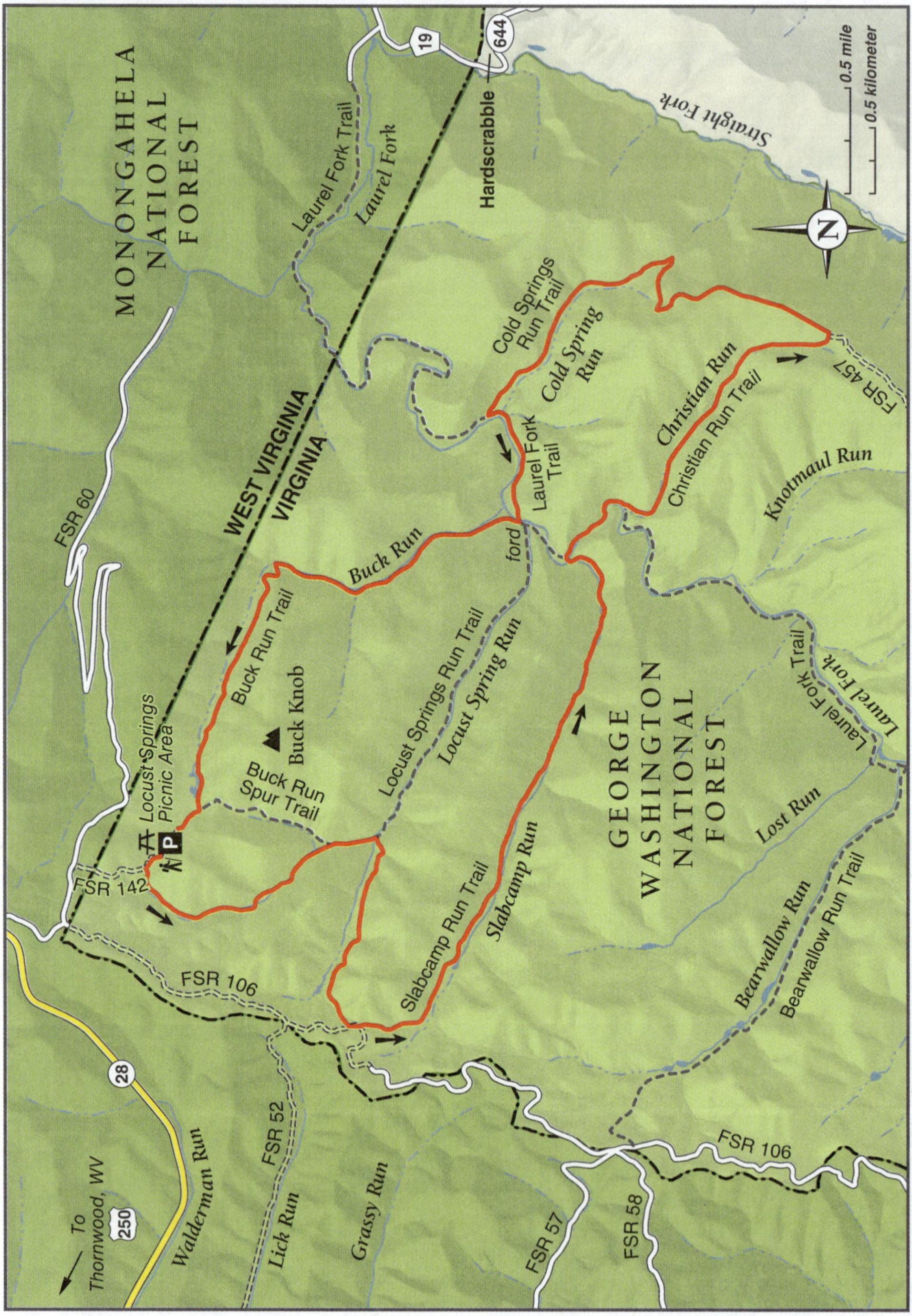

MONONGAHELA NATIONAL FOREST
GEORGE WASHINGTON NATIONAL FOREST
WEST VIRGINIA
VIRGINIA
19
644
Hardscrabble
Straight Fork
0.5 mile
0.5 kilometer
N
Laurel Fork Trail
Laurel Fork
Cold Springs Run Trail
Cold Spring Run
Christian Run
Christian Run Trail
FSR 457
Knotmaul Run
FSR 60
Buck Run
Buck Run Trail
ford
Buck Knob
Locust Springs Run Trail
Locust Spring Run
Locust Springs Picnic Area
P
Buck Run Spur Trail
FSR 142
Slabcamp Run Trail
Slabcamp Run
Lost Run
Bearwallow Run
Bearwallow Run Trail
FSR 106
28
FSR 52
Walderman Run
Lick Run
Grassy Run
FSR 57
FSR 58
To Thornwood, WV
250

junction of US 250 and WV 28 near Thornwood, West Virginia. Make a right, following WV 28 for 6.7 miles to turn right onto FSR 106 (a sign will identify the Locust Springs Picnic Area). In 0.5 mile, bear left onto FSR 60, and make a right onto FSR 142 in another 0.3 mile. Continue on FSR 142 for 0.4 mile to the picnic area. If you are arriving late in the day you will be happy to know that camping is permitted here.

Route Description

Facing the picnic area, walk to the right and take the Locust Springs Run Trail {FS 633}, descending gradually past the spring on a wide, old railroad grade in a forest of birch, beech, red spruce, pine, and mountain laurel. The trail is grassy and soft from years of dropped evergreen needles, and the songbirds and sound of the brook make for relaxing walking. In order to avoid a couple of stream crossings and some muddy spots, a high-water trail goes off to the left at 0.6 mile. The main route crosses the stream before going by the Buck Run Spur Trail {FS598A} coming in from the left at 1.1 miles. Stay right, enjoying the peace, beauty, and solitude of the high altitude through which you are walking. Continue downstream, crossing the run a few more times before stepping over a side stream and making a right to ascend steeply on the Locust Springs Run Spur Trail {FS 633A} at 1.6 miles.

When the pathway begins following an old railroad grade at 1.7 miles, the gain in elevation is so gradual that you'll put forth little effort to achieve it. It is often worthwhile to leave the route, searching for shreds of evidence from the days when steam engines ran up and down these narrow valleys. At 2.0 miles, depending on the current beaver population, you may see beaver dams and their resulting ponds that have flooded the valley below. From where you are standing, it may be possible to make out the individual sticks in the dams, but if you don't mind climbing back up, it's more interesting to drop to the valley floor for an even closer look at the beavers' handiwork. After felling a tree, a beaver trims off its branches in convenient sizes and carries them with its teeth to the dam or lodge site. Dam construction is adapted to local conditions—to lessen the pressure from a fast-moving creek, the dam will be bowed upstream, and in times of high water, the beaver will fashion temporary spillways. Although beaver ponds can be a nuisance to humans by flooding agricultural fields or blocking the route of a pathway, they also provide a place for insects to lay eggs, supporting a fish population that feeds on the insect larvae. In turn, the fish provide nourishment for osprey, mink, bears, and other birds and mammals.

At 2.5 miles, you must be alert for, and take, the blue-blazed pathway ascending steeply to the left. (If you miss the turn, you will eventually come to FSR 106, where you need to make a left and continue for several hundred yards to rejoin this route description.) At the top of the narrow ridgeline at 2.8 miles is a small parking area just off FSR 106; you, however, want to continue straight across the ridge, dropping on Slabcamp Run Trail {FS 600} and keeping to the left when passing through an old gate. The beaver ponds on your right and the open fields of wildflowers the trail passes through will leave no doubt in your mind that you are walking in a transplanted section of New England's Great North Woods. Cross the stream at 3.1 miles and enter an evergreen forest, where the pathway shows so little evidence of use that you could swear you are walking on an animal track. In summer, the display of wood sorrel is simply outrageous—its small, pink-veined petals and green leaves cover literally every inch of boulders and ground close to the creek.

You may have to adjust your stride a bit to adapt to the spacing of the "ripples" on the pathway when you begin following the railroad grade at 3.8 miles. This stretch of uneven ground is the result of the railroad track and its ties being removed when logging operations ceased. However, at one time, so many trees were being felled in this hollow that it required two tracks to haul them out. Look to the opposite side of the valley and you can see the contour of the other railroad grade.

Eventually the grade you are following will deteriorate to the point that you might as well give up trying to stay dry; just continue downstream, rock-hopping from one spot to the next. It really doesn't matter if you get your feet damp because they are going to get soaked when you ford Laurel Fork, a native brook trout stream, at 5.5 miles.

After wading through the run, turn right onto the Laurel Fork Trail {FS 450} and walk through tunnels of rhododendron. (If you wish to shorten this hike by 4.0 miles, you could make a left on Laurel Fork Trail and continue for about half a mile to rejoin this hike description at the 10.4-mile point.) At 5.8 miles, bear left to ascend the Christian Run Trail {FS 599}.

A heavy growth of almost neon green moss appears on the rocks and boulders as you ascend the railroad grade next to Christian Run. By the time you cross the run at 6.8 miles, the stream has become nothing more than a trickle and the landscape flattens out, with ferns lining the less steep and rocky pathway. The trail may become faint in the meadow at 7.2 miles. If so, aim for the depression slightly to your left. Upon reaching the gap, turn left onto the dirt roadbed of Cold Springs Run Trail {FS 634} and continue to ascend for a distance. At 7.9 miles, be sure to take the right fork and descend. Pay attention at 8.6 miles, where you do not continue straight but instead make a left to keep on Cold Springs Run Trail. This narrow valley is an exceptionally beautiful repeat of the other small hollows you've traveled—a multitude of wood sorrel moss, rhododendron, and railroad tie "ripples."

Reaching Laurel Fork at 9.9 miles, turn left to follow it upstream and, in June, look for pink lady's slippers. The valley gradually widens as you come to an obviously large campsite on your right at 10.4 miles. You can either spend the night here or, if you don't want to face a river crossing first thing in the morning, ford the stream now to find a tent site on the opposite side.

Once you are across Laurel Fork, the Locust Springs Trail is a short distance upstream from the large campsite; the Buck Run Trail {FS 598} is the old railroad grade that begins to ascend the mountain just a short distance downstream. Follow the Buck Run Trail as it goes by tens of thousands of richly green wood-sorrel leaves. So many little shamrock shapes spread across the forest floor that you probably wouldn't be surprised if you happened upon a leprechaun propped up against a moss-covered rock. After crossing the stream at 12.0 miles, swing left to continue the ascent, soon crossing it again and bearing left. You'll head downstream for a short distance before climbing via switchbacks. Upon coming into an open area at 13.2 miles, make an abrupt left onto a pathway through a planted evergreen forest. Turn right onto a grassy roadbed, pass through a gate to bear left onto a dirt road, and return to the picnic area at 14.0 miles.

Visiting and exploring places such as Laurel Fork can help to refresh and revitalize our spirits, enabling us to truly understand what Emerson meant when he wrote, "In the woods is perpetual youth."

Late fall is a great time for hiking along Laurel Fork. photo: Johnny Molloy

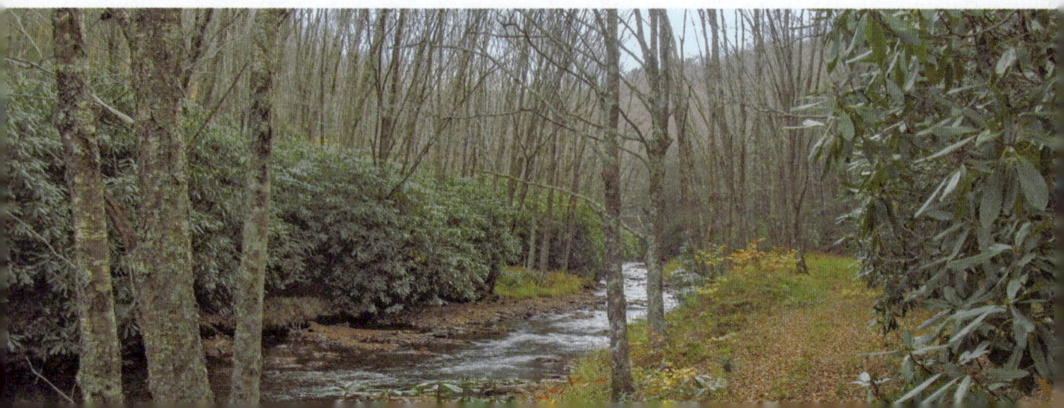

46 Hidden Valley

- **GPS:** N38.1043688 W79.8126466
- **TOTAL DISTANCE (circuit):** 4.3 miles
- **HIKING TIME:** 2.25 hours
- **VERTICAL RISE:** 100 feet
- **MAPS:** USGS *Warm Springs; U.S. Forest Service Hidden Valley Trail System map; National Geographic Trails Illustrated Map #791 Staunton/Shenandoah Mountain*
- **CONTACT:** Warm Springs Ranger District
  422 Forestry Road
  Hot Springs, VA 24425
  540-839-2521
  fs.usda.gov/gwj

The Hike at a Glance

1.3 Leave open meadows and enter woods
2.1 Cross Muddy Run
2.3 Left to cross bridge over Jackson River; then turn left onto Jackson River Gorge Trail
4.1 Left onto FSR 241 and cross Jackson River
4.3 Return to automobile

Hidden Valley has changed so little since the Warwick Mansion was built here in the mid-1800s that the area was used to film the 993 post–Civil War movie *Sommersby*. According to publicity releases, after a search in 15 states, Hidden Valley was chosen because "its rugged and remote hill overlooking the pristine Jackson River presented an unspoiled, stark but picturesque setting. . . . You could shoot 360 degrees and not know you were in the 20th century."

Happily, this was not merely Hollywood hype—and is still the case today. In any direction you gaze, there are no high-power utility lines cutting across the hillsides or communication towers and radio dishes rising above the ridges. In fact, other than the Warwick Mansion and its few outbuildings; a couple of forest service structures; an old, overgrown fenceline; and a dirt road that part of the hike follows, there is scant evidence of humans ever having been in the valley.

Archaeological digs indicate the presence of Native Americans in the valley more than 8,000 years ago. The first settlement by European immigrants wasn't established until 1740, but only the most skilled researcher could find any trace of this small community that was abandoned after being burned in 1754 during the French and Indian War. In 1788, Jacob Warwick obtained the property in Hidden Valley that was to be passed onto his grandson, Judge James Warwick. The judge, using the labor of slaves, had his mansion built out of bricks formed from mud along the Jackson River, and his plantation, known as Warwickton, endured until he and his wife passed away in the late 1890s. The land and mansion went through a number of owners, eventually falling into disrepair by the 1960s. However, a renovated Warwickton is now once again a working farm (on a smaller scale) and was opened to the public as a bed-and-breakfast in 1993.

DIRECTIONS At the intersection of US 220 and VA 39 near Warm Springs, follow VA 39 westward for 3.3 miles, turn right on VA 621, go an additional 0.9 mile to bear left onto Hidden Valley Road (FSR 241), and bypass the Hidden Valley Campground in another 1.6 miles. The parking area is on the right in an additional 0.5 mile.

Route Description

Begin the hike on the Hidden Valley Trail {FS 481}, an old woods road, into the open meadows and fields along the Jackson River that are more or less encircled by Back Creek Mountain and the long, heavily forested ridgelines of Cobbler, Warwick, and Little Mountains.

Enjoy the walk through these quiet meadows of grasses and a wide variety of wildflowers,

Hidden Valley

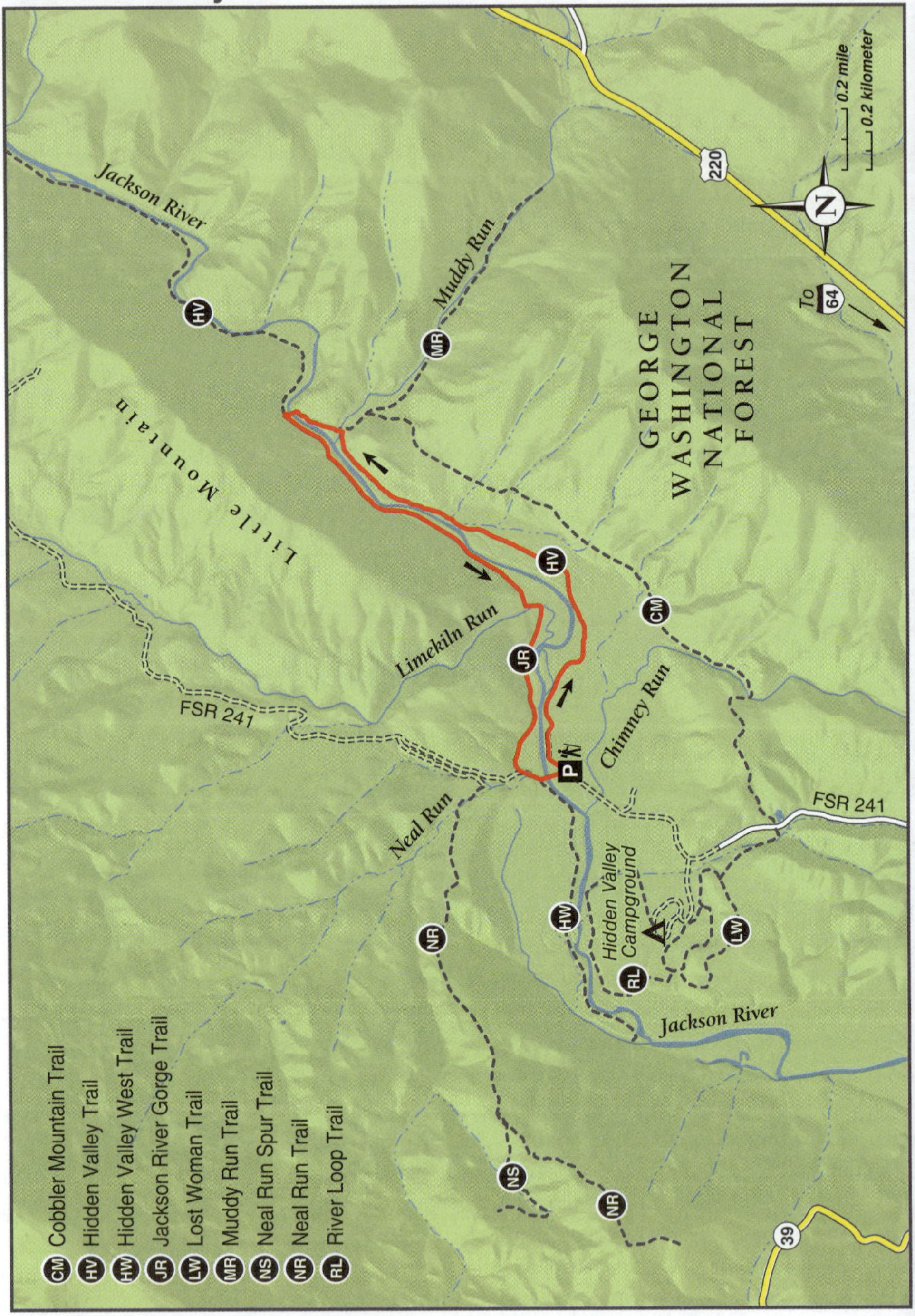

ncluding chicory, black-eyed Susan, yarrow,)eptford pink, and crown vetch. The abun-lant milkweed also attracts a multitude of utterflies. The open views of the meadows ade when the roadway (which may be muddy n wet weather) enters the woods at 1.3 miles, oon coming close to the Jackson River. Look long ground-hugging rhododendron limbs nd on rocks in the moist draws of the hillside nd you just might spy a lizardlike, red-spotted ewt. Spending a great portion of their lives in he water, newts, like salamanders, may wan-ler miles from their home stream but almost lways return to breed. Researchers say that he nervous systems in some newts are able to levelop a "map" of the terrain they cross and hat the information can be recalled when it is ime to return. The red-spotted newts have an dditional mechanism at their disposal—they an detect the Earth's magnetic field and are ble to use it as a directional reference!

Just before crossing Muddy Run at 2.1 niles, many anglers make use of the route earing to the right, the 1.0-mile Muddy Run rail {FS 481B}, and come back with reports of a ealthy population of trout in this side stream. Jnless you are going to do some exploring p Muddy Run, keep to the left on the road-vay, crossing the Jackson River on a superbly esigned and constructed suspension bridge t 2.3 miles. On the far side of the bridge, the Hidden Valley Trail bears right; you'll turn left nto Jackson River Gorge Trail {FS 481D} on a liffside above the river.

By the very nature of the terrain and vegeta-on this riverside route travels, it may often be frustrating pathway to negotiate. At times it ises along the steep hillside on a narrow path-vay that may not have been brushed out for uite some time; quick-growing briars, bram-les, and other entangling plants may leave vidence on your skin as you walk through 1em. If you find the trail in such condition nd not to your liking, you may want to retrace our steps back to the parking area, but if you re feeling adventurous and don't mind a little it of adversity, continue onward.

At one time, the trail descended into the very damp and moist bottomland, where its route became difficult to determine. However, it now rises over a low ridgeline to begin following an old woods road where deer tracks may be seen in the soft soil.

At 4.1 miles, make a left onto what is the main throughway through the valley, FSR 241. Passing the Greek Revival–style Warwick Mansion (placed on the National Register of Historic Places), cross the Jackson River and come into the area that served as Vine Hill, Tennessee, while the 1993 film *Sommersby* was in production. In a matter of just a few months, the movie company built a small community of about a dozen structures, filmed the movie, and then dismantled the set, leaving (at the forest service's request) several outbuildings next to the mansion as the only evidence of their activities. The hike comes to an end when you return to your car at 4.3 miles.

Warwick Mansion

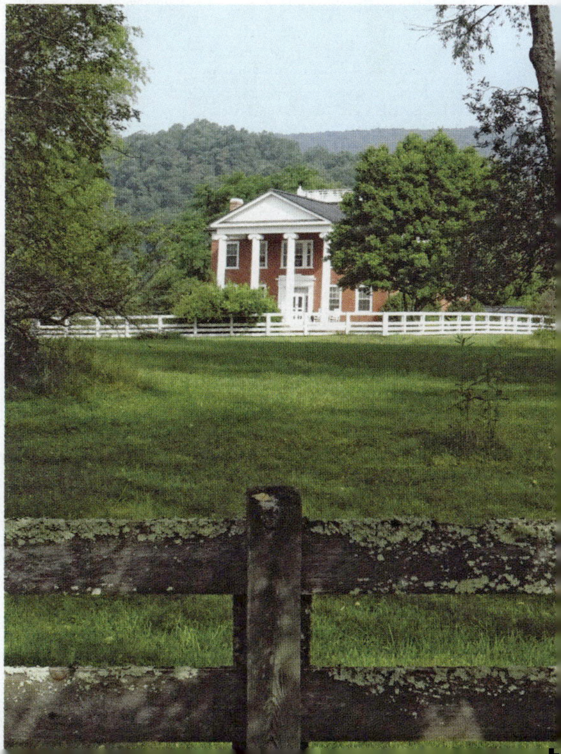

Lake Moomaw: Greenwood Point Trail

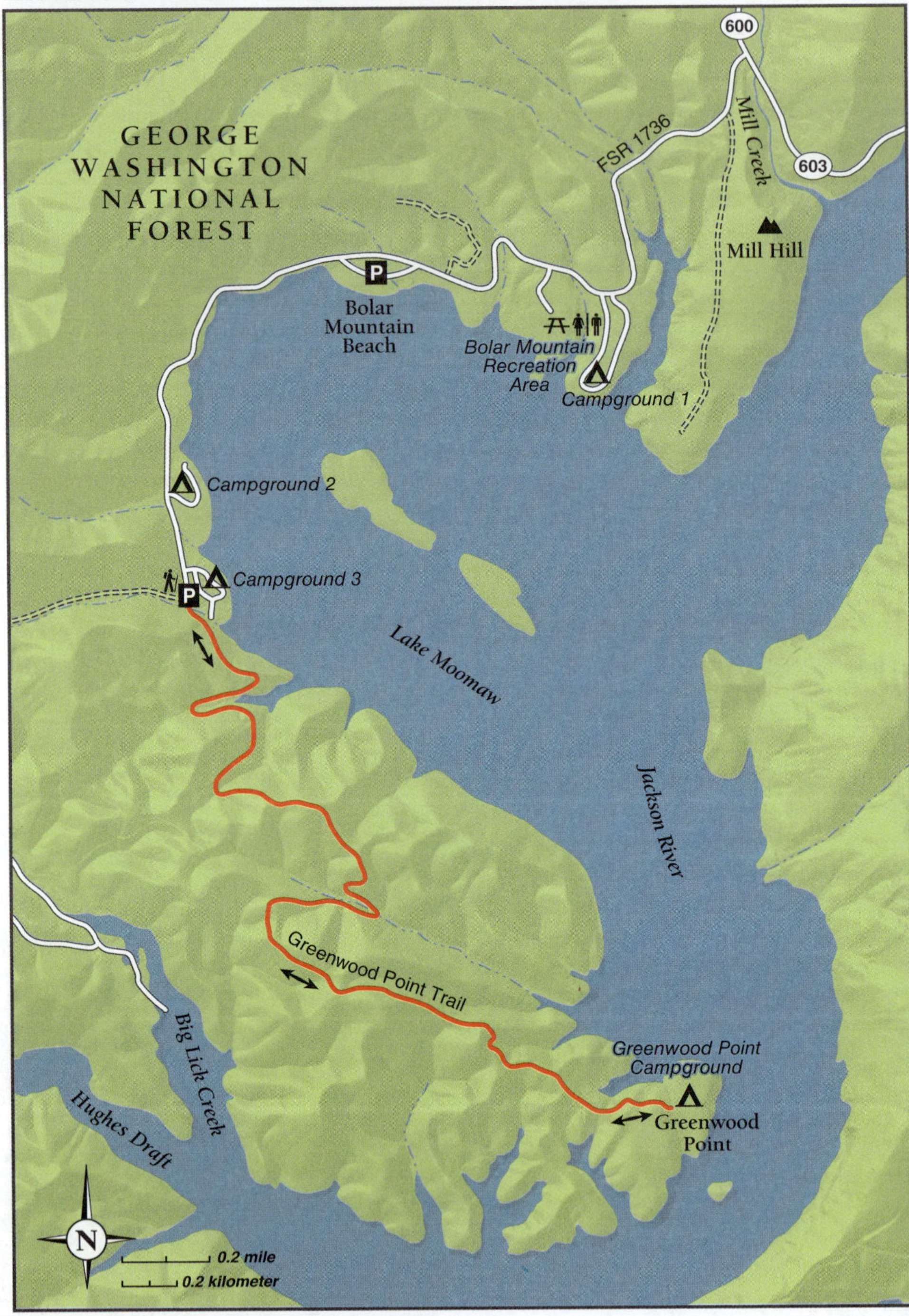

47 Lake Moomaw: Greenwood Point Trail

- **GPS:** N37.9757580 W79.9856846
- **TOTAL DISTANCE (round-trip):** 6.6 miles
- **HIKING TIME:** 4.5 hours
- **VERTICAL RISE:** 1,700 feet
- **MAPS:** USGS *Falling Springs; National Geographic Trails Illustrated Map #788 Covington/Alleghany Highlands*
- **CONTACT:** Warm Springs Ranger District
  422 Forestry Road
  Hot Springs, VA 24425
  540-839-2521
  fs.usda.gov/gwj

The Hike at a Glance

0.9 Cross ridgeline
1.3 Cross another ridgeline
3.3 Greenwood Point Campground; retrace steps
6.6 Return to automobile

There are few places in Virginia where you can legally camp on public land next to a large lake and not be situated in an often crowded and noisy developed campground. The primitive campsites at Greenwood Point on Lake Moomaw can be reached only by boat or by hiking the moderately strenuous 3.3-mile Greenwood Point Trail—thereby limiting the number of people who will put forth the effort needed in order to camp close to you. You will be rewarded with a quieter camp of much less human activity, where you can enjoy golden sunrises and pink sunsets reflected in the lake and secluded coves in which to take a leisurely swim (no lifeguards, so take care) or idly read a book. This isolation does bring some responsibilities your way, though. There are portable sanitary facilities at the site but no potable source of water, so you will have to carry in all that you're going to need. Also, be aware that there are only five authorized campsites at Greenwood Point, and during the summer vacation months these are often filled quickly by boaters. Start your hike early enough in the day so that if you find all the sites filled, you have enough time to walk back to one of the developed campgrounds.

The building of Lake Moomaw and its dam was originally authorized by Congress in 1947, but construction by the U.S. Army Corps of Engineers didn't begin until 1965. With completion of the work in 1981, the lake reached its present length of 12.0 miles and width (at its widest) of 2.5 miles, with a surface area of 2,530 acres enclosed by more than 43.0 miles of shoreline. The Army Corps retains the responsibility of managing flood control and water quality and maintains a visitor center at the dam, but the forest service administers the surrounding lands.

Spread around the lake are numerous developed campgrounds, picnic areas, swimming beaches, boat-launching ramps, marinas, and fishing access sites. Among other fish, the lake contains bass, trout, northern pike, catfish, and crappie. The Bolar Mountain Recreation Area on the northern side of the lake is one of the most developed spots, and in addition to the Greenwood Point Trail {FS 720}, the area has the approximately 2-mile Grouse Point Overlook Loop Trail {FS 721}, providing a couple of good views of the lake.

DIRECTIONS To reach the Bolar Mountain Recreation Area, follow VA 39 westward from the intersection of US 220 and VA 39 near Warm Springs, passing VA 621 (access to Hidden Valley, see Hike 46) in 3.3 miles. Continue up and over Back Creek Mountain to make a left onto VA 600, which you follow to its intersection with VA 603. Make a right onto the forest service road to arrive at the recreation area, a US Fee Area. (You will need to pay the fee to camp, either at the campground entrance or at the marina, depending on the time of year.) The Greenwood Point Trail begins in campground 3.

Route Description

Start an immediate ascent on steep switchbacks, attaining the ridgeline in less than 300 yards. With views of the lake through the vegetation, you will be on a downward trend on the grassy ridge when the trail makes an abrupt switchback to the right. The route soon follows an old road for less than 300 feet before switchbacking left off the roadway to gain elevation on a steep grade, only to cross the ridgeline at 0.9 mile and descend by dogwood, maple, hickory, oak, and abundant cancer root. A parasite upon the roots of trees, especially oak, cancer root has amazingly small yellow flowers. But the flower is probably not what will catch your eye at first—it will be the stem. It produces no chlorophyll—the substance that gives plants their green color—so its entire stalk is a sort of yellowish brown. Because the scalelike leaves resemble a pinecone, its Latin name (*Conopholis*) is derived from the Greek words *conos,* meaning "cone," and *pholis,* meaning "scale." Cancer root was used by Native American women to treat menstrual disorders.

Climb steeply out of a narrow draw to cross another ridgeline at 1.3 miles, only to drop down and repeat this process again. Having attained the final ridge, which will deliver you to Greenwood Point, there will be an old trail coming in from the right at 2.0 miles, where you will bear left onto a wide and well-built pathway in a mixed hardwood forest. As it does in cancer root during the summer months, the absence of chlorophyll plays a part in the look of the woods in the fall. Not only does chlorophyll give the leaves their green color, but it also produces simple sugars to nourish the trees. The leaves also contain yellow pigments—carotenoids—that are masked by the chlorophyll. Cooler temperatures and less daylight signal the leaves to quit making the sugars, and as the chlorophyll breaks down, the green fades and the yellows, browns, and oranges emerge. Autumn's reds and purples come from other pigments called anthocyanins, which develop in the sap of leaves as a result of a complex interaction between sugars, phosphates, and other chemicals. An early fall of bright, sunny days and cool nights (but not below freezing) will produce the most brilliant colors.

Continuing along the ridge, descend gradually to arrive at the Greenwood Point Campground at 3.3 miles. Pitch the tent, have a little lunch break, and then go exploring—there are many miles of shoreline from which to fish and acres of trailless woodlands waiting to be discovered. And, if you strike up a friendly conversation with some of your neighbors who arrived by boat, you may get a free ride around the lake or a chance to try your luck at a bit of waterskiing. In a day or two, or three, or whenever you finally decide to go home, simply retrace your route back to campground 3.

Greenwood Point Campground on Lake Moomaw photo: Johnny Molloy

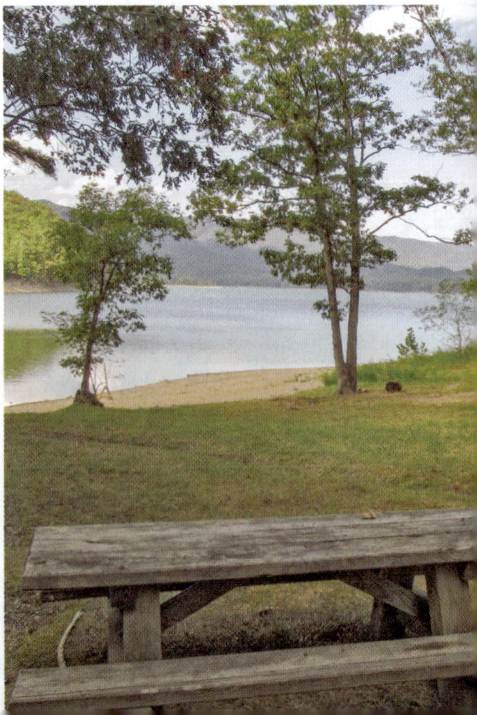

48 Rich Hole Wilderness

- **GPS:** N37.8698881 W79.6249995
- **TOTAL DISTANCE (one-way):** 5.8 miles
- **HIKING TIME:** 3.5 hours
- **VERTICAL RISE:** 980 feet
- **MAPS:** USGS *Longdale Furnace and Nimrod Hall; National Geographic Trails Illustrated Map* #788 *Covington/Alleghany Highlands*
- **CONTACT:** James River Ranger District
  801-A Madison Ave.
  Covington, VA 24426
  540-962-2214
  fs.usda.gov/gwj

The Hike at a Glance

0.6 Viewpoint
1.1 Reach Brushy Mountain ridgeline
2.3 Cross North Branch for the first time
5.8 Return to shuttled car

In May 1988, more than 6,000 acres on and around Mill and Brushy Mountains were designated as the Rich Hole Wilderness. Like Saint Mary's Wilderness (see Hike 34), Rich Hole is a beneficiary of the 1975 national law that permits places where the evidence of human activity is gradually being reclaimed by natural processes to fit within the definition of a wilderness.

In 1827, Colonel John Jordon built an iron-producing furnace in Longdale, about a mile from the present-day boundary of the wilderness. Due to America's voracious appetite for materials with which to build its expanding cities and transportation systems, the colonel's business thrived. Roads soon ribboned the hillsides so that iron ore could be mined and hardwood trees could be harvested for timber and charcoal to fuel the furnaces. By the time the factory closed in the early 1900s, only the steepest and most inaccessible areas of what are now Rich Hole had escaped this activity.

Recognizing these nearly pristine spots as rather unique and rare in the eastern United States, the U.S. Forest Service has managed them as a primitive area since it acquired the property in 1935; the logged and mined areas that are included in the wilderness have now had well over three-quarters of a century to return to a somewhat more natural state.

In one of nature's interesting twists of fate, even the unlogged areas are not as they once were. Many of the tall trees you see today were a part of the understory until the chestnut blight of the 1930s. The death of the American chestnuts liberated the oaks and hickories to become the dominant species. In turn, some of these trees were damaged or killed in the massive Easter ice storm of 1978, changing the look of the forest again.

Despite a gain of nearly 1,000 feet in a little more than 1 mile at the beginning, the rest of the walk is a moderate one. Although the outing is relatively short, there is so much to see, enjoy, and experience in Rich Hole that you should consider making this an overnight hike and not just a day trip. Either way, don't pass up this chance to hike into a lush and green part of Virginia where, more than likely, you will not see another person or even signs of other people the entire time you are on the trail. Do remember that this is a wilderness area, so the trail will not be blazed and may be overgrown in places. In addition, there are numerous stream crossings that are usually easy to do but could be more difficult in the spring or after heavy rains.

You are, however, almost guaranteed to see evidence of black bears. In 1958, an inspection team from the Wilderness Society recommended the suitability of Rich Hole as a wild area based almost exclusively on its large bear population. Of course, that was several decades ago, and bears move about from year to year, but each time I've been to Rich Hole I've seen

Rich Hole Wilderness

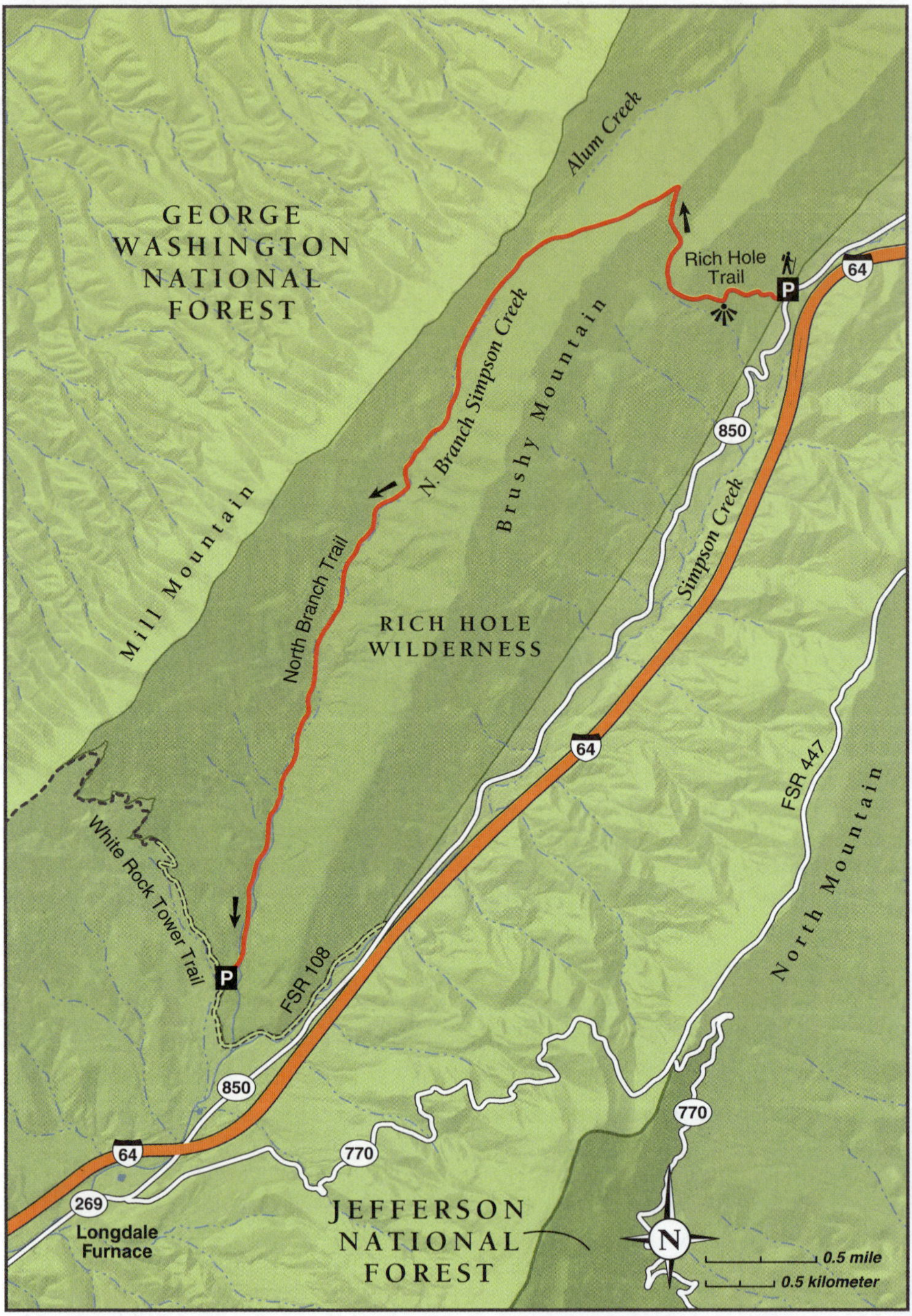

more piles of scat per mile than in any other place I've hiked. Other signs that will help you identify whether there are any bears around are tree trunks marked by long, scraping claw marks and rocks and boulders that have been overturned as the bears searched for grubs, termites, and other insects.

DIRECTIONS Unless you want to walk several miles on VA 850 after completing this hike, it will be necessary to have two cars for a shuttle. Take I-64 Exit 35 at Longdale Furnace, going east on VA 850 about 1.5 miles to a left turn onto FSR 108. Come to the trailhead on the right in 1.5 miles and leave one car in the small parking area. Return to and continue east on VA 850 for 3.6 miles to a small, graveled parking lot on the left with a sign identifying the Rich Hole Wilderness.

Route Description

Begin the Rich Hole Trail {FS 464} by leaving the parking area to walk on a blazed old forest service road. In 0.1 mile your route begins a series of switchbacks, ascending the mountain at a more than 10% grade. The forest is a mixture of chestnut oak, red oak, white oak, and sugar maple. Evergreens become more numerous for a short distance as the trail grade moderates a bit at 0.3 mile.

In the rhododendron and mountain laurel shrubs found at 0.6 mile from leaving the trailhead, a rock outcrop to the left provides lofty views to the south of 3,000-foot North Mountain and motor vehicles speeding along I-64, paralleling Simpson Creek in the valley below.

At 0.7 mile, the trail steepens once more; you may find it worthwhile to leave the trail at 0.9 mile to explore the natural bowl to your left. Rich Hole receives its name from the deep, fertile, organic soils found in heads of drainage systems such as this. Amid the mature black locust, it is possible to find remnants of a former homestead. Old apple trees are the most obvious signs, but you might also locate a cabin's crumbling foundation, a decaying farm implement, or a rusting metal pail.

After a short, steep climb at an almost 50% grade, Brushy Mountain's ridgeline, separating North Branch from Alum Creek, is reached at 1.1 miles. There are no official pathways dropping down into the Alum Creek drainage to the right, yet this area contains one-third to one-half of Rich Hole's acreage and promises an excellent wilderness experience for those equipped with backcountry skills and appropriate maps.

Your trail begins its descent from the ridge into large stands of rhododendron. A good, but waterless, camp could be made where the trail crosses a level spur ridge at 1.6 miles. Other campsites can be found on the moist land the trail passes through at 1.9 miles. A spring, the source of North Branch, will provide water in all but the driest of seasons.

A club moss, sometimes known as crow's foot, grows prolifically in the middle of the pathway at 2.2 miles. You will recognize this point because the ground will be covered by what appear to be miniature evergreen trees.

Cross North Branch for the first time at 2.3 miles; cross the creek again in 200 feet and then again in 500 more feet.

The next 2.0 miles of scenery the rough and rocky trail passes through make any walking or hardships you have had to endure all worth it. Tall, straight poplar trees vie for dominance with red maples and several different kinds of oaks, and elegant fern fronds dance in the breeze over neon green moss-covered rocks in the creek. Although there is a plethora of spots suitable for great tent sites, there are almost no traces of anyone ever having camped here. This apparent lack of use is even more amazing in light of the fact that the forest service classifies North Branch as a native trout stream.

Be alert at 3.0 miles; the trail makes a sudden switchback to the right to cross the creek. The route crosses the stream 12 more times before the hike comes to an end. Abundant spring runoff may make these crossings a little tricky, and an interesting situation develops in the fall when the flow of the creek diminishes: The hardwood trees drop so many leaves onto standing pools of water that it becomes next to impossible to distinguish solid ground from liquid creekbed. Pick your steps carefully or you will end up with wet feet.

Wintergreen, with its evergreen leaves (and rich red berries in the fall), is a major part of the ground cover; a small cave can be found in the rock facing to the right at 3.7 miles. Rocky treadway is replaced by a wide, grassy woods road at 4.4 miles, and pines become numerous once again as the road brings you to your shuttled car, FSR 108, and the end of the hike at 5.8 miles.

Lightly utilized White Rock Tower Trail {FS 466} basically starts from this point and could be used to extend your trip for another 7–8 miles, but it is best to contact the forest service about its present condition and accesses before setting out to walk it. Excellent nearby hikes are in Douthat State Park (see Hikes 49 and 50) and Dry Run (see Hike 51) near Clifton Forge and Covington, each just several miles to the west via I-64.

You can see North Mountain and I-64 from the Rich Hole Wilderness.

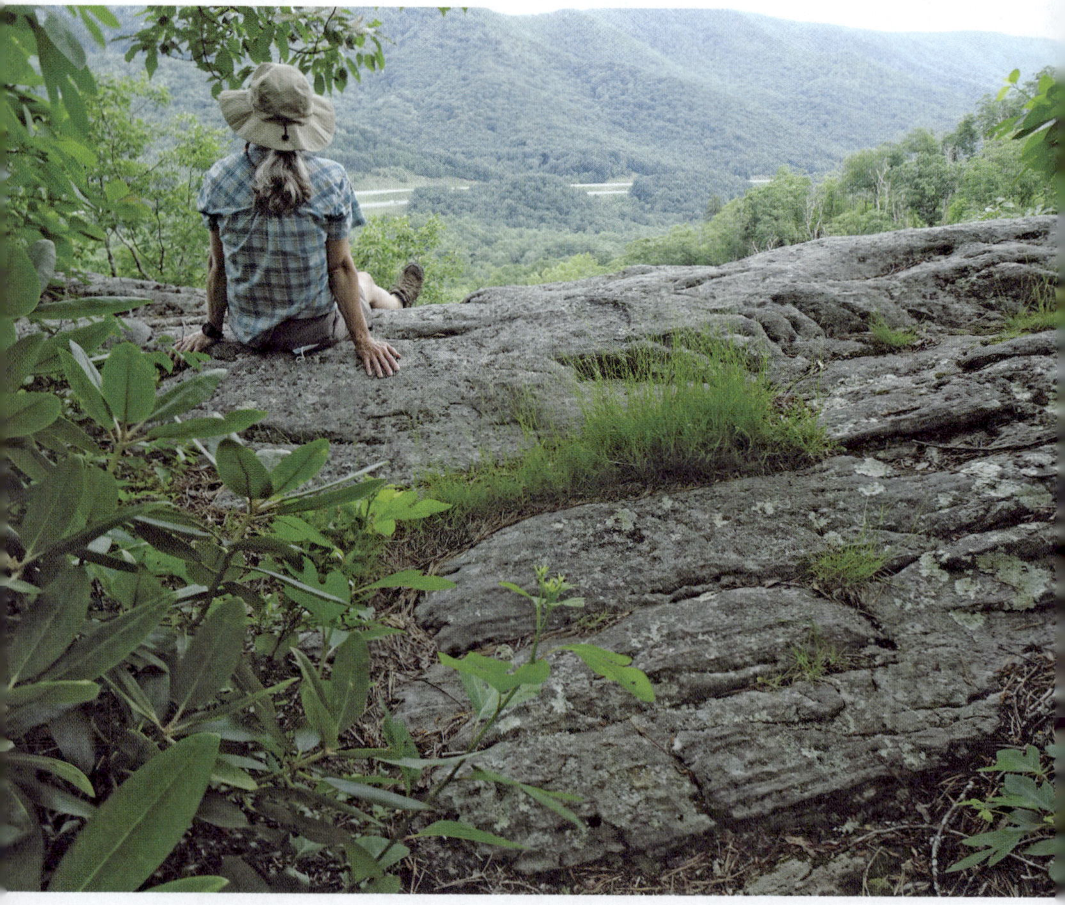

49 Douthat State Park: Beards Mountain

- **GPS:** N37.8958515 W79.8014058
- **TOTAL DISTANCE (circuit):** 7.1 miles
- **HIKING TIME:** 4.5 hours
- **VERTICAL RISE:** 1,360 feet
- **MAPS:** USGS *Healing Springs; Douthat State Park map; National Geographic Trails Illustrated Map #788 Covington/Alleghany Highlands*
- **CONTACT:** Douthat State Park
  14239 Douthat State Park Road
  Millboro, VA 24460
  540-862-8100
  dcr.virginia.gov/state-parks/douthat

The Hike at a Glance

1.2 Left onto Mountain Top Trail

1.7 Buck Hollow Trail comes in from the left; keep right. Keep right again in a few feet when Mountain Side Trail comes in from the left

3.8 Ross Camp Trail comes in from the right; keep left to begin following Mountain Side Trail

5.1 Junction of Mountain Top Trail and Buck Hollow Trail; make hard right to follow Buck Hollow Trail

6.6 Left onto Wilson Creek Trail; soon Wilson Creek Trail ends. Follow gravel road

7.1 Return to the beginning of the hike

Rising north of Clifton Forge and attaining heights of more than 2,600 feet above sea level, blueberry bush–covered Beards Mountain separates the Cowpasture River Valley from the Wilson Creek Valley. Situated on Beards Mountain's western slopes and the eastern edge of Middle Mountain and nestled along Wilson Creek is 4,545-acre Douthat State Park. Six hundred men of the Civilian Conservation Corps (CCC)—stationed at three separate campsites—worked on developing the park, fabricating cabins and other buildings, along with roads, bridges, trails, and a 50-acre lake contained by a rock spillway dam. One of the six original state parks in Virginia, Douthat was opened to the public on June 15, 1936. Its blend of recreational opportunities makes use of many of the still-standing CCC constructions, and the park therefore was designated a National Registered Historic Landmark in 1986. The park offers interpretive programs during the usual heavy-use months, rental cabins (plus large lodge-cabins with five and six bedrooms), campgrounds, hot showers, a camp store, a restaurant (check ahead of time to see if it's open), dumping stations, swimming, boat rentals, and picnic areas and shelters. Douthat Lake and Wilson Creek are stocked (times vary by season) with trout, and licenses are available in the park, so bring the rod and reel. (Fishing the stocked area requires a special daily permit.)

DIRECTIONS Take I-64 Exit 27 east of Clifton Forge and follow VA 629 north about 5 miles to the park office.

Route Description

With a system of interconnecting trails totaling more than 40 miles (more than any other state park in Virginia), almost countless circuit hikes can be taken. This hike along Beards Mountain provides an opportunity to get away from the crowds at the lake and campgrounds, study a mountaintop environment, and explore numerous, isolated hollows. Be aware that the park has become very popular with mountain bikers. In fact, I have encountered more cyclists than hikers on my recent visits.

Begin by walking behind the park office, picking up blue-blazed Beards Gap Trail, and passing the park's maintenance building compound. Enter the woods and cross the stream the first of nine times as you ascend the narrow valley. The narrower side hollows that you pass invite off-trail explorations. It's hard to get lost if you stay close to these mini valleys' small streams, in which you might find a frog or a salamander. Salamanders, like frogs, are

Douthat State Park: Beards Mountain

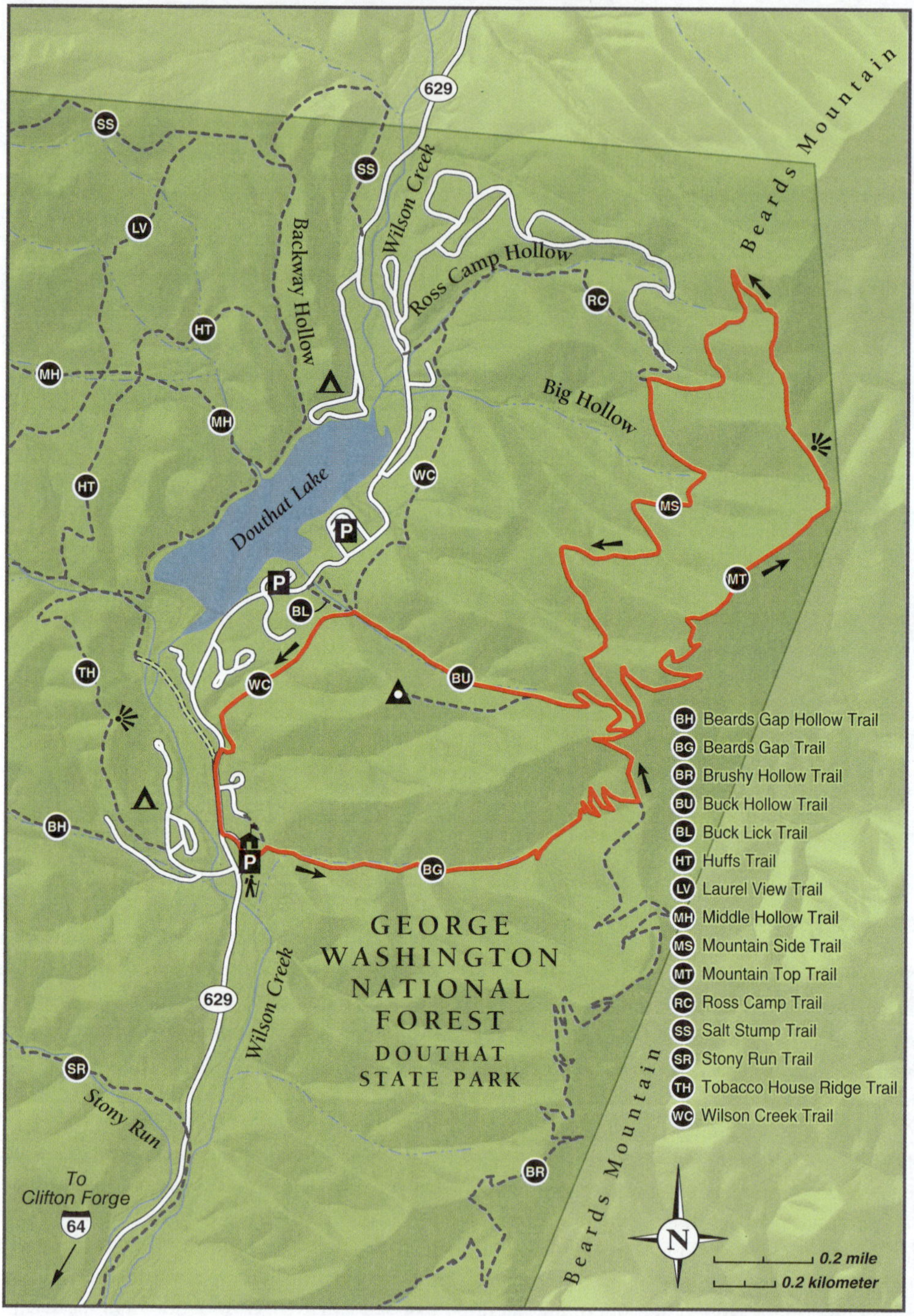

amphibians, not lizards, and must keep their skin damp, so you will never find them far from some source of moisture. And, although they spend very little time in water, you may see a box turtle poking along one of the streams. There is no mistaking this reptile because, of all the turtles in the United States, this is the only one able to "box" itself in completely by closing its shell. Continuing on the main pathway, there is a good wintertime view of Middle Mountain on the western border of the park from a switchback at 1.1 miles.

Upon reaching Beards Gap at 1.2 miles, orange-blazed Brushy Hollow Trail goes right for 3.5 miles to VA 629 near the park entrance. You want to bear left and rise on yellow-blazed Mountain Top Trail. Now on the crest of Beards Mountain, come to the junction at 1.7 miles with blue-blazed Buck Hollow Trail. Since you are going to make use of this pathway later in the hike, keep right on yellow-blazed Mountain Top Trail. In just a few feet, keep right again when passing the white-blazed Mountain Side Trail. After encountering a view of Middle Mountain and the 1,000-foot-higher Warm Springs Mountain rising behind it, attain a knob at 2.4 miles, with a wintertime view of pastoral Cowpasture River Valley to the east. With its headwaters far to the north near the Highland-Bath county line, the Cowpasture River has created one of the most visually pleasing valleys in western Virginia. The river joins the Jackson River (which is dammed near the West Virginia–Virginia border, creating Lake Moomaw—see Hike 47) southeast of Clifton Forge to form the James River.

The reason this trail was named Mountain Top is obvious as you continue along the crest of the ridgeline to another knob at 2.8 miles. Yet here on the park's border with the George Washington and Jefferson National Forests, you will leave the heights and follow your route when it drops steeply to the left for a short distance before descending at a more gradual rate. At 3.8 miles, keep to the left and begin following white-blazed Mountain Side Trail. (Orange-blazed Ross Camp Trail descends right 0.7 mile to VA 629.) The Mountain Side Trail winds in and out of small draws, keeping on an almost even contour of about 2,000 feet and reaching its termination at the junction with Mountain Top and Buck Hollow Trails at 5.1 miles.

Make a hard right, descending the switchbacked, blue-blazed Buck Hollow Trail to take the side trail to the left at 5.6 miles. Once again, this viewpoint overlooking the interior of the park may be overgrown, but it is still an enjoyable walk through a mixed hardwood forest and an additional chance to see one of the park's many white-tailed deer. Returning to the main trail, continue the descent as the hollow becomes wider and you cross a couple of small (possibly dry) water runs.

Buck Hollow Trail comes to an end when it runs into white-blazed Wilson Creek Trail at 6.6 miles. VA 629 is just a few feet in front of you, but make a left onto Wilson Creek Trail, following it across a wooden footbridge and past the Buck Lick Trail on the right. Ascend on a woods road, passing cabins and leaving the utility line right-of-way to enter the woods on the left. Crossing another set of utility lines, keep to the right; don't follow the right-of-way to the left. Soon, Wilson Creek Trail terminates at VA 629 (next to the stone chimney that was once a part of a CCC dining hall), but to avoid walking the paved roadway, keep to the left on a gravel road, returning to your car at 7.1 miles.

Don't leave the park just because you've finished the hike. If it is a hot day, your best bet is to head to the lake for a refreshing dip. If you have been walking in a cold rain, sipping a cup of coffee in the restaurant will warm your insides. And, if you've used a little foresight, your tent is already set up in the campground and waiting for you to crawl in to get a good night's sleep before taking off on tomorrow's hike.

Douthat State Park: Tuscarora Overlook

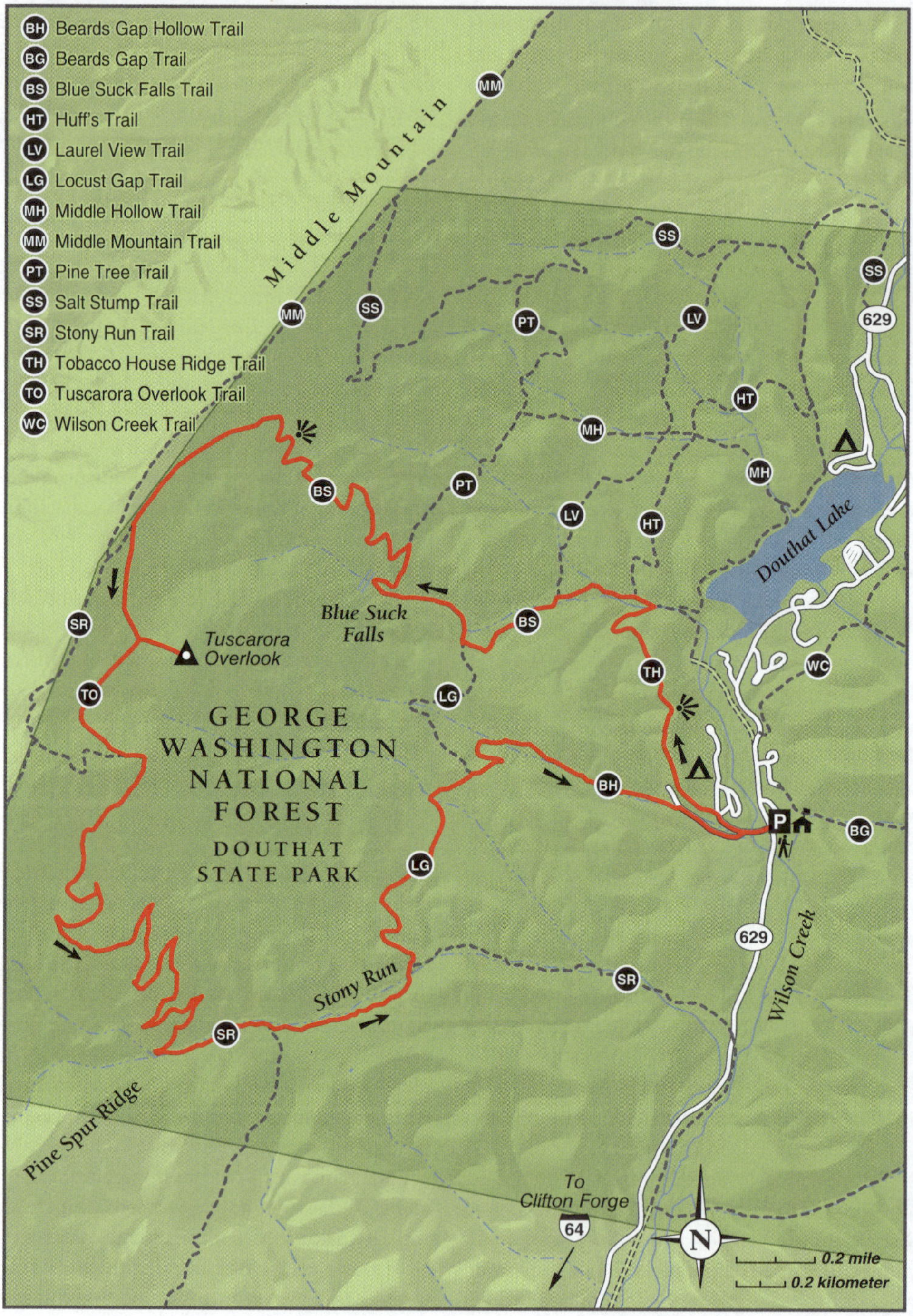

50 Douthat State Park: Tuscarora Overlook

- **GPS:** N37.8958515 W79.8014058
- **TOTAL DISTANCE (circuit):** 9.6 miles
- **HIKING TIME:** 6.0 hours
- **VERTICAL RISE:** 2,180 feet
- **MAPS:** USGS *Healing Springs; Douthat State Park* map; *National Geographic Trails Illustrated Map #788 Covington/Alleghany Highlands*
- **CONTACT:** Douthat State Park
14239 Douthat State Park Road
Millboro, VA 24460; 540-862-8100
dcr.virginia.gov/state-parks/douthat

The Hike at a Glance

0.9 Left onto Blue Suck Falls Trail

1.0 Huff's Trail comes in from the right; keep left

1.2 Laurel View Trail comes in from the right; keep left

1.5 Locust Gap Trail comes in from the left; keep right

2.0 Pine Tree Trail comes in from the right; keep left

2.7 Take side trail to Lookout Rock; retrace steps to intersection and turn left to continue hike

3.6 Trail to right heads into George Washington and Jefferson National Forests; go left onto Tuscarora Overlook Trail

4.0 Take side trail left to Tuscarora Overlook; retrace steps to intersection and turn left to continue hike

4.6 Tuscarora Overlook Trail ends; turn onto Stony Run Trail

6.9 Cross Stony Run, turn right on side trial to Stony Run Falls, then retrace steps to intersection and turn left to continue hike

7.7 Bear left onto Locust Gap Trail

8.6 Bear right onto Beards Gap Hollow Trail

9.3 Turn right onto dirt service road, then keep left when another road joins it in a few feet. Cross footbridge and turn right onto paved campground road

9.6 Return to your car

This excursion into the western and southern regions of Douthat State Park is probably best done in the early spring. Not only will the trees still be leafless so that the views will be more extensive, but the two waterfalls you encounter will also be running at their highest and most impressive volume.

DIRECTIONS Take I-64 Exit 27 east of Clifton Forge and follow VA 629 north about 5 miles to the park office.

Route Description

Leave your car at the entrance parking area of White Oak Campground (C) and walk across Wilson Creek on the low-water bridge into the campground and past Beards Gap Hollow Trail (on which you will be returning). Across from the bathhouse, make a left into a woods of pine and oak on yellow-blazed Tobacco House Ridge Trail. Some of the trees and shrubs you pass may have galls on them. Galls form on almost every plant in the world and are not a cancer or some other disease but the plant's reaction to an attack by a parasite (which could be a bacterium, fungus, eelworm, mite, or insect). Rarely will a plant be affected by the formation of a gall. Rather, this abnormal increase in the number or size of cells isolates the parasite and helps to localize any poisons it may produce.

A break in the vegetation at 0.5 mile provides a pleasant spot, especially early in the morning when songbirds are most active, to overlook Douthat Lake. The Tobacco House Ridge Trail comes to an end upon meeting blue-blazed Blue Suck Falls Trail at 0.9 mile. This trail descends right to VA 629, but it also ascends to the left and that is the direction in which you need to turn. Early settlers noticed that wildlife was attracted to the salt from high-sulfur-content springs in the area of Douthat State Park and that the animals would stand above the springs to inhale the vapors—thus the name "suck."

At 1.0 mile, gold-blazed Huff's Trail bears right toward the northern portion of the park; keep left on Blue Suck Falls Trail. Keep left again when white-blazed Laurel View Trail comes in from the right at 1.2 miles. Conversely, bear right upon reaching the junction with yellow-blazed Locust Gap Trail at 1.5 miles. (You could follow Locust Gap Trail left for about a mile and rejoin this hike description at the 8.6-mile point. This would shorten your hike by about 6 miles, but you'd miss the waterfalls and views.)

Continuing to ascend on Blue Suck Falls Trail, which is now steep and rocky, come to the falls, which drop about 50 feet down a rock facing lined by mountain laurel and rhododendron. Your route crosses the stream just below the falls and swings around the side of the mountain on a pathway still supported by rock cribbing constructed in the 1930s by the Civilian Conservation Corps (CCC). Keep left at 2.0 miles, when yellow-blazed Pine Tree Trail comes in from the right; pass by two excellent views of Wilson Creek valley bordered by Beards Mountain. The stone bench at 2.5 miles provides a place to rest and enjoy the view, but take the short side trail to the right to Lookout Rock at 2.7 miles for an even better vantage point on this vista of wave after wave of undulating Virginia ridgelines.

Returning to the main trail, continue to the end of Blue Suck Falls Trail at 3.6 miles. A short pathway to the right provides access to George Washington and Jefferson National Forests' Middle Mountain Trail {FS 458}. You want to bear left, descending on yellow-blazed Tuscarora Overlook Trail, taking the side pathway left to Tuscarora Overlook at 4.0 miles for a view unsurpassed anywhere else in the park. Douthat Lake sparkles more than 1,000 feet below you, and now that you are high above the elevation to which Beards Mountain to the east attains, you can see far beyond it—into Cowpasture River Valley and all the way out to Rough and Mill Mountains, well over 10 miles from where you're standing. To the southeast it is even possible to see a bit of four-lane I-64 snaking toward Lexington. The rustic cabin at the overlook was originally built by the CCC and later used as a fire warden's station; it was restored in the late 1980s. It is not available for overnight stays and should only be used in case of an emergency. Because the Tuscarora people inhabited North Carolina (and later New York and Ontario) and not Virginia, it must be assumed that this overlook is named for the Tuscarora sandstone that forms the upper layer of the mountains in the region.

Returning to the main trail, make a left and contour along the mountain in an upland environment of hardwoods and mountain laurel to where the Tuscarora Overlook Trail ends at 4.6 miles. A portion of orange-blazed Stony Run Trail ascends right to connect with the Middle Mountain Trail. However, you will follow its orange blazes as they descend to the left. Be alert at 5.0 miles! Do not take the old trail straight ahead, but bear left to swing around the ridgeline and begin a series of long, well-graded switchbacks down the steep slope of the mountain. After entering a rhododendron tunnel at 6.9 miles, cross scenic Stony Run and bear right onto a 100-foot-long side trail to Stony Run Falls. This is a great place to stop and relax on a warm, dry day. Tiny bits of mist from the falls add moisture to the air, and thick rhododendron shrubs block the sunlight to provide dark patches of shade. It's interesting to see how the rhododendron is affected by its environment; in some places it grows tall and straight, while in others it is twisted and gnarled.

Return to the main trail to continue downstream as the valley becomes wider and more open. At 7.7 miles, Stony Run Trail continues right for 1.5 miles to VA 629. You'll bear left onto yellow-blazed Locust Gap Trail, swinging around several spur ridges with little change in elevation to the next intersection at 8.6 miles. Locust Gap Trail continues left for about a mile to intersect Blue Suck Falls Trail; you should bear right to drop quickly along white-blazed Beards Gap Hollow Trail, crossing the water run several times. Keep a sharp eye out at 9.2 miles and you might notice an old telegraph wire connector in an evergreen tree. In the days before wireless radios and phones, the only contact with isolated outposts—such as the cabin at Tuscarora Overlook—was by way of telegraph lines. If you watch closely when hiking in Virginia on a pathway going to the site of an old lookout station, you will likely find some kind of evidence of this form of communication.

Turn right onto a dirt service road at 9.3 miles, keeping left when another road joins it in a few hundred feet. After crossing a wooden footbridge, turn right onto the paved campground road. If you are near the campground in early morning or evening, there's a good chance of seeing a raccoon or an opossum. The opossum is the only marsupial (meaning it carries its young in a pouch) in the United States. When the young are born they weigh less than a tenth of an ounce each, measure about one-half to two-thirds the size of a honeybee, and an entire litter of 13 could easily fit into a tablespoon. Opossums live in abandoned burrows or hollow trees and are often seen walking along a tree's lower limbs; clawed feet and a strong prehensile tail make them excellent, if somewhat clumsy, climbers.

Follow the campground road across Wilson Creek and to your car, ending the hike at 9.6 miles. If you have also done the Beards Mountain hike (see Hike 49), you've now completed an exploration of some of the eastern, western, and southern portions of Douthat State Park. Take a look at the park handout map and you will see that by combining the Salt Stump, Pine Tree, Middle Hollow, Heron Run, and Backway Hollow Trails you can accomplish an approximately 4-mile discovery trip into a segment of the park's northern district.

Mountain laurel's delicate blooms are a highlight of this hike.

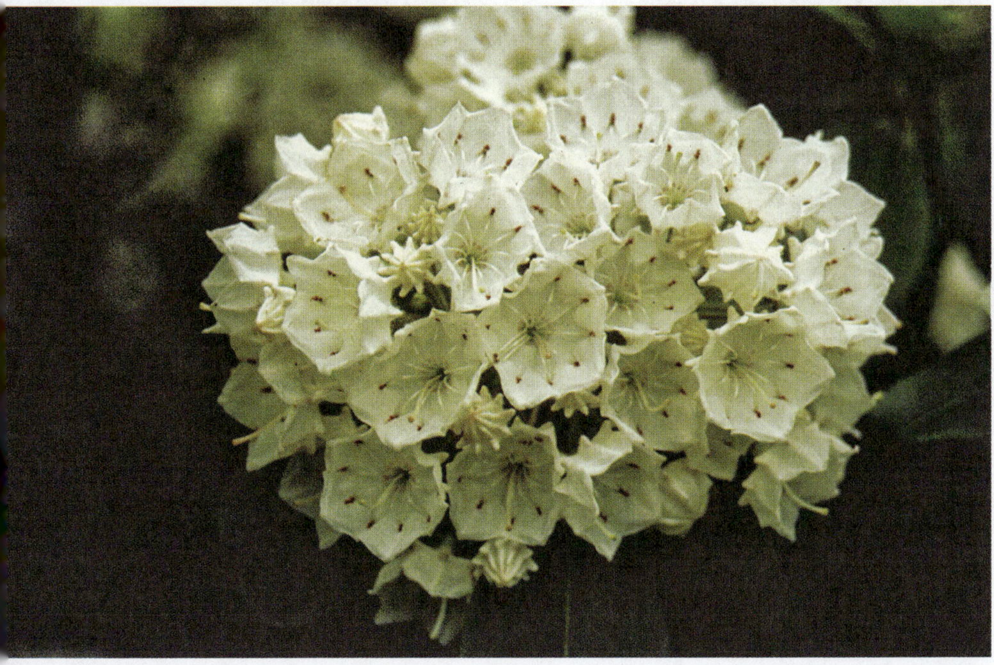

Dry Run

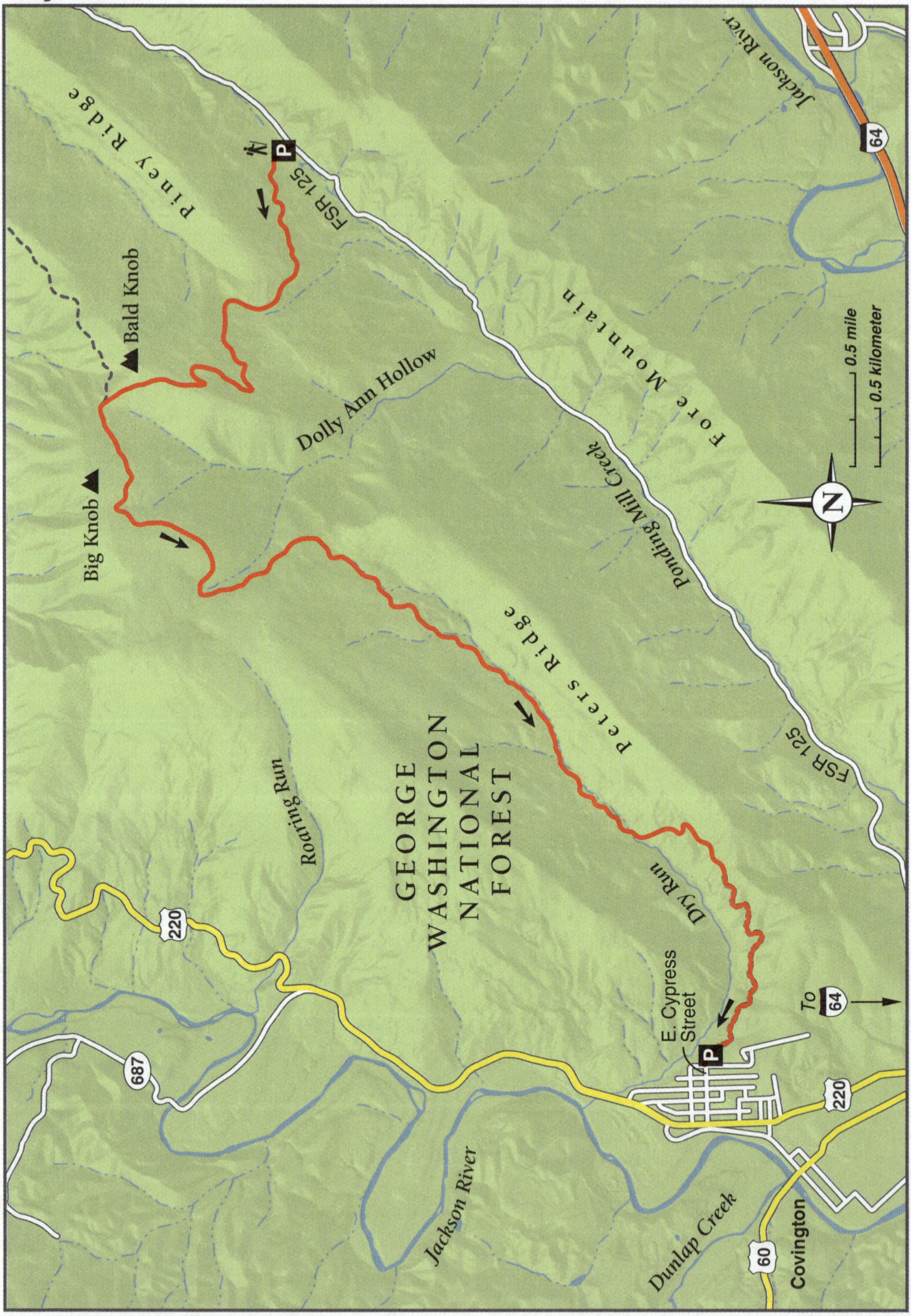

Piney Ridge
Bald Knob
Big Knob
Dolly Ann Hollow
FSR 125
Jackson River
64
Fore Mountain
Ponding Mill Creek
0.5 mile
0.5 kilometer
N
Peters Ridge
GEORGE WASHINGTON NATIONAL FOREST
Roaring Run
Dry Run
220
E. Cypress Street
To 64
687
Jackson River
Dunlap Creek
60
Covington

51 Dry Run

- **GPS:** N37.8014558 W79.9844240 **(Cypress St. Trailhead)**
  N37.8329970 W79.8952404 **(FR 125 Trailhead)**
- **TOTAL DISTANCE (one-way):** 9.7 miles
- **HIKING TIME:** 6.25 hours
- **VERTICAL RISE:** 1,640 feet
- **MAPS:** USGS *Covington; U.S. Forest Service Fore Mountain Trail/Dry Run Trail map; National Geographic Trails Illustrated Map #788 Covington/Alleghany Highlands*
- **CONTACT:** James River Ranger District
  801-A Madison Ave.
  Covington, VA 24426
  540-962-2214
  fs.usda.gov/gwj

The Hike at a Glance

- **2.3** Pass through gate
- **4.0** Side trail to right to overlook (not maintained); stay left on Dry Run Trail
- **4.2** Spring
- **6.1** Cross Dry Run
- **7.6** Turn left and recross Dry Run; soon begin walking on FSR 339
- **8.6** View of pulp mill in Covington
- **9.7** End of hike

A moderately easy ascent of Warm Springs Mountain, passage close to Big Knob and Bald Knob—two of the highest points in the Allegheny Mountains of Virginia—and a pleasurable descent along tumbling Dry Run make this excursion a good choice for a long day trip or an overnight hike.

A number of years ago, the U.S. Forest Service officially combined what were known as the Skyline and Dry Run Trails into the Dry Run Trail, and portions of these two pathways are used for this hike.

DIRECTIONS Because this is a one-way walk, a car shuttle will be necessary. Take I-64 Exit 16 at Covington and follow US 60 toward downtown. In 1.4 miles, US 60 forks left; take US 220 to the right. Watch for East Cypress Street in another 1.4 miles, where you turn right to follow it 0.3 mile to its dead end with the gate for FSR 339. Park one car (there is very little room, so be sure you are off the pavement) and retrace your route back toward the interstate. Be watching for the left turn you need to make onto East Dolly Ann Drive (VA 625), 0.9 mile before you would return to the interstate exit. Paved VA 625 becomes dirt FSR 125 in 1.0 mile. Continue on FSR 125 for 4.6 miles to a trailhead sign for the Dry Run {FS 417} directly across the road from gated FSR 448. Be sure to watch your odometer; the trailhead sign may be obscured, removed, or possibly, by the time you take your walk, replaced with a sign designating this as the Dry Run Trail. Leave your car here, being sure not to block any roadways.

Route Description

Two roads diverge from the large parking area. Do not take the level, gated road to the right. Your hike route begins by following the ungated, rough, four-wheel-drive road that ascends to the left. The first few feet are a little steep, but soon the road takes on a gradual and gentle grade.

At 1.1 miles, and again in a few hundred feet, roads come in from the right. Keep to the left on the main road at both spots.

Come to a T-intersection at 1.3 miles. Bald Knob is visible to the right (no views from its summit, though). Bear left and continue to ascend, staying on the main roadway when old roads come in from the right and then the left.

The road makes its first major switchback to the right at 1.8 miles.

Reach the top of the ridgeline at 2.3 miles, where the road becomes gated. Look toward the northwest for a view of Big Bald before crossing through the gate. Now the slightly undulating road, receiving no regular motorized traffic, takes on a completely different feel. There are fewer ruts or potholes, leaves and other decaying vegetation make the walking a little softer, and bushes and other underbrush lining the roadway appear healthier and more abundant.

Begin to descend at 2.5 miles. To the right of the trail is a large outcrop that invites exploration. Enjoy this natural "jungle gym," but there are cracks, crevices, and drop-offs, so keep an eye on the children.

Before the two trails were combined, the Skyline Trail officially ended as you come into a wildlife clearing. Posted signs about 300 feet to the right let you know that the land is private property. Look for blazes to your left, which mark the former beginning of the Dry Run Trail. Follow the blazes along a short pathway for 200 feet, turn left, and ascend along an old woods road. The route takes on a different feel again. The terrain is more rugged; rock outcrops and jumbles of boulders are on both sides of the roadway. Stop for a few moments to enjoy the isolation you have obtained. With the possible exception of a passing airplane, you will probably hear no other signs of human life. Listen for the wind coming across the ridgeline from the west, rustling leaves and creaking tree branches. In an area this quiet, the sounds made by tiny squirrels hopping through dry leaves on the ground may become exaggerated and be perceived as the movements of larger animals, such as foxes, bobcats, or deer, which also make their home in this forest.

At 3.2 miles, the route levels out somewhat as you slab the mountainside just below the ridgeline. Where the road makes a swing to the left at 3.4 miles, several small, flat spots could provide a campsite for an overnight stay.

A side trail to the right at 4.0 miles leads, in 1.0 mile, to an overlook to the west. This trail is not well marked or maintained and should

You may see deer on the Dry Run Trail.

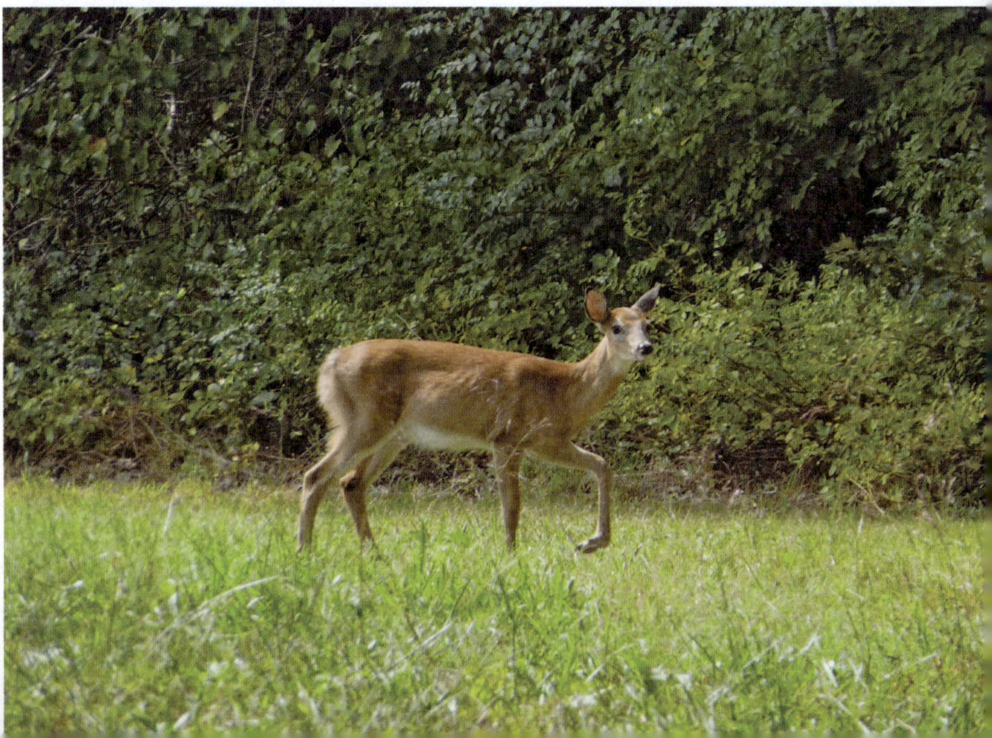

probably be followed only by the adventurous. I suggest checking on its current condition at the ranger station in Covington before deciding whether or not you want to take this side trip.

A well-flowing spring is located on the right at 4.2 miles. Cross the ridgeline at 4.8 miles and begin the descent to Dry Run. The route narrows; laurel has begun to reclaim the edges of the roadway. Pass through a draw in the mountainside at 5.3 miles; this is actually the headwater area of Dry Run.

Fallen trees at 5.6 miles show the great expanse of root systems that are required to sustain the life of a tree. The route becomes a well-built, narrow, sidehill pathway supported by rock-wall cribbing. You are walking high above Dry Run, which you can hear working its way down the hollow.

Swing right at 5.9 miles to begin descending along a spur ridge to come to a grove of hemlocks lining Dry Run. Groves such as this often become favorite places for those who walk through forests on hot, humid days. Hemlocks are very tolerant of the shade of taller trees or of those growing higher up on the mountainside. As a result, the sun is blocked by both the overstory trees and the spreading branches of the hemlocks, making temperatures sometimes 10 or more degrees cooler than those in the surrounding woods. (Sadly, many of the hemlocks may have succumbed to infestations of the hemlock woolly adelgid by the time you hike here.) This area is also a good place to look for opportunities to cool yourself in the many inviting wading pools of the run.

Cross Dry Run at 6.1 miles and continue downhill, paralleling the stream. Evidently, in times of high water the trail becomes part of the stream; the pathway is rough, rocky, and a little faint at 6.5 miles. Just continue descending along the same side of the stream and you will eventually find blazing to mark your route. Small campsites can be found along this stretch.

Pay very close attention to the blazing at 7.6 miles, where you should not continue to go straight on an obviously well-used trail. This may be alright for hunters and anglers who wish to continue to follow Dry Run, but the trail you need to take makes an abrupt turn to the left and recrosses Dry Run.

Switchback uphill, eventually working your way high above the stream. The route again takes on another kind of feeling. The pathway is soft from a cushiony layer of moss. Hardwoods and pines have replaced the hemlocks around the creek (which can no longer be heard), and galax and trailing arbutus help stabilize the soil that was disturbed by construction of the trail.

Come onto wide, graveled FSR 339 for the final descent. Although walking along a road littered with the rusting remains of every kind of modern appliance you can think of—stoves, refrigerators, washers, dryers, microwave ovens, televisions, and more—may not be the best way to end a hike, it is still possible to appreciate the natural surroundings. Sumac grows well and is one of the first trees to leaf out in early spring. About this same time coltsfoot adds its bit of yellow along the roadway. Later, in early fall, the sumac's leaves turn a crimson red several weeks before other leaves begin to change color. Honeysuckle and greenbrier seem to be doing their best to overtake the edge of the forest.

A bend in the road at 8.6 miles permits views of the pulp mill in Covington and of the mountains to the west and south. The hike ends at 9.7 miles as you come to the gate. Your shuttled automobile sits on Cypress Road ready to whisk you away to your next exploration of Virginia's natural wonders. Happy trails.

Suggested Readings and Field Guides

Abercrombie, Jay. *Weekend Walks on the Delmarva Peninsula: Walks and Hikes in Delaware, and the Eastern Shore of Maryland and Virginia.* New York: Countryman Press, 2006.

Adkins, Leonard M. *All About the Appalachian Trail* (for ages 9-13). Indianapolis, IN: Blue River Press, 2020.

———. *Fifty Hikes in Maryland: Walks, Hikes, and Backpacks from the Allegheny Plateau to the Atlantic Ocean.* New York: Countryman Press, 2013.

———. *Fifty Hikes in West Virginia: From the Allegheny Mountains to Ohio River.* New York: Countryman Press, 2013.

———. *Hike Virginia South of US 60: 51 Hikes from the Cumberland Gap to the Atlantic Coast.* Birmingham, AL: Menasha Ridge Press, 2022.

———. *Hiking and Traveling the Blue Ridge Parkway: The Only Guide You Will Ever Need, Including GPS, Detailed Maps, and More.* Chapel Hill, NC: University of North Carolina Press, 2018.

———. *Nature of the Appalachian Trail.* Birmingham, AL: Menasha Ridge Press, 2021.

———. *Wildflowers of the Appalachian Trail.* Birmingham, AL: Menasha Ridge Press, 2017.

———. *Wildflowers of the Blue Ridge and Great Smoky Mountains.* Birmingham, AL: Menasha Ridge Press, 2005.

Beane, Jeffrey C., Alvin L. Braswell, Joseph C. Mitchell, William M. Palmer, and James R. Harrison. *Amphibians and Reptiles of the Carolinas and Virginia.* Chapel Hill: University of North Carolina Press, 2010.

Brill, David. *As Far as the Eye Can See: Reflections of an Appalachian Trail Hiker.* Knoxville: University of Tennessee Press, 2013.

Brooks, Maurice. *The Appalachians.* Morgantown, WV: Seneca Books, 1995.

Bull, John, and John Farrand Jr. *The Audubon Society Field Guide to North American Birds: Eastern Region.* New York: Knopf, 2000.

Byrd, Nathan, ed. *A Forester's Guide to Observing Animal Use of Forest Habitat in the South.* Atlanta, GA: U.S. Department of Agriculture, Forest Service, 1981.

Constantz, George. *Hollows, Peepers, and Highlanders: An Appalachian Mountain Ecology.* Morgantown: West Virginia University Press, 2004.

Fletcher, Colin, and Chip Rawlins. *The Complete Walker IV.* New York: Knopf, 1984, 2002.

Graf, Irma, and Brian King. *Appalachian Trail Guide to Central Virginia.* Harpers Ferry, WV: Appalachian Trail Conservancy, 2014.

Gupton, Oscar W., and Fred C. Swope. *Trees and Shrubs of Virginia.* Charlottesville: University of Virginia Press, 1989.

———. *Wildflowers of the Shenandoah Valley and Blue Ridge Mountains.* Charlottesville: University of Virginia Press, 1982.

Kephart, Horace. *Our Southern Highlanders.* Knoxville: University of Tennessee Press, 1987.

Little, Elbert L. *The Audubon Society Field Guide to North American Trees: Eastern Region.* New York: Knopf, 1994.

Peterson, Roger T. *A Field Guide to Eastern Birds: A Field Guide to Birds East of the Rockies.* Boston, MA: Houghton Mifflin, 1984.

Peterson, Roger T., and Margaret McKenny. *A Field Guide to Wildflowers of Northeastern and North-Central North America.* Boston, MA: Houghton Mifflin, 1998.

Petrides, George A. *A Field Guide to Trees and Shrubs.* Boston, MA: Houghton Mifflin, 1998.

Simpson, Marcus B., Jr. *Birds of the Blue Ridge Mountains: A Guide for the Blue Ridge Parkway, Great Smoky Mountains, Shenandoah National Park, and Neighboring Areas.* Chapel Hill: University of North Carolina Press, 1992.

Slone, Harry. *Trout Streams of Virginia: An Angler's Guide to the Blue Ridge Watershed.* 3rd ed. New York: Countryman Press, 2006.

Stokes, Donald W. *The Natural History of Wild Shrubs and Vines.* New York: Harper and Row, 1989.

Waterman, Laura, and Guy Waterman. *Wilderness Ethics: Preserving the Spirit of Wildness.* New York: Countryman Press, 2014.

Webster, William D., et al. *Mammals of the Carolinas, Virginia and Maryland.* Chapel Hill: University of North Carolina Press, 2004.

White, Christopher P. *Chesapeake Bay: Nature of the Estuary, A Field Guide.* Atglen, PA: Shiffer Publishing, 2009.

———. *Appalachian Trail Guide to Central Virginia.* Harpers Ferry, WV: Appalachian Trail Conservancy, 2019.

———. *Appalachian Trail Guide to Maryland and Northern Virginia.* Harpers Ferry, WV: Appalachian Trail Conservancy, 2015.

———. *Appalachian Trail Guide to Shenandoah National Park.* Vienna, VA: Potomac Appalachian Trail Club, 2016.

Index

G *(continued)*

H

I

J

K

L

O *(continued)*

P

Q

R

S

W *(continued)*

Y

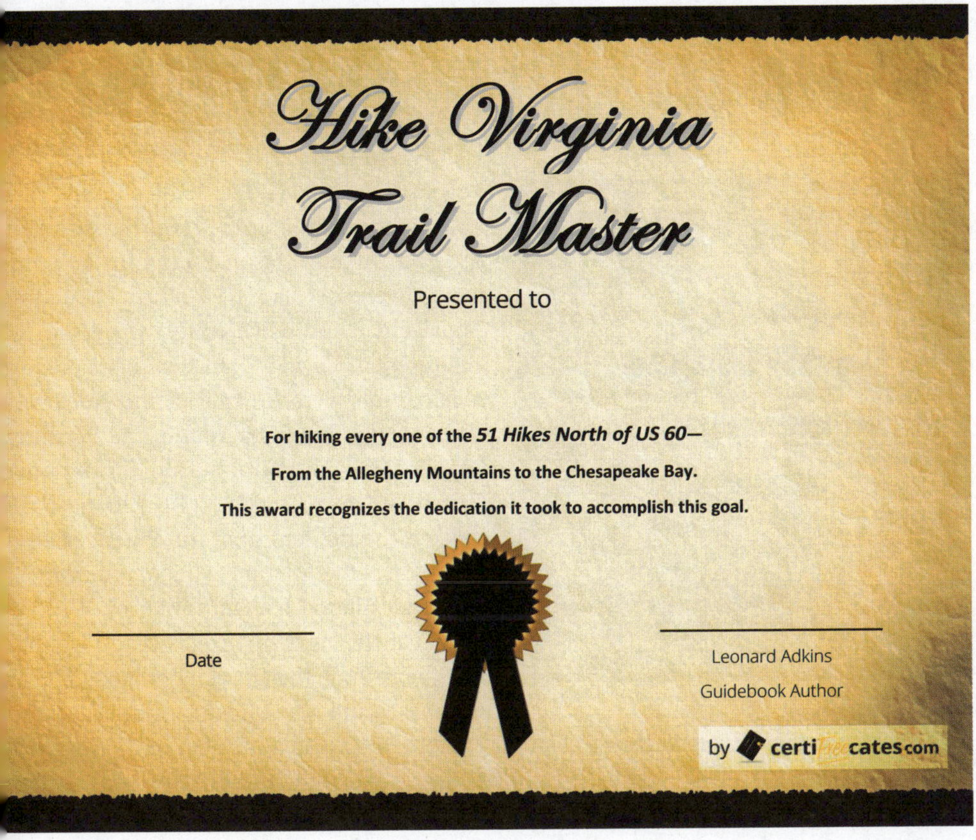

Become a Hike Virginia Trail Master

Become a recognized Hike Virginia Trail Master by hiking every one of the trips in this book. Simply keep a record of the date of each of your hikes and write a report (no more than one or two sentences) for each trail, providing your feelings about the hike, its condition, and if anything has changed since this book was published. In return, receive the Hike Virginia Trail Master certificate of recognition. Join a very elite club—as of the publication of this book, the author, Leonard M. Adkins, is the only person to have reported having done all of the hikes. Send reports to habitualhiker@verizon.net.

About the Author

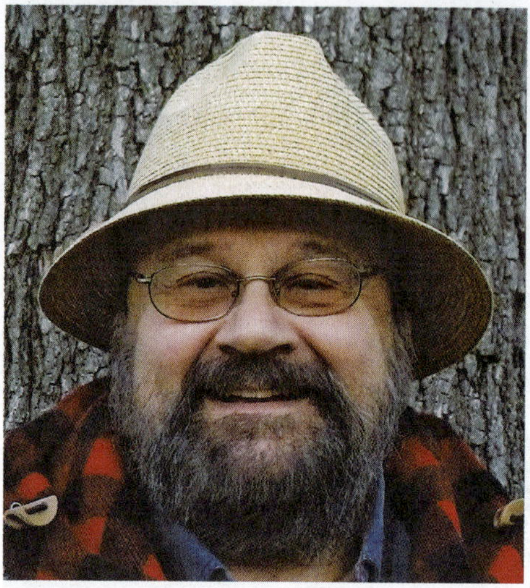

Leonard M. Adkins has logged more than 20,000 miles hiking the world's backcountry. Each hiking season finds him on some new adventure. He has hiked the entire Appalachian Trail five times; traversed the Continental Divide Trail from Canada to Mexico; followed the full Pacific Northwest Trail through Montana, Idaho, and Washington; and walked several hundred miles upon Canada's Great Divide Trail. He has also trekked the full length of the Pyrenees High Route from the Atlantic to the Mediterranean and has explored Iceland's interior. With his wife, Laurie, he has hiked West Virginia's Allegheny Trail, the Ozark Highlands Trail in Arkansas, and the Mid-Atlantic's Tuscarora Trail. Together, they tramped New Zealand's Milford Track and a number of the country's other Great Walks. And, of course, he has hiked every one of the trails in this book—along with many other pathways to determine which ones were the best to include. In addition he walked each of these routes with a surveyor's measuring wheel to ensure the accuracy of the mileage and the description.

Leonard is the author of more than 20 books and over 200 articles on the outdoors, nature, and travel and is the walking columnist for *Blue Ridge Country* magazine. His writing has received numerous awards, including the National Outdoor Book Award and SATW Foundation's Lowell Thomas Travel Journalism Award. He has also been a Ridge Runner and a Natural Heritage Monitor for the Appalachian Trail Conservancy helping to observe and protect rare and endangered plants, and has been on the boards of directors of two Appalachian Trail maintenance clubs. He and his wife currently live in North Chesterfield, Virginia.